# Health Risks
# of Energy
# Technologies

*AAAS Selected Symposia Series*

# Health Risks of Energy Technologies

Edited by *Curtis C. Travis*
*and Elizabeth L. Etnier*

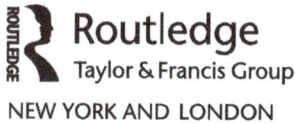

Routledge
Taylor & Francis Group

NEW YORK AND LONDON

First published in 1983 by Westview Press

Published in 2021 by Routledge
605 Third Avenue, New York, NY 10017
2 Park Square, Milton Park, Abingdon, Oxon OX14 4RN

*Routledge is an imprint of the Taylor & Francis Group, an informa business*

Library of Congress Catalog Card Number 82-61813
ISBN 0-86531-520-5

ISBN 13: 978-0-3670-1965-5 (hbk)
ISBN 13: 978-0-3671-6952-7 (pbk)

# About the Book

Public apprehension about nuclear power has contributed to the virtual halt in licensing and construction of nuclear reactors while continued reliance on coal-fired power plants has raised concern about the occupational safety of workers and the risks posed by increasing air pollution. The authors of this volume examine occupational, public health, and environmental risks of the coal fuel cycle, the nuclear fuel cycle, and unconventional energy technologies. They also explore in detail the relationship between energy economics and risk analysis, assess the problems of applying traditional cost-benefit analysis to long-term environmental problems (such as global carbon dioxide levels), and consider questions about the public's perception and acceptance of risk.

The book includes an examination of the global risks associated with current and proposed levels of energy production and consumption from all major sources. Perhaps the most uncertain of the risks associated with energy technologies, these global risks are also among the most important; they affect relationships among nations and may thus have a direct impact on the probability of war.

# About the Series

The *AAAS Selected Symposia Series* was begun in 1977 to provide a means for more permanently recording and more widely disseminating some of the valuable material which is discussed at the AAAS Annual National Meetings. The volumes in this *Series* are based on symposia held at the Meetings which address topics of current and continuing significance, both within and among the sciences, and in the areas in which science and technology impact on public policy. The *Series* format is designed to provide for rapid dissemination of information, so the papers are not typeset but are reproduced directly from the camera-copy submitted by the authors. The papers are organized and edited by the symposium arrangers who then become the editors of the various volumes. Most papers published in this *Series* are original contributions which have not been previously published, although in some cases additional papers from other sources have been added by an editor to provide a more comprehensive view of a particular topic. Symposia may be reports of new research or reviews of established work, particularly work of an interdisciplinary nature, since the AAAS Annual Meetings typically embrace the full range of the sciences and their societal implications.

WILLIAM D. CAREY
*Executive Officer*
*American Association for*
*the Advancement of Science*

# Contents

# About the Editors and Authors

Curtis C. Travis, *an applied mathematician, is head of the Exposure Analysis Group in the Health and Safety Research Division at Oak Ridge National Laboratory, Oak Ridge, Tennessee. His major research has involved the development and evaluation of mathematical models to estimate human health effects of energy technologies. He has also studied the health effects of a large coal liquefaction facility and of hazardous chemical incineration; the health and safety aspects of wood-burning stoves; and the environmental transport, dosimetry, and health effects of tritium and cadmium.*

Elizabeth L. Etnier *is on the staff of the Exposure Analysis Group at Oak Ridge National Laboratory. Her research has focused on the occupational and public health and safety aspects of non-nuclear energy technologies, including solar, tar sands, oil shale, unconventional gas recovery, coal liquefaction, and wood burning; and the assessment of the nuclear fuel cycle, in particular the environmental transport and dosimetry of tritium.*

Kent B. Anderson, *a graduate student at the University of California, Berkeley, has specialized in the economic and environmental impacts of energy supply and conservation.*

David S. Brookshire, *a specialist in resource and environmental economics, is associate professor of economics at the University of Wyoming, Laramie. In the last five years he has been a principal motivator in the development of techniques for valuing non-market goods for use in environmental policy assessments. His other research interests have included analysis of boomtowns, wildlife resources, distributional impacts of environmental policies and valuation of natural hazards information.*

Peter M. Deibler *is a policy analyst for the Governor's Office of Appropriate Technology in Sacramento, California.*

*He has done environmental assessments of different energy technologies, in particular unconventional natural gas, and he has worked on the development of alternatives to land disposal of hazardous waste.*

**Ralph C. d'Arge,** *a specialist in resource economics, is John S. Bugas Distinguished Professor of Economics at the University of Wyoming, Laramie. The founder and joint managing editor of* The Journal of Environmental Economics and Management, *he is coeditor of the volume* Progress in Resource Management and Environmental Planning *(with T. O'Riordan; Wiley, 1979) and coauthor of* Economics of the Environment: A Materials Balance Approach *(with A. V. Kneese and R. U. Ayres; Resources for the Future/Johns Hopkins Press, 1970). In 1981 he served as president of the Association of Environmental and Resource Economists.*

**Baruch Fischhoff** *is research associate at Decision Research (a branch of Perceptronics, Inc.) in Eugene, Oregon; visiting associate professor of psychology at the University of Oregon at Eugene; and visiting scientist at the Medical Research Council/Applied Psychology Unit in Cambridge, England. A specialist in risk analysis and in decision making and judgment under uncertainty, he has written numerous articles on risk perception, public values and technology management, and the quality of scientific judgment. He is senior author of* Acceptable Risk *(with S. Lichtenstein et al.; Cambridge University Press, 1981).*

**Peter H. Gleick** *is a research specialist with the Energy and Resources Group at the University of California, Berkeley. His research has focused on the environmental consequences of energy production and use, the occupational and public health and safety aspects of energy use, and on the comparative risks of various energy systems. Since July 1981 he has served as Deputy Assistant for Energy and Environment to Governor Jerry Brown of California.*

**Reginald L. Gotchy** *is currently an administrative judge (technical) on the Atomic Safety and Licensing Appeal Panel of the U.S. Nuclear Regulatory Commission. Formerly a senior radiobiologist in the NRC's Office of Nuclear Reactor Regulation, he has done extensive analyses of the potential health and environmental effects associated with nuclear and alternative fuel cycles, radiation dose assessment, and environmental radiological monitoring.*

**John P. Holdren** *is professor of energy and resources at the University of California, Berkeley, a principal investigator for the Energy and Environment Division,*

*Lawrence Berkeley Laboratory, and a faculty consultant to the Magnetic Fusion Energy Division, Lawrence Livermore Laboratory. He has written numerous publications on energy technology and policy, including the environmental and sociopolitical impacts of fusion and fission energy, the environmental aspects of renewable energy sources, the potential role of renewable energy sources in the United States, and the role of energy in international conflict. His books include* **Ecoscience: Population, Resources, Environment** *(with P. R. and A. H. Ehrlich; W. H. Freeman, 1977) and* **Energy: A Crisis in Power** *(with P. Herrera; Sierra Club Books, 1971).*

**Sarah Lichtenstein** *is a research associate at Decision Research (a branch of Perceptronics, Inc.) in Eugene, Oregon, and adjunct professor of psychology at the University of Oregon, Eugene. Her research interests are judgment and decision making, decision aids, and risk assessment, and she is a coauthor of* **Acceptable Risk** *(with B. Fischhoff et al.; Cambridge University Press, 1981).*

**Irving M. Mintzer** *is associate research specialist with the Energy and Resources Group, University of California, Berkeley. His specialties include environmental risk assessment and the technological and policy issues raised by renewable resource utilization, and he has published on the environmental impacts of photovoltaic power systems and the impacts of photovoltaic deployment on electric utilities.*

**Gregory P. Morris** *is a research specialist with the Energy and Resources Group at the University of California, Berkeley. A specialist in synthetic fuels and biomass energy, he has published on the environmental implications of renewable energy sources and on the environmental impacts and optimal use of biomass energy resources.*

**Samuel C. Morris** *is a research scientist in the Department of Energy and Environment at Brookhaven National Laboratory and an adjunct associate professor of engineering and public policy at Carnegie-Mellon University. A specialist in risk assessment, he has been concerned with the health and environmental effects of various energy technologies. He has published on the health effects of coal synfuels, the health effects of air pollution from coal combustion, and the health and environmental implications of the National Energy Plan.*

**William D. Schulze** *is currently professor of economics at the University of Wyoming, Laramie. The author of more than 60 papers and reports, he has done his principal research on issues related to energy, including solar and geothermal,*

*natural resources, and the environment.  He has done statis-
tical analyses of the health effects of air pollution and
benefit analyses of reducing health risks from toxic substances.  His other research interests include nuclear waste
storage, water quality, earthquake hazards, and boomtown
impacts.*

*Paul Slovic is research associate at Decision Research
(a branch of Perceptronics, Inc.) in Eugene, Oregon, and
adjunct professor of psychology at the University of Oregon,
Eugene.  His specialties include judgment, decision making,
and risk assessment, and he has coauthored numerous publications on these topics.  He is a council member of the Society
for Risk Analysis, a fellow of the American Psychological
Association, and a member of the editorial boards of several
professional journals.*

*Frank von Hippel, a theoretical physicist, is a senior
research physicist at the Center for Energy and Environmental
Studies at Princeton University.  His interests include nuclear energy policy, nuclear arms policy, energy efficiency,
and the rights and responsibilities of scientists.  He is
coauthor of* Advice and Dissent:  Scientists in the Political
Arena *(with J. Primack; Basic, 1974), and in 1977 he received
the American Physical Society Forum Award for Promoting the
Understanding of the Relationship Between Physics and Society.*

_____ *Curtis C. Travis, Elizabeth L. Etnier*

# Introduction

Health and environmental risks associated with energy production have become a matter of increasing public concern. Apprehension regarding nuclear power has been responsible for a virtual halt in the licensing and construction of nuclear reactors. At the same time, the option of increased reliance on coal-fired power plants raises concern regarding occupational safety of coal workers, and public health risks linked to air pollution. The need for greater public and scientific participation in the decision making processes regarding energy production necessitates a clear presentation of the issues.

All energy technologies have inherent health and environmental risks associated with their use. The origins and potential magnitude of these risks are as varied as the technologies themselves. The most obvious, and readily quantifiable, risks are those related to occupational health and safety. However, many energy systems produce categories of social and environmental harm that are highly resistant to quantification: global climate change, acid rain, nuclear proliferation, and radioactive waste disposal are but a few examples. It may well be that the most important impacts of energy production are those most difficult to quantify. Given the complexity of the situation, a complete and comprehensive comparison of risks from the various existing and proposed energy technologies is not currently possible. Such a comparison would require identification and quantification of all risks in each of the respective fuel cycles. For emerging technologies such as solar power, synfuels, or fusion energy, data necessary to quantify the totality of risk do not exist. Even for well-defined technologies, such as coal-fired power plants, incomplete and uncertain data preclude definitive analysis.[1] Despite these problems, decisions on energy policy cannot be delayed. A systematic distillation of available information

*1*

concerning technology-related risks should be of benefit to
policymakers in formulating these decisions.

This book presents a state-of-the-art compilation of
the occupational and public health risks associated with
coal and nuclear power generation, as well as some of the
less conventional energy technologies. We consider such
aspects as mining, processing, construction, power generation, waste disposal, and transportation. Unconventional
energy technologies discussed include solar power, biomass,
and municipal and animal wastes.

Decisions concerning the management of hazardous technologies often hinge on societal acceptance of the risks
involved. Public perception and acceptance of risk are
influenced by a number of factors. Public familiarity with
the technology involved is of primary importance. A Commission of European Communities (CEC, 1980) report cites a study
showing that the risk of rail travel, highly unacceptable
to the general public 150 years ago, has become accepted
with the passage of time even though the absolute level of
risk has changed very little. A second factor involved in
societal acceptance is the "degree of choice" in exposure
to risk. For example, smokers voluntarily accept the risk
of lung cancer resulting from inhalation of cigarette smoke,
whereas most people will not accept the much lower, but
involuntary, risk of death from radiation linked to nuclear
power generation [a risk about five orders of magnitude
lower (Cohen and Lee, 1979)]. A third factor involves fear
of catastrophic accidents. The public is inherently fright-
ened by this possibility, even when such accidents have a
low probability of occurrence; they are much more willing
to accept common hazards that injure one person at a time,
but which occur at a high frequency (for instance, automobile accidents). Since risk perception is one of the key
issues in deciding the acceptability of a particular national
energy policy, it is an area deserving greater attention.

The first chapter, by Fischhoff, Slovic, and Lichtenstein, addresses the disparity between expert opinion and
public perception of risk. Studies by the authors suggest
that a number of reasons exist for differences between
expert and lay opinion. Most important is a *communication
gap* between the experts and the public, in which pertinent
information relating to the risk of a technology may be
omitted for fear of misunderstanding. It seems that lay
people may be better informed and more educable than is
generally believed by experts. Secondly, there appears to
be a *perception gap*, possibly due in part to the lack of
adequate technical data regarding the probabilities and consequences of accidents. When lay people appear irrational

in their decisions, they may only have been poorly informed or solving a different problem than that assumed by the experts. Fischoff and his co-authors conclude that more respectful and balanced relationships between the expert and lay communities would promote better communication. Nonexperts should attempt to be better informed and to rely less on preconceived judgments, while experts need to recognize their shortcomings in assessing risk, and give greater attention to the psychological aspects of risk perception.

The energy technology that is viewed most negatively by the public is, without doubt, nuclear energy. A possible explanation for the public's unique lack of confidence in nuclear power as an energy alternative is that it scores low in most factors of societal risk acceptance. The newness of nuclear technology, in conjunction with the possibility of a catastrophic accident and the involuntary nature of the associated risk, all contribute to public concern over widespread adoption of this technology.

In the chapter on health risks from the nuclear fuel cycle, Reginald Gotchy presents estimates of the health risks associated with the nuclear fuel cycle, including normal operation and accidents. He considers the entire fuel cycle starting with uranium mining and milling, following it through fuel fabrication and electric power generation by nuclear reactors, and finally looks at the risks associated with the transportation, storage, and disposal of radioactive wastes. Gotchy lists occupational deaths and range of injuries per gigawatt electric year [GW(e)-year] as 0.22 and 7-20, respectively, for the nuclear fuel cycle. These deaths and injuries result primarily during the uranium mining process, and are nonradiological in nature. Radiological risk from the nuclear fuel cycle may also cause health effects in present and future generations. Gotchy presents estimates of radiologically induced health risk for 100- and 1000-yr time periods. The total cancer and genetic risk over the next century from normal operation of the nuclear fuel cycle (including reprocessing and waste disposal) is about equally divided between workers (0.25 and 0.17) and the general public (0.20 and 0.17)[2], respectively. If risk from catastrophic accidents is included, the total cancer and genetic risk to the general public is increased to 0.24 and 0.25, respectively. To place this risk in perspective, the total cancer risk from nuclear power over the next century per GW(e)-year is 10,000 times less than the expected cancer risk to the U. S. population from natural background radiation. Gotchy discusses the uncertainties associated with predictions of future risk including the difficulty in making accurate population projections, and the dependence of potential radiation risk on the characteristics of

society.  He attempts to put in perspective the comparative
public health risk of the nuclear fuel cycle, other sources
of radiation exposure, and normal annual risk of mortality
from everyday events (smoking, driving, fires, falls, etc.).

In May 1979, the U. S. Department of Energy issued a
revised version of the National Energy Plan.  This plan was
an attempt to define the government's long-term goals for
guiding the nation past its current energy crisis.  A primary
thrust of this plan was a projected increased reliance on
the use of coal to meet the nation's energy needs.  This
reliance will of necessity result in increased health and
environmental problems.  Occupational health risks associated
with coal technologies include, but are not limited to,
fatalities and injuries during the mining of coal, chronic
lung disease found in coal miners, accidental deaths from
increased coal transportation activities, and injuries and
deaths during power generation.  Coal burning also promotes
adverse health effects among the general public.  The
increased effects of air pollution from coal combustion are
difficult to quantify, but nevertheless may prove significant.  In the third chapter of this book, Samuel Morris
addresses the health risk of coal technologies from extraction to ultimate energy consumption.  He estimates occupational deaths and injuries per GW(e)-year as 1.3 and 96.6,
respectively.  Underground coal mining contributes the bulk
of these occupational impacts.  The primary public health
impact from the coal fuel cycle, 10-21 deaths/GW(e)-year,
results from air pollution.  Even though this latter risk
is involuntary in nature, and approximately 100 times greater
than the comparable risk from nuclear energy, the public
appears more willing to accept it.  Again, this reflects
public acceptance of risk resulting from familiar technologies, and fear of the unknown or unpredictable, i.e.,
catastrophic nuclear accidents, nuclear waste disposal and
proliferation.

Many renewable energy sources are viewed by the general
public as having no direct public health impacts.  Perhaps
this is because they produce no pollutants during normal
operation.  Energy sources such as solar, wind, ocean thermal, and hydropower fall in this category.  However, these
energy technologies produce health impacts during their
fabrication and construction, and also through the materials
supply sectors required to support them.  There are many
technical and conceptual problems associated with making
estimates of the health and safety impacts of the less conventional energy technologies.  However, estimates of the
health risks associated with these energy technologies must
be made if we are to have a clear presentation of the issues.
John Holdren and his co-authors survey risk from renewable

energy technologies and conclude that some of the renewable options have particular promise for reducing health and environmental costs, per unit of energy delivered, to well below levels associated with the use of oil and coal.

In making choices among different energy technologies, we tend to focus on local risks from pollution or accidents. However, several energy technologies have consequences which are global in nature. Examples are the possibility of nuclear war due to the proliferation of nuclear materials, and the production of acid rain from sulfates and nitrates formed in the atmosphere after coal combustion. Another problem associated with coal combustion is the possibility of global climate modification caused by atmospheric accumulations of carbon dioxide given off during combustion of fossil fuels. The so-called "greenhouse effect" has caused substantial concern that increased reliance on coal as an energy source will result in critical global temperature changes. A fundamental issue in the energy debate is the long range risk to the future health of our economy and environment implied by the priority given to investments in new energy supply technologies at the expense of investments in energy efficiency improvements. For example, the nation might better spend its' resources retooling automobile production plants to make much more fuel efficient automobiles than building new synthetic fuel plants. Frank von Hippel discusses these and other global issues associated with energy production.

Health risk associated with energy generation is but one factor which must be considered in determining a national energy policy. Economic considerations must, of necessity, be given a high priority. The last chapter of this book, written by Schulze, Brookshire, and d'Arge, explores in detail the relationship between economics and risk analysis. The importance of the selection of an appropriate ethical criterion upon which to base benefit-cost analysis is stressed. The authors also discuss the shortcomings of traditional benefit-cost analysis when applied to such long-term environmental problems as carbon dioxide-induced climate changes. For example, complete loss of the world's gross national product in 100 years, growing at 3%, would be worth about one million dollars today if discounted at recent prime rates. Thus, future catastrophic environmental losses may be almost valueless to the present generation. The bias introduced when current ethical values are imposed on future generations is discussed. It is argued that the appropriate social rate of discount varies substantially depending on the underlying ethical beliefs of society. Some ethical beliefs lead to discounting future effects to zero, while

others require valuing future effects at more than present
costs or benefits.

The field of comparative risk assessment is in its
infancy. However, the multitude of complex technological
problems facing our country necessitates its early maturity.
This book represents an attempt to highlight the methodological and conceptual difficulties inherent in estimating and
comparing risks of energy production. Despite the difficulties and uncertainties involved, the authors provide a comprehensive compilation of risk resulting from energy technologies. The book also provides insight into the impact
of public perception and economic considerations on decisions
related to risk management.

We hope that this book will enhance communication
between policy makers, scientists, and the general public
as they search for an acceptable solution to the Nation's
energy needs.

## Acknowledgements

Work on this manuscript was performed at the Oak Ridge
National Laboratory, operated by Union Carbide Corporation
under contract W-7405-eng-26 with the U. S. Department of
Energy. The editors wish to thank Robin Smith for her contributions to the typing of this volume. Special gratitude
goes to Wilma Minor for her competence and extreme patience
in preparing the many revisions and final camera-ready copy
of the manuscript herein.

## Notes

[1] A more complete discussion of the data limitations
and uncertainties associated with risk analysis can be
found in House et al. (1981); Holdren, Morris, and Mintzer
(1980); and Whipple (1981).

[2] Cancer risk is measured in deaths/GW(e)-year, and
genetic risk is measured as genetically or irregularly
inherited disorders/$10^6$ liveborn.

## References

Cohen, B. L. and I-S Lee. 1979. A catalog of risk.
    *Health Phys.* 36:707-722.

Commission of the European Communities (CEC). 1980.
    *Nuclear and Non-Nuclear Risk — An Exercise in Compar-
    ability.* EUR-6417. Pollution Preventions (Consul-
    tants) Ltd., Crawley, England. CEC, Luxenbourg.

Holdren, J. P., G. Morris, and I. Mintzer. 1980. Environmental aspects of renewable energy sources. *Ann. Rev. Energy* 5:241-91.

House, P. W., J. A. Coleman, R. D. Shull, R. W. Matheny, and J. C. Hock. 1981. *Comparing Energy Technology Alternatives from an Environmental Perspective.* DOE/EV-0109. U. S. Department of Energy, Washington, D.C.

Whipple, C. 1981. Energy production risks: what perspective should we take? *Risk Anal.* 1(1):29-36.

*Baruch Fischhoff, Paul Slovic,*
*Sarah Lichtenstein*

# 1. Judging the Health Risks of Energy Systems

## Introduction[1]

Over the next few decades, the success of energy production policies will depend vitally on public attitudes. It
has gradually come to be recognized that energy decisions
cannot be determined by technical criteria alone. Social,
psychological, and political issues are also crucial in
deciding on national energy policies. Involved with these
decisions are such questions as: "What kinds of risks should
be accepted in exchange for what kinds of benefits? With
how much uncertainty of specific kinds does the public care
to live? How does one weigh the substantial routine impact
of some technologies (for example, burning coal) with the
small chance of a big disaster associated with others. . . ."
(Holdren, 1976, p. 22).

Despite the importance of these questions, we are only
beginning to understand the social and psychological factors
(goals, values, criteria, etc.) that determine public
responses to technological risks in general and from energy
systems in particular. This is both because the problems in
this area are difficult and because relatively little time,
effort, and research funding have been applied to them. One
reason for this neglect is the fact that scientists and
policymakers have been slow to recognize the importance of
public attitudes and perceptions. Writing in the *American
Scientist*, Alvin Weinberg (1976) observed:

"As I compare the issues we perceived during
the infancy of nuclear energy with those that have
emerged during its maturity, the public perception
and acceptance of nuclear energy appears to be the
question that we missed rather badly. . . This
issue has emerged as the most critical question concerning the future of nuclear energy" (p. 19).

In place of systematic research, one often finds unsubstantiated assertions about what the public wants, knows, and is capable of understanding. However, like speculations about chemical reactions, speculations about human behavior need to be disciplined by fact. Because those speculations make important statements about people and their capabilities, failure to validate them may mean arrogating to oneself considerable political power. Such happens, for example, when one says that people are so poorly informed (and uneducable) that they might be better off surrendering some political rights to technical experts. It also happens, at the other extreme, when one claims that people are so well informed (and offered such freedom of choice) that one need not ask them anything at all about their desires; to know what they want, one need only observe their behavior in the marketplace. It also happens when we assume that people are consummate hedonists, rational to the extreme in their consumer behavior, but totally uncomprehending of broader economic issues, so that we can impose effective fiscal policies on them without being second guessed.

There are several reasons for survival of such simplistic and contradictory positions. One reason is political convenience. For some people it is politically convenient that the lay public be described as competent and that they be encouraged to participate actively in hazard management decisions; others need an incompetent public to legitimate an expert elite. A second reason is theoretical convenience. It is hard to build models of people who are sometimes wise and sometimes foolish, sometimes risk-seeking and sometimes risk averse. A third reason is that it is relatively easy to produce anecdotal information to support one's personal speculations about human nature. Indeed, good social theory may be so rare precisely because poor social theory is so easy.

Fortunately, a flurry of research activity in recent years has provided some insight into the sociopsychological dynamics of societal risk taking. What follows is a brief review of that work and the tentative conclusions that it allows. It starts with a discussion of difficulties that people experience when attempting to estimate risks. With this as background, the remainder of the chapter discusses perception and acceptance of risks from energy systems, with particular emphasis being placed on responses to nuclear power.

## Coping Intellectually with Risk

Evaluation of the risks from energy systems requires, of experts and lay people alike, an appreciation of the probabilistic nature of the world and an ability to think intelligently about unlikely, but consequential events. As Weinberg (1976) noted in the context of nuclear power, ". . . we certainly accept on faith that our human intellect is capable of dealing with this new source of energy" (p. 21). The message resulting from much of the research into human judgment and decision processes is to question that faith.

## Risk Perception

Because of its importance to decision making, the question of how people assess the probabilities of uncertain events has become a focus of research interest. This research indicates that intelligent people systematically violate the principles of rational decision making when judging probabilities, making predictions, or otherwise attempting to cope with uncertainty. Frequently, these violations can be traced to the use of judgmental heuristics, mental strategies by which people reduce difficult judgments to simpler ones (Tversky and Kahneman, 1974). These heuristics are useful guides in some circumstances, but in others they lead to large and persistent biases with serious implications for decision making (Slovic, Kunreuther, and White, 1974; Slovic, Fischhoff, and Lichtenstein, 1977; Tversky and Kahneman, 1974).

One such heuristic that may have special relevance to energy decisions is the "availability heuristic," whereby an event is judged likely or frequent if it is easy to imagine or recall instances of it. Generally, instances of frequent events are easier to recall than instances of less frequent events and likely occurrences are easier to imagine than unlikely ones. Thus availability is often an appropriate cue for judging frequency and probability. However, availability is also affected by numerous factors unrelated to likelihood. As a result, reliance on it may lead people to exaggerate the probabilities of events that are particularly recent, vivid, or emotionally salient.

Availability bias is illustrated by several recent studies in which college students and members of the League of Women Voters were asked to judge the frequency of various causes of death, such as smallpox, tornadoes, and heart disease (Lichtenstein et al., 1978). In one study (depicted in Figure 1), they were first told the annual death toll for motor vehicle accidents in the United States (50,000) and then asked to estimate the frequencies of forty other causes of death. In another study, participants were given two causes of death and were asked to judge which of the two was more frequent.

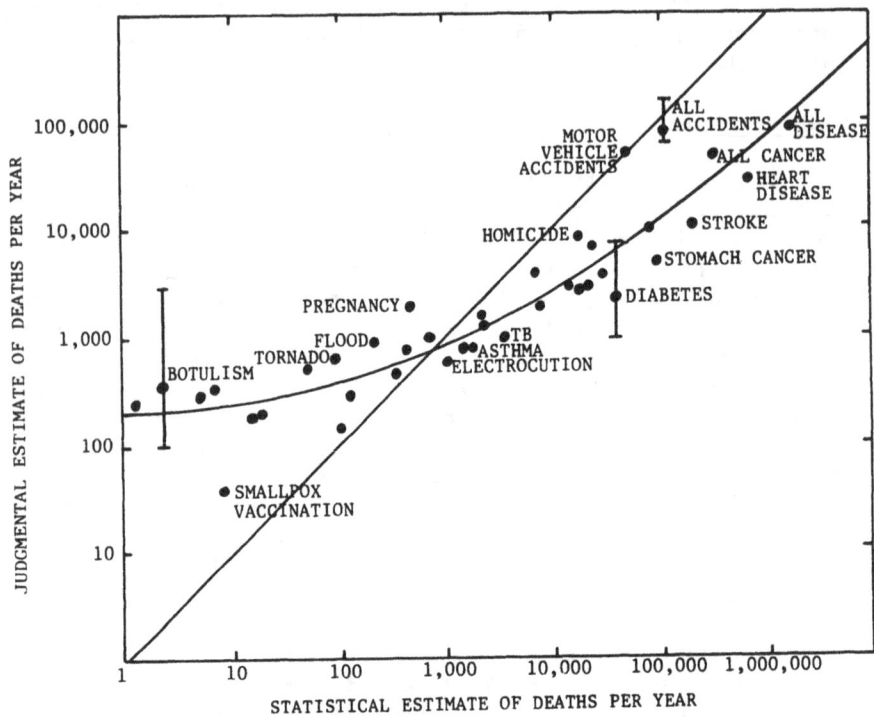

Figure 1.  Relationship between judged frequency and
the actual number of deaths per year for 41 causes of death.
If judged and actual frequencies were equal, the data would
fall on the straight line.  The points, and the curved line
fitted to them, represent the averaged responses of a large
number of lay people.  Although people were approximately
accurate, their judgments were systematically distorted.
To give an idea of the degree of agreement among subjects,
vertical bars are drawn to depict the 25th and 75th percen-
tile of individual judgment for botulism, diabetes, and
all accidents.  Fifty percent of all judgments fall between
these limits.  The range of responses for the other 37 causes
of death are similar.  Source:  Slovic, Fischhoff, and
Lichtenstein (1979).

Table 1.  Bias in judged frequency of death

| Most overestimated | Most underestimated |
| --- | --- |
| All accidents | Smallpox vaccination |
| Motor vehicle accidents | Diabetes |
| Pregnancy, childbirth and | Stomach cancer |
|   abortion | Lightning |
| Tornadoes | Stroke |
| Flood | Tuberculosis |
| Botulism | Asthma |
| All cancer | Emphysema |
| Fire and flames | |
| Venomous bite or sting | |
| Homicide | |

Adapted from Lichtenstein et al., 1978.

Both studies showed people's judgments to be moderately accurate in a global sense; that is, people usually knew which were the most and least frequent lethal events.  Moreover, several different ways of asking people to assess these risks produced highly similar subjective orderings of their magnitude, indicating a consistent internal scale of frequency.  However, within this global picture, people made serious misjudgments, many of which seemed to reflect availability bias.  For example, accidents were judged to cause as many deaths as diseases, whereas diseases actually take about fifteen times as many lives.  Homicides were incorrectly judged to be more frequent than diabetes and stomach cancer.  Homicides were also judged to be about as frequent as stroke, although the latter actually claim about eleven times as many lives.  Frequencies of death from botulism, tornadoes, and pregnancy (including childbirth and abortion) were also greatly overestimated.

Table 1 lists the lethal events whose frequencies were most poorly judged in our studies.  In keeping with availability considerations, overestimated items were dramatic and sensational, whereas underestimated items tended to be unspectacular events that claim one victim at a time and are common in nonfatal form.  A follow-up study showed that newspaper coverage of the various causes of death was biased in much the same way as were people's judgments (Combs and Slovic, 1979).

Was the performance of people's judgments in these studies good or bad?  One possible summary is that it may be about as good as can be expected, given that these people were neither specialists in the hazards considered, nor exposed to a representative sample of information.

Such accurate perception of misleading samples of information might also underlie another apparent judgmental bias, people's predilection for exaggerating their personal immunity from many hazards. The vast majority of individuals believe themselves to be better than average drivers, more likely than average to live past 80, less likely than average to be injured by tools they operate, and so on (Weinstein, 1980). Although such perceptions are obviously unrealistic, from the perspective of each individual's experience, the risks do look very small. Consider automobile driving: despite driving too fast, tailgating, etc., poor drivers make trip after trip without mishap. This personal experience may demonstrate to them their exceptional skill and safety. Moreover, their indirect experience via the media shows them that when accidents happen, they happen to others. One could hope that people would see beyond the limits of their own minds and information, but inability to do so need not render them imcompetent to make decisions in their own behalf.

## Confidence

A particularly pernicious aspect of heuristics is that people are typically very confident about judgments based on them. For example, in a follow-up to the study on causes of death, participants were asked to indicate the odds that they were correct in their judgments about which of two lethal events was more frequent (Fischhoff, Slovic, and Lichtenstein, 1977). Odds of 100:1 or greater were given often (25% of the time). However, about one out of every eight answers associated with such extreme confidence was wrong (fewer than 1 in 100 would have been wrong had the odds been appropriate). About 30% of the judges gave odds greater than 50:1 to the incorrect assertion that homicides were more frequent than suicides. The psychological basis for this unwarranted certainty seems to be people's insensitivity to the tenuousness of the assumptions upon which their judgments are based. In this case, the erroneous assumption may have been the validity of the availability heuristic. In other cases, other assumptions might be implicated. Such overconfidence is dangerous. It indicates that we often do not realize how little we know and how much additional information we need about the various problems we face.

Overconfidence manifests itself in other ways as well. A typical task in estimating failure rates or other uncertain quantities is to set upper and lower confidence bounds so that there is a 98% chance that the true value lies between them. Experiments with diverse groups of people making many different kinds of judgments have shown that, rather than 2% of true values falling outside the 98% confidence bounds, 20-50% do so (Lichtenstein, Fischhoff, and Phillips, 1982). People think that they can estimate such values with much greater precision than is actually the case.

Unfortunately, experts may be as prone to overconfidence as lay people. Hynes and Vanmarcke (1976) asked seven "internationally known" geotechnical engineers to predict the height of an embankment that would cause a clay foundation to fail and to specify confidence bounds around this estimate that were wide enough to have a 50% chance of enclosing the true failure height. None of the bounds specified by these experts actually did enclose the true height. (The fact that some were too high and others too low indicates that this was not just a trick question.) The Reactor Safety Study (USNRC, 1975), in assessing the probability of a core melt in a nuclear reactor, used a procedure for setting confidence bounds that has been found in experiments to produce a particularly high degree of overconfidence. Related problems led a review committee to conclude that the Reactor Safety Study greatly overestimated the precision with which it had assessed the probability of a core melt (USNRC, 1978).

Another case in point is the 1976 collapse of the Teton Dam. The Committee on Government Operations has attributed this disaster to the unwarranted confidence of engineers who were absolutely certain they had solved the many serious problems that arose during construction (U.S. Government, 1976). In routine practice, failure probabilities are not even calculated for new dams even though about 1 in 300 fails when the reservoir is first filled. Further anecdotal evidence of overconfidence may be found in many other technical risk assessments (Fischhoff, 1977). Table 2 offers some common ways in which experts may overlook or misjudge pathways to disaster.

## Conflicting Views

A characteristic feature of many risk debates is the confrontation between polarized views held with great confidence (and perhaps overconfidence). For example, some people view nuclear power as extraordinarily safe, whereas others view it as a catastrophe in the making. It would be comforting to believe that these divergent beliefs would converge toward one "appropriate" view as new evidence was presented. Unfortunately, this is not likely to be the

Table 2. Some problems in structuring risk assessments

| Problem | Example | Reference |
|---------|---------|-----------|
| Failure to consider the ways in which human errors can affect technological systems. | Due to inadequate training and control room design, operators at Three Mill Island repeatedly misdiagnosed the problems of the reactor and took inappropriate actions. | Sheridan, 1980; U. S. Government, 1979. |
| Overconfidence in current scientific knowledge. | Use of DDT came in widespread and uncontrolled use before scientists had even considered the possibility of the side effects that today make it look like a mixed and irreversible blessing. | Dunlap, 1978. |
| Failure to appreciate how technological systems function as a whole. | The DC-10 failed in several early flights because its designers had not realized that decompression of the cargo compartment would destroy vital control systems. | Hohenemser, 1975. |

Table 2. (continued)

| Problem | Example | Reference |
| --- | --- | --- |
| Slowness in detecting chronic, cumulative effects. | Although accidents to coal miners have long been recognized as one cost of operating fossil-fueled plants, the effects of acid rains on ecosystems were slow to be discovered. | Rosencranz and Wetstone, 1980. |
| Failure to anticipate human response to safety measures. | The partial protection afforded by dams and levees gives people a false sense of security and promotes development of the flood plain. Thus, although floods are rarer, damage per flood is so much greater that the average yearly dollar loss is larger than before the dams were built. | Burton, Kates and White, 1978. |
| Failure to anticipate "common-mode failures" which simultaneously afflict systems that are designed to be independent. | Because electrical cables controlling the multiple safety systems of the reactor at Browns Ferry, Alabama, were not spatially separated, all five emergency core cooling systems were damaged by a single fire. | U. S. Government, 1975; Jennergren and Keeney, in press. |

case. A great deal of research suggests that people's beliefs change slowly, and are extraordinarily persistent in the face of contradictory evidence (Mahoney, 1979; Ross, 1977). Once formed, initial impressions tend to structure and distort the way in which subsequent evidence is interpreted. New evidence appears reliable and informative if it is consistent with one's initial beliefs; contradictory evidence is dismissed as unreliable, erroneous, or unrepresentative. Ross (1977) concluded his review of this phenomenon as follows:

> "Erroneous impressions, theories, or data processing strategies, therefore, may not be changed through mere exposure to samples of new evidence. It is not contended, of course, that new evidence can *never* produce change — only that new evidence will produce *less* change than would be demanded by any logical or rational information-processing model" (p. 210).

Examples of information being interpreted so as to enhance the polarization of views, rather than bring about their convergence, are easy to find in risk debates. Three Mile Island "proved" the possibility of a catastrophic meltdown to some, while to others, it demonstrated the reliability of multiple containment systems. The existence of those containment systems shows the safety consciousness of the industry to some, the inherent hazardousness of nuclear power to others.

## Assessing Values

Once the facts of an issue have been estimated and communicated, it is usually held that lay people should (in a democracy) be asked about their values. What do they want, after the experts have told them what they can (conceivably) have? Such questions would seem to be the last redoubt of unaided intuition. Who knows better than an individual what he or she prefers? When one is considering simple, familiar events with which people have direct experience, it may be reasonable to assume that they have well-articulated opinions. Regarding the novel, global consequences potentially associated with $CO_2$-induced climatic change, nuclear meltdowns, or genetic engineering, that may not be the case. Our values may be incoherent, not thought through. In thinking about acceptable levels of risk, for example, we may be unfamiliar with the terms in which issues are formulated (e.g., social discount rates, minuscule probabilities, megadeaths). We may have contradictory values (e.g., a strong aversion to catastrophic losses of life and a realization that we're no more moved by a plane

crash with 500 fatalities than one with 300). We may
occupy different roles in life (parents, workers, children)
each of which produces clear-cut, but inconsistent values.
We may vacillate between incompatible, but strongly held
positions (e.g., freedom of speech is inviolate, but should
be denied to authoritarian movements). We may not even know
how to begin thinking about some issues (e.g., the appropriate trade-off between the benefits of dyeing one's hair
and a minute risk of cancer 20 years from now). Our view
may undergo changes of time (say, as we near the hour of
decision or of experiencing the consequence) and we may not
know which view should form the basis of our decision.

When people do not know, or have difficulty appraising
what they want, the way a question is posed may significantly affect the values expressed, or apparently expressed,
in the responses they elicit. As a result, scientists,
politicians, merchants, and the media may be able to represent issues so as to induce random error (by confusing the
respondent), systematic error (by hinting at what the
"correct" response is), or unduly extreme judgments (by
suggesting clarity and coherence of opinions that are not
warranted). In such cases, the method becomes the message.
If elicited values are used to guide policy, they may lead
to decisions not in the decision maker's best interest, to
action when caution is desirable (or the opposite), or to
the obfuscation of poorly formulated views that need careful
development and clarification (Fischhoff, Slovic, and Lichtenstein, 1980; Payne, 1952).

Judgments are sensitive to elicitation procedure
because formulating a response always involves an inferential process. When confronted with an issue for which
neither habit nor tradition dictates our answer, we must
decide which of our basic values are relevant to that situation, how they are to be interpreted, and what weight each
is to be given. Unless one has thought deeply about the
issue, it is natural to turn to the questioner for hints as
to what to say. Table 3 summarizes the elicitor's opportunities. The first is to decide that there is something to
question. In this fundamental way, the elicitor impinges on
the respondent's values. By asking about the desirability
of premarital sex, interracial dating, daily prayer, freedom
of expression, or the fall of capitalism, the elicitor may
legitimate events that were previously viewed as unacceptable or cast doubts on events that were previously unques-
tioned. Opinion polls help set our national agenda by the
questions they do and do not ask (Marsh, 1979). Advertising
helps set our personal agendas by the questions it induces
us to ask ourselves (two-door or four-door?) and those it
tacitly answers (more is better).

Table 3.  Ways that an elicitor may affect a respondent's
          judgments of value

---

Defining the issue

   Is there a problem?
   What options and consequences are relevant?
   How should options and consequences be labeled?
   How should values be measured?
   Should the problem be decomposed?

Changing the respondent's perspective

   Altering the salience of perspectives.
   Altering the importance of perspectives.
   Choosing the time of inquiry.
   Changing the confidence in expressed values.
   Changing the apparent degree of coherence.

Changing the respondent

   Destroying existing perspectives.
   Creating perspective.
   Deepening perspectives.

---

Source:  Fischhoff, Slovic and Lichtenstein, 1980.

Table 4.  Two formulations of a choice problem

---

Imagine that the United States is preparing for the outbreak
of an unusual Asian disease, which is expected to kill 600
people.  Two alternative programs to combat the disease
have been proposed.  Assume that the consequences of the
programs are as follows:

| Lives saved | Lives lost |
|---|---|
| If Program A is adopted, 200 people will be saved. | If Program C is adopted, 400 people will die. |
| If Program B is adopted, there is a 1/3 probability that 600 people will be saved, and 2/3 probability that no people will be saved. | If Program D is adopted, there is a 1/3 probability that nobody will die, and 2/3 probability that 600 people will die. |

Which of the two programs would you favor?

---

Source:  Tversky and Kahneman, 1981.

Once the issue has been evoked, it must be given a label.  In the absence of hard, evaluative standards, such symbolic interpretations may be very important (Marks, 1977).  Although the facts of abortion remain constant, individuals may vacillate in their attitude as they attach and detach the label of "murder."  The use of economic, psychological, or anthropocentric terminology may evoke particular modes of thought and ethical standards (Ashcraft, 1977).  Table 4 shows a labeling effect that produced a reversal of preference with practicing physicians, most pre-ferred Program A over Program B, and Program D over Program C, despite the formal equivalence of A and C and of B and D.  The labels, saving lives and losing lives, afforded very different perspectives on the same problem.

It would be comforting to be able to say which way of phrasing value questions is the right one.  Indeed, there are norms and procedures for spotting deliberately confusing or biased formulations (Payne, 1952; Zeisel, 1980).  How-ever, no procedure can guarantee a polished product when respondents start with an incoherent opinion or none at all. Different perspectives may continue to evoke opinions that refuse to converge.  Indeed, life is too involved for anyone to have articulated preferences on every issue that might be posed by a pollster or a decision-making specialist or the political process or the marketplace.

When the questioner must have an answer (say, because public input is statutorily required), there may be no sub-stitute for an elicitation procedure that educates respond-ents about how they might look at the question and expli-cates the practical implications and logical concomitants of various possible perspectives.  The possibilities for manip-ulation in such interviews are obvious, as anyone who has had their values articulated by interaction with a used car salesperson knows.  Indeed, protracted interactions with respondents are anathema to many surveyors.  However, one cannot claim to be serving respondents' best interests (let-ting them speak their minds) by asking a question or posing a choice that touches only one facet of a complex and incom-pletely formulated set of views.

## Forecasting Public Response Towards Energy Systems

People respond to the hazards they perceive.  The basic research cited above, supplemented by studies of perceptions of specific energy systems, could deepen our understanding of how and why people form attitudes towards those systems and what are the possibilities for greater societal consen-sus.  Any attempt to plan the role of nuclear power, in par-ticular, in the nation's energy future must consider the

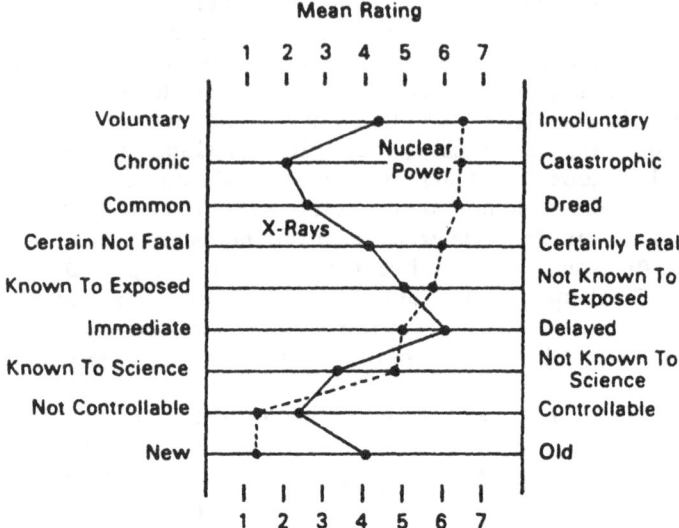

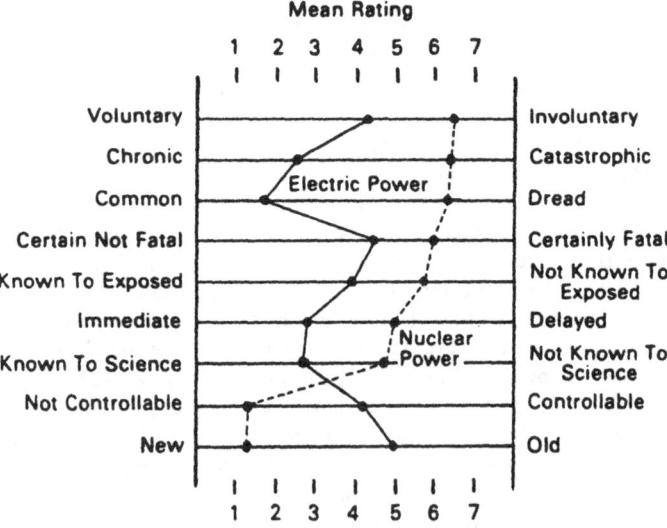

Figure 2.   Characteristics of risk for nuclear power and related technologies, as noted by members of the Eugene, Oregon, League of Women Voters.   Reprinted by permission from Fischhoff et al., "How Safe is Safe Enough?   A Psychometric Study of Attitudes Towards Technological Risks and Benefits," *Policy Sciences* 9:127-152 (1978).

determinants of the opposition it has evoked. One clue lies
in research showing that the images of potential nuclear
disasters formed in the minds of the anti-nuclear public are
remarkably different from the assessments put forth by most
technical experts.

Although questions of safety dominate the nuclear
debate, and figure prominently in the research cited here,
it is important to recognize that opposition to nuclear
power is an organized political movement fueled by many
other concerns besides safety (Bronfman and Mattingly, 1976;
Otway, Maurer, and Thomas, 1978). Although some nuclear
opponents are motivated primarily by fear of routine or
catastrophic radiation releases, others are disenchanted
with growth, centralization, corporate dominance, technology, or government. These latter individuals may argue
about safety because they view the hazardousness of nuclear
power as its "Achilles heel." The discussion that follows
is not directly concerned with this larger political context, but it does highlight the special qualities of nuclear
power that cause (or allow) political opposition to be
focused around considerations of risk.

## Basic Perceptions

Opponents of nuclear power tend to believe both that
its benefits are quite low and its risks are unacceptably
great (Fischhoff et al., 1978; Slovic, Fischhoff, and
Lichtenstein, 1980). On the benefit side, people do not see
nuclear power as a vital link in the meeting of basic energy
needs (Pokorny, 1977). Many believe it to be merely a sup-
plement to other sources of energy which themselves are
adequate (or could be made adequate by conservation).

On the risk side, nuclear power appears to evoke
greater feelings of dread than almost any other technological activity (Fischhoff et al., 1978). Some have attributed
this reaction to fear of radiation's invisible and irreversible contamination, threatening cancer and genetic damage.
However, use of diagnostic X rays, another radiation technology that incurs similar risks, is not similarly dreaded.
If anything, people underestimate its risks. Other judgments of nuclear power's subjective property may provide
additional clues. Figure 2 contrasts the risk profile of
nuclear with that of X rays and non-nuclear energy, as
judged by members of a middle-aged civic group with anti-
nuclear leanings. As the top figure shows, nuclear power is
viewed as being unlike X rays by virtue of having risks that
are uncontrollable, lethal, and potentially catastrophic.
The bottom figure shows the ways in which it is not seen as
just another energy source, vis-a-vis, its risks.

These views are also reflected in studies asking people opposed to nuclear power to describe their mental images of a nuclear accident and its consequences. We have found a widely held expectation that a serious reactor accident is likely within one's lifetime and could result in hundreds of thousands, even millions, of deaths (Slovic, Lichtenstein, and Fischhoff, 1979). In addition, such an accident is expected to cause severe, irreparable environmental damage over a vast geographic area. These expectations contrast dramatically with the nuclear industry's official view that multiple safety systems will limit the damage in the (extremely unlikely) event of a major accident. The accident sequences described by these lay people do not seem to differ qualitatively from those described by experts (e.g., even opponents of nuclear power did not indicate the belief that nuclear power plants could explode like atomic bombs). However, their respective scenarios differed quantitatively in their judged likelihood of occurrence.

One inevitable consequence of this "perception gap" is uncertainty and distrust on the part of a public that suspects that the risks are incomparably greater than the experts' assessments (Kasper, 1979). The experts, in turn, question the rationality of the public and decry the "emotionalism" stymying technological progress. Bitter and sometimes violent confrontations result.

Recognition of this perception gap has led many experts to claim that the public must be "educated" about the "real" risks from nuclear power. One public opinion analyst (Pokorny, 1977) put the matter as follows:

> "The biggest problem hindering a sophisticated judgment on this question is basic lack of knowledge and facts. Within this current attitudinal milieu, scare stories, confusion, and irrationality often triumph. Only through careful education of facts and knowledge can the people know what the real choices are" . . . (p. 12).

Although we agree that public education campaigns are vital, we feel that they face major obstacles, which need to be overcome if such efforts are to be successful. Some of these are technical, others psychological, and still others reside in the ways in which expert and lay communities view one another.

## Technical Problems

The focus of many people's concern seems to be the catastrophic potential of nuclear power. Yet the technical reality is that there are few cut-and-dried facts regarding the probabilities of such mishaps. The technology is so new and the probabilities in question are so small that risk estimates cannot rely entirely on empirical observations. Instead, such assessments must be derived from complex mathematical models, such as the fault trees and event trees used in the Reactor Safety Study (USNRC, 1975) to assess the probability and consequences of a loss-of-coolant accident. Despite an appearance of objectivity, risk assessments are inherently subjective. Someone, relying on judgment, must structure the analysis to determine the ways that failure might occur, their relative importance, and their logical interconnections.

The difficulties of performing risk assessments have led many critics to question their validity (Bryan, 1974; Fischhoff, 1977; Primack, 1975). One major concern is that important initiating events or pathways to failure may be omitted, causing risks to be underestimated. If omissions are as common and difficult to detect as some critics believe, then underestimation may be substantial. Another problem in assessing the reliability of reactor designs is the difficulty of taking proper account of "common-mode failures." To insure greater safety, many technological systems are highly redundant. Should one crucial part fail, there are others designed to do the same job or to limit the resulting damage. Since the probability of each part failing is very small, the probability of all failing, thereby creating a major disaster, should be minuscule. This reasoning is valid only if the various components are independent (so whatever causes one part to fail will not automatically cause the others to fail). "Common-mode failure" occurs when the independence assumption does not hold. For example, because electrical cables controlling the redundant safety systems at a reactor in Browns Ferry, Alabama, were not spatially separated, all five emergency core cooling systems were rendered inoperative by a single fire (U.S. Government, 1975; Jennergren and Keeney, in press). Developing models that take proper account of such contingencies is a very difficult enterprise.

One critic's skepticism regarding the defensibility of assessments of rare catastrophies summarizes the technical problem concisely:

". . . the expert community is divided about the conceivable realism of probability estimates in the range of one in ten thousand to one in one billion per reactor year. I am among those who believe it to be impossible *in principle* to support numbers as small as these with convincing theoretical argu-

ments . . . . The reason I hold this view is
straightforward: nuclear power systems are so complex that the probability the safety analysis contains serious errors . . . is so big as to render
meaningless the tiny computed probability of accident" (Holdren, 1976, p. 21).

## Communication Problems

Once the best possible technical estimates have been
derived, they must still be communicated. We have noted
some of the ways in which lay people may misinterpret the
information they receive. However, it takes two to communi-
cate. There are a number of ways in which the experts may
fail in their responsibility to inform the public. One is
obviously by not telling the whole story about the hazards
they know best, because they fear that the information would
make the public anxious, because dissemination is not their
job, or because they have a vested interest in keeping
things quiet (Hanley, 1980).

If listeners realize that the tale an expert tells is
incomplete, they may discredit the expert and perhaps exaggerate the presentation's incompleteness ("if I caught that
omission, how many others are there that I didn't catch?").
For that to happen, however, the omission must be dis-
covered. Some evidence suggests that more typically what is
out of sight is effectively out of mind. For example,
Fischhoff, Slovic, and Lichtenstein (1978) presented various
versions of a fault tree describing ways in which a car
might fail to start. These versions differed in how much of
the full tree was left out. When asked to estimate degree
of completeness, respondents were very insensitive to
deletions; even omission of major, commonly known components, such as the ignition and fuel systems, led to only
minor decreases in perceived completeness. Perhaps surprisingly (perhaps disturbingly) similar insensitivity was
found with a group of expert mechanics.

Experts may also exacerbate any tendency people have to
deny or ignore the uncertainty associated with hazardous but
beneficial technologies (Borch, 1968; Kahneman and Tversky,
1979; Kates, 1962; Lichtenstein and Slovic, 1973). In order
to reduce this uncertainty, people may insist on statements
of fact, not probability. Thus, just prior to hearing a
blue-ribbon panel of scientists report being 95% certain
that cyclamates do not cause cancer, former Food and Drug
Administration Commissioner Alexander Schmidt said, "I'm
looking for a clean bill of health, not a wishy-washy, iffy
answer on cyclamates" (*Eugene Register-Guard*, 1976). Like-
wise, when asked about the health effects of pollutants,

Edmund Muskie called for "one-armed" scientists who do not respond, ". . . on the one hand, the evidence is so, but on the other hand . . ." (David, 1975). Lord Rothschild (1978) has noted that the BBC does not like to trouble its listeners with hearing about the confidence intervals surrounding technical estimates. In this atmosphere, unduly confident, one-fisted debators, ready to make definitive statements beyond the available data, may unjustifiably win the day from more even-handed scholars. The temptation may be very great to give people the simple answers they often seem to want.

Social as well as psychological processes help to make balanced presentations an endangered genre. The constraints of legal settings (Bazelon, 1980; Piehler et al., 1974), the exigencies of the political arena, and the provocations of the news media all encourage adversarial encounters that are inhospitable to properly qualified scientific evidence (Mazur, 1973). Lay people viewing such shouting matches may begin to wonder about these "experts" or may feel, "since they can't agree, my guess may be as good as theirs" (Handler, 1980). One positive repercussion of Three Mile Island was that for a time the public was educated in plain English about the process of nuclear power generation and the sources of technical disputes, not just presented with conflicting assertions about overall safety.

## Search for Rationality

In studying people's behavior, perhaps the most reasonable assumption is that there is some method in any apparent madness. For example, Zentner (1979) berates the public because its rate of concern about cancer is increasing faster than the cancer rate. One rational explanation would be that people believe that too little concern has been given to cancer in the past (e.g., our concern for acute hazards like traffic safety and infectious disease allowed cancer to creep up on us). A second is that people may realize that some forms of cancers are the only major cause of death whose rate is increasing. Just as it is counterproductive for lay people to view technology promoters as evil on the basis of insufficient or misinterpreted evidence, it is counterproductive for promoters to view lay people as misinformed and irresponsible on similar grounds.

Other apparently irrational behavior can be attributed to the rational pursuit of officially unreasonable objectives. This can happen when one rejects the problem definition deemed reasonable by the presenting body. Consider, for example, an individual who is opposed to increased energy consumption but is asked only about which energy

source to adopt or where to site proposed facilities.  The
answers to these narrow questions provide a de facto answer
to the broader question of growth.  Such an individual may
have little choice but to fight dirty, engaging in uncon-
structive criticism, poking holes in analyses supporting
other positions, or ridiculing opponents who adhere to the
more narrow definition.

Indeed, some participants in technology debates are in
it for the fight.  Many approaches to determining accept-
able-risk levels (e.g., cost-benefit analyses) make the
political-ideological assumption that our society is sufficiently cohesive and common-goaled that its problems can be
resolved by reason and without struggle.  Although such a
"get on with business" orientation will be pleasing to many,
it will not satisfy all.  For those who do not believe that
society is in a fine-tuning stage, a technique that fails to
mobilize public consciousness and involvement has little to
recommend it (Fischhoff et al., 1981).  Their strategy may
involve a calculated attack on what they interpret as
narrowly defined rationality.

Even when experts and lay people have the same goals,
they may be solving different problems.  For example, lay
people are often maligned for their failure to wear seat
belts.  However, their formulation of the problem may be
quite different from that of the safety expert.  The latter
sees the tens of thousands of lives that might be saved from
the small statistical reduction in each trip's probability
of ending in death.  Drivers may see only that minute probability and view the benefits of buckling up too small to
justify the minimal benefits (Slovic, Fischhoff, and Lichtenstein, 1978).

Still other apparent disagreements may reflect no more
than differences in semantics.  Data that we have collected
suggest that the word "risk" has somewhat different connota-
tions to experts and lay people.  Experts seem to interpret
risk as something akin to annual fatalities.  Lay people can
judge "annual fatalities," and indeed produce estimates that
are quite similar to those of experts.  However, when asked
about "risk," they give a judgment that reflects annual
fatalities *and* other considerations, such as threat to
future generations and catastrophic potential.

## Implications

More respectful and balanced relations between the
expert and lay communities (to which any expert belongs
except for a narrow range of problems) are good not only for
science, but also for society.  In many, if not most, cases,

effective energy systems and their incumbent health risk
management require the cooperation of a large body of lay
people.  These people must agree to do without some things
and accept substitutes for others; they must vote sensibly
on ballot measures and choose legislators who will serve as
surrogate hazard managers; they must obey safety rules and
use the legal system responsibly.  Even if the experts were
much better judges of risk than lay people, giving experts
an exclusive franchise for hazard management would mean sub-
stituting short-term efficiency for the long-term effort
needed to create an informed citizenry.

For non-experts, these findings pose an important
series of challenges:  to be better informed, to rely less
on unexamined or unsupported judgments, to be aware of the
qualitative dimensions that strongly condition risk judgments, and to be more open to new evidence; in short, to
realize the potential of being just as educable as the
experts.

For experts, these findings pose what may be a more
difficult challenge:  to recognize and admit one's own cognitive limitations, to temper risk assessments with the
important qualitative aspects of risk that influence the
responses of lay people, and to create continuing and
respectful relations with the public.

What do we do if disagreements persist between the
experts and the public (treating them for the moment as
corporate bodies)?  In a democratic system, "we" don't do
anything.  The political process resolves the issue, for
better or for worse.  Elected representatives, through their
votes, appointees and bureaucracy, do what needs to be done
to balance the public will, the public weal, and their own
needs for popularity, fulfillment, etc.

Assume, however, that there is a dispassionate institu-
tion entrusted with resolving such disagreements (or that
our courts or legislatures or civil service constitute such
institutions).  Could it responsibly act in accordance with
the public's "fears" rather than upon the experts' "facts?"
The answer could be "yes" if one (or more) of three conditions holds:

(a)  The lay public knows something that the experts
     do not.  In that case, the dispassionate insti-
     tution should change its best estimate of what
     the facts are.

(b)  The lay public does not know anything
     special, but has good reason not to be all

that convinced by the evidence supporting the experts' testimony.  In such situations, it may be appropriate to leave the best estimate unchanged, but to increase substantially the confidence intervals around it.  The result might be delay, hedging of bets, or even switching to a more certain course of action.

(c) The public is truly unreasonable, but has a deep emotional investment in its beliefs. There are costs to a society for overriding the strong wishes of its members; these include anomie, alienation, resentment, distrust, sabotage, stress and even psychosomatic effects (whose impact is physical even when their source is illusory).  Such costs could tip the balance against the action indicated by the experts' best guess.

## Acknowledgement

This research was supported by the Technology Assessment and Risk Analysis Program of the National Science Foundation under Grant PRA79-11934 to Clark University under subcontract to Perceptronics, Inc.  Any opinions, findings and conclusions or recommendations expressed in this publication are those of the authors and do not necessarily reflect the views of the National Science Foundation.

## Notes

[1]This article is a composite of material appearing in B. Fischhoff, P. Slovic and S. Lichtenstein.  Lay foibles and expert fables in judgements about risk.  In T. O'Riordan and R. K. Turner (Eds.), *Progress in Resource Management and Environment Planning, Vol. 3*, Chichester:  Wiley, 1981, and P. Slovic, B. Fischhoff, and S. Lichtenstein.  Perception and acceptability of risk from energy systems.  In A. Baum and J. Singer (Eds.), *Advances in Environmental Psychology 3.* Hillsdale, N. J.:  Erlbaum, 1981.

## References

Ashcraft, R.  1977.  Economic metaphors, behavioralism, and political theory:  Some observations on the ideological uses of language.  *Western Political Quart.* 30:313-328.

Bazelon, D. L.  1980.  Science, technology, and the court. *Science* 208:661.

Borch, K.  1968.  *The Economics of Uncertainty.*  Princeton University Press, Princeton, N. J.

Bronfman, L. M. and T. J. Mattingly Jr.  1976.  Critical mass:  Politics, technology, and the public interest. *Nucl. Saf.* 17:539-549.

Bryan, W. B.  1974.  Testimony before the Subcommittee on State Energy Policy, Committee on Planning, Land Use, and Energy, California State Assembly.

Burton, I., R. W. Kates, and G. F. White.  1978.  *The Environment as Hazard.*  Oxford University Press, New York.

Combs, B. and P. Slovic.  1979.  Causes of death:  Biased newspaper coverage and biased judgments.  *Journalism Quart.* 56:837-843.

David, E. E.  1975.  Editorial.  *Science* 189:891.

Dunlap, T. R.  1978.  Science as a guide in regulating technology:  The case of DDT in the United States.  *Soc. Stud. Sci.* 8:265-285.

*Eugene Register-Guard.*  1976.  Doubts linger on cyclamate risks.  January 14, 1976, p. 9.

Fischhoff, B.  1977.  Cost-benefit analysis and the art of motorcycle maintenance.  *Policy Sciences* 8:177-202.

Fischhoff, B., S. Lichtenstein, P. Slovic, S. Derby, and R. Keeney.  1981.  *Acceptable Risk.*  Cambridge University sity Press, New York.

Fischhoff, B., P. Slovic, and S. Lichtenstein.  1977.  Knowing with certainty:  The appropriateness of extreme confidence.  *J. Exper. Psychol.: Human Perception and Performance* 3:552-564.

Fischhoff, B., P. Slovic, and S. Lichtenstein.  1978.  Fault trees:  Sensitivity of estimated failure probabilities to problem representation.  *J. Exper. Psychol.: Human Perception and Performance* 4:330-344.

Fischhoff, B., P. Slovic, and S. Lichtenstein.  1980.  Knowing what you want:  Measuring labile values.  In *Cognitive Processes in Choice and Decision Behavior.* T. Wallsten (Ed.).  Erlbaum, Hillsdale, N. J.

Fischhoff, B., P. Slovic, S. Lichtenstein, S. Read, and B. Combs.  1978.  How safe is safe enough?  A psychometric study of attitudes towards technological risks and benefits.  *Policy Sciences* 9:127-152.

Handler, P.  1980.  Public doubts about science.  *Science* 208:1093.

Hanley, J.  1980.  The silence of scientists. *Chem. Eng. News* 58:5.

Hohenemser, K. H.  1975.  The failsafe risk.  *Environ.* 17:6-10.

Holdren, J. P.  1976.  The nuclear controversy and the limitations of decision making by experts.  *Bull. At. Sci.* 32:20-22.

Hynes, M. and E. Vanmarcke.  1976.  Reliability of embankment performance predictions.  *Proceedings of the ASCE Engineering Mechanics Division Specialty Conference.* University of Waterloo Press, Waterloo, Ontario, Canada.

Jennergren, L. P. and R. L. Keeney.  (In press).  Risk assessment.  In *Handbook of Applied Systems Analysis.* IIASA, Laxenburg, Austria.

Kahneman, D. and A. Tversky.  1979.  Prospect theory. *Econometrica* 47:263-292.

Kasper, R. G.  1979.  Perceived risk:  Implications for policy.  In *Energy Risk Management.*  G. Goodman and W. D. Rowe (Eds.).  Academic Press, London.

Kates, R. W.  1962.  *Hazard and Choice Perception in Flood Plain Management.*  University of Chicago, Department of Geography, Research Paper No. 78, Chicago, Illinois.

Lichtenstein, S., B. Fischhoff, and L. D. Phillips.  1982. Calibration of probabilities:  The state of the art to 1980.  In *Judgment Under Uncertainty: Heuristics and Biases.*  D. Kahneman, P. Slovic and A. Tversky (Eds.).  Cambridge University Press, New York.

Lichtenstein, S. and P. Slovic.  1973.  Response-induced reversals of preference in gambling:  An extended replication in Las Vegas.  *J. Exper. Psychol.* 101:16-20.

Lichtenstein, S., P. Slovic, B. Fischhoff, M. Layman, and B. Combs.  1978.  Judged frequency of lethal events. *J. Exper. Psychol.: Human Learning and Memory* 4:551-578.

Mahoney, M. J.  1979.  Psychology of the scientist:  An evaluative review.  *Soc. Stud. Sci.* 9:349-375.

Marks, B. A.  1977.  Decision under uncertainty:  The narrative sense.  *Admin. and Soc.* 9:379-394.

Marsh, C.  1979.  How would you say you felt about political opinion surveys?  Would you say you were very happy, fairly happy or not too happy?  Prepared for BSA/SSRC Conference on *Methodology and Techniques of Sociology,* Lancaster, England.

Mazur, A. 1973. Disputes between experts. *Minerva* 11: 243-262.

Otway, H. J., D. Maurer, and K. Thomas. 1978. Nuclear power: The question of public acceptance. *Futures* 10: 109-118.

Payne, S. L. 1952. *The Art of Asking Questions.* Princeton University Press, Princeton, N. J.

Piehler, H. R., A. D. Twerski, A. Weinstein, and W. A. Donaher. 1974. Product liability and the technical expert. *Science* 186:1089-1093.

Pokorny, G. 1977. *Energy Development: Attitudes and Beliefs at the Regional/National Levels.* Cambridge Reports, Cambridge, Mass.

Primack, J. 1975. Nuclear reactor safety: An introduction to the issues. *Bull. At. Sci.* 31:15-17.

Rosencranz, A. and G. S. Wetstove. 1980. Acid precipitation. *Environment* 22(5):6-20; 40-41.

Ross, L. 1977. The intuitive psychologist and his short-comings: Distortions in the attribution process. In *Advances in Experimental Social Psychology.* L. Berkowitz (Ed.). Academic Press, New York.

Rothschild, N. M. 1978. Rothschild: An antidote to panic. *Nature* 276:555.

Sheridan, T. B. 1980. Human error in nuclear power plants. *Technol. Rev.* 82:23-33.

Slovic, P., B. Fischhoff, and S. Lichtenstein. 1977. Behavioral decision theory. *Ann. Rev. Psychol.* 28:1-39.

Slovic, P., B. Fischhoff, and S. Lichtenstein. 1978. Accident probabilities and seat belt usage: A psychological perspective. *Accident Analysis and Prevention* 10:281-285.

Slovic, P., B. Fischhoff, and S. Lichtenstein. 1979. Rating the risks. *Environment* 21:14-20, 36-39.

Slovic, P., B. Fischhoff, and S. Lichtenstein. 1980. Perceived risk. In *Societal Risk Assessment: How Safe is Safe Enough?* R. Schwing and W. A. Albers (Eds.). Plenum Press, New York.

Slovic, P., H. Kunreuther, and G. F. White. 1974. Decision processes, rationality, and adjustment to natural hazards. In *Natural Hazards, Local, National and Global.* G. F. White (Ed.). Oxford University Press, New York.

Slovic, P., S. Lichtenstein, and B. Fischhoff. 1979. Images of disaster: Perception and acceptance of risks from nuclear power. In *Energy Risk Management*. G. Goodman and W. D. Rowe (Eds.). Academic Press, London.

Tversky, A. and D. Kahneman. 1974. Judgment under uncertainty: Heuristics and biases. *Science* 185:1124-1131.

Tversky, A. and D. Kahneman. 1981. The framing of decisions and the psychology of choice. *Science* 211:453-458.

U.S. Government. 1975. Hearings, 94th Congress, 1st Session. *Browns Ferry Nuclear Plant Fire*. September 16. U. S. Government Printing Office, Washington, D. C.

U.S. Government. 1976. *Teton Dam Disaster*. Committee on Government Operations, Washington, D. C.

U.S. Government. 1979. *Accident at Three Mile Island*. Report of the President's Commission. U. S. Government Printing Office, Washington, D. C.

U.S. Nuclear Regulatory Commission. 1975. *Reactor Safety Study: An Assessment of Accident Risks in U.S. Commercial Nuclear Power Plants*. WASH 1400 (NUREG-75/014). USNRC, Washington, D. C.

U.S. Nuclear Regulatory Commission. 1978. Risk assessment review group to the U.S. Nuclear Regulatory Commission. NUREG/CR-0400. USNRC, Washington, D. C.

Weinberg, A. M. 1976. The maturity and future of nuclear power. *Amer. Sci.* 64:16-21.

Weinberg, A. M. 1979. Salvaging the atomic age. *The Wilson Quart.* Summer, 88-112.

Weinstein, N. D. 1980. Unrealistic optimism about future life events. *J. Person. Soc. Psychol.* 39:806-820.

Zeisel, H. 1980. Lawmaking and public opinion research: The President and Patrick Caddell. *Amer. Bar Found. Res. J.* 1: 133-139.

Zentner, R. D. 1979. Hazards in the chemical industry. *Chem. Eng. News* 57:25-27, 30-34.

# 2. Health Risks from the Nuclear Fuel Cycle

## Introduction[1]

In the present state of knowledge, all health risk assessments of energy systems contain fairly large uncertainties. Some parts of the assessments, such as risk of accidental death among uranium miners, can be estimated reasonably well based on recent experience. Other parts, such as the potential risk associated with serious accidents in nuclear power plants, can only be estimated to within perhaps one or two orders of magnitude due to the absence of actual experience. Although many of the numerical values of health effects presented later in this chapter will be given to more than one significant figure, it should be recognized that this is not an indication that these effects are known with even that degree of precision. Nevertheless, it is in the vital interest of the nation that such assessments be made and updated as new information becomes available. How else can policy and decision makers, and the public (scientists and citizens) hope to make decisions that are in the best interests of society?

In this discussion, as in those in Chapter 3, all health risk estimates are normalized to the annual operation of a modern, light-water-cooled, power plant that generates 1,000 megawatt-years of electric power [i.e., a GW(e)-yr]. Thus, the reader can extrapolate the risks to any number of nuclear power plants over any period of time simply by multiplying by the total projected electric power for these plants. A similar unit is defined in the Code of Federal Regulations, Title 10, Part 51, as a reference reactor year, or RRY, and represents the estimated releases of radioactivity from generating 0.8 GW(e)-yr of electric power [i.e., a 1,000 MW(e) plant operating at 80% of capacity for one year].

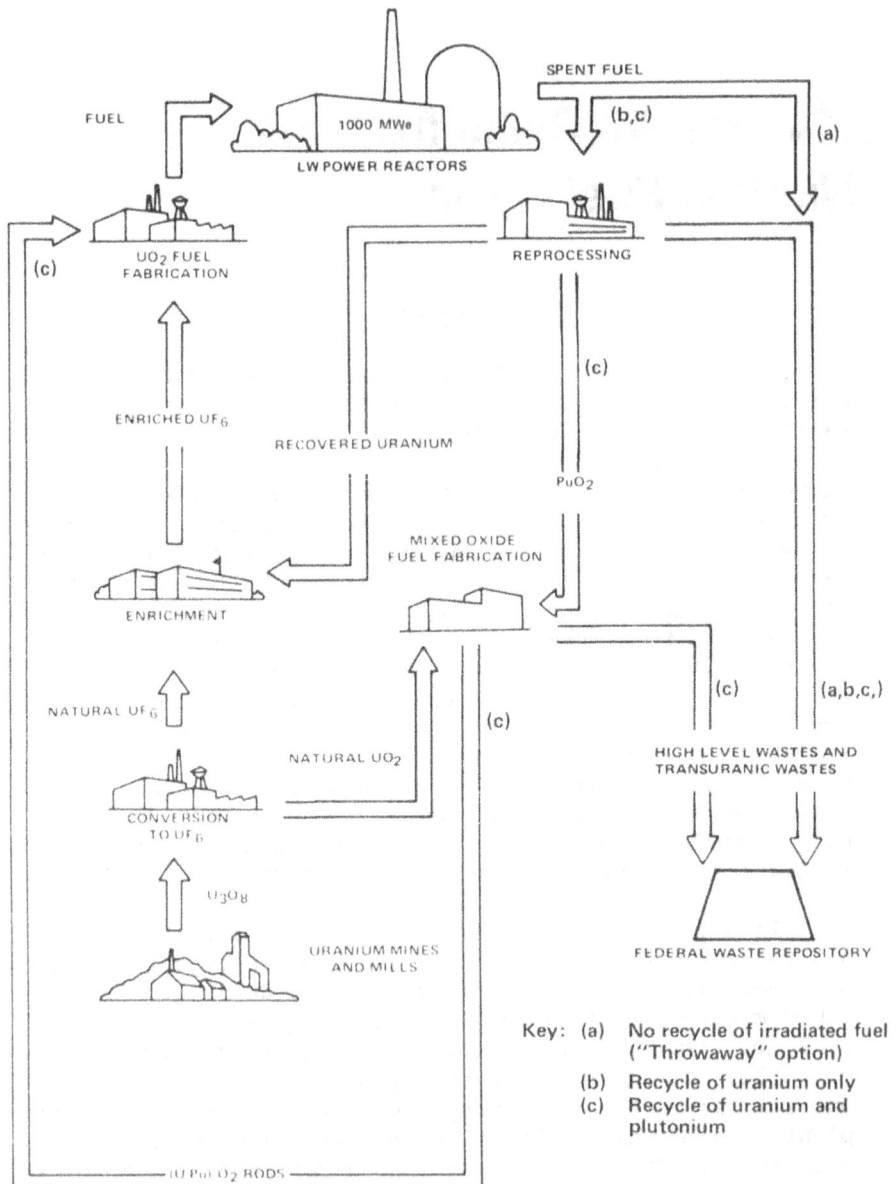

Figure 1.   Current options for the nuclear fuel cycle.

A diagram of the nuclear fuel cycle is shown in Figure 1 to assist the reader in understanding the discussions that follow.

## Radiological Effluents

The radiological effluents estimated for the supporting fuel cycle (i.e., everything except the power reactor itself) for one RRY are specified in the *Code of Federal Regulations*, Title 10, Part 51, Table S-3 (CFR, 1981). These effluents represent the sum of the maximum probable releases occurring from reprocessing, waste management and transportation of wastes for either of the two options: no recycle of uranium or plutonium (the so-called throwaway option), or recycle of uranium only. A third option, recycle of uranium and plutonium, results in population doses that are somewhat less but not significantly different from those for recycle of uranium only.

These effluents (gaseous and liquid) were selected from detailed studies, such as the generic environmental statement on mixed oxide fuel (GESMO) (USNRC, 1976a), and the extensive Table S-3 Rule Hearings, conducted over a several year period by the U.S. Nuclear Regulatory Commission (USNRC), which resulted in the current rule. Detailed bases are provided in GESMO (USNRC, 1976a), WASH-1248 (USNRC, 1974), NUREG-0116 (USNRC, 1976b), and NUREG-0216 (USNRC, 1977a), and in the record of the final rulemaking pertaining to Uranium Fuel Cycle Impacts from Spent Fuel Reprocessing and Radioactive Waste Management (USNRC, 1977b).

Because the GESMO study represented only a 26-year period (1975 to 2000), and the environmental dose commitment period was limited to 40 years for each year of the 26-year period, it was necessary to extend the time integral for $^{222}$Rn emissions from uranium mines and mill tailings piles to cover the maximum period of time which the inherent uncertainties in such projections reasonably permit. A detailed discussion of those uncertainties follows later in this chapter. However, the $^{222}$Rn issue has been studied thoroughly and debated soundly in numerous reactor licensing hearings,[2] and in a recent generic decision which supports the approach used in this assessment.[3] The $^{222}$Rn source terms selected for this assessment represent a reasonable range of releases which might occur over periods of 100 to 1000 years into the future. These estimates are based on a recent reevaluation of this question by the USNRC, and the reader is referred to that report for details on the methods used for estimating $^{222}$Rn releases (USNRC, 1981a).

The radiological effluents used in this assessment are shown in Table 1. It should be stressed that, for the time periods examined (i.e., up to 1,000 years into the future), actual releases are expected to be lower than those shown in Table 1. This is particularly true for tritium (H-3), krypton-85 (Kr-85), and carbon-14 (C-14) because engineering and technological improvements appear likely to reduce these releases significantly.[4]

## Environmental Transport Models

To estimate the radiation doses to populations, it is necessary to use environmental transport models that describe the dispersion, deposition, and resuspension of hundreds of radionuclides released by the fuel cycle during normal and accident conditions. The models used for normal operations are described in detail in GESMO (USNRC, 1976a) and in the S-3 Hearing transcripts and reports (USNRC, 1976b, 1977a, 1977b).[5] The environmental transport model for gaseous releases (from normal and abnormal occurrences) is a so-called "wedge" model that permits vertical dispersion to a maximum height of 1000 m (typical for non-buoyant, near-surface releases). After several miles of transport from the point of release, a fairly uniform cross-sectional concentration for the balance of the "first pass" across the United States results.

Once the plume exits the United States, the volatile radionuclides of sufficiently long radiological half-life are assumed to mix uniformly in the world's atmosphere or hydrosphere. Thus, longer lived nuclides like $^3$H (12-year half-life), $^{14}$C (5,700-year half-life), and $^{85}$Kr (10-year half-life) have at least two exposure modes to consider: first-pass exposure and subsequent exposures. Global dispersion of $^{85}$Kr is simple to model since it is known to mix fairly uniformly in the world's atmosphere (3.8 x 10$^{21}$ liters) over a period of time that is short relative to its half-life. However, $^3$H and $^{14}$C are more difficult to model. After the first pass, tritium was reasonably assumed to mix in the earth's circulating water volume (2.7 x 10$^{19}$ liters), while $^{14}$C was assumed to mix initially in the world's atmosphere where it is gradually removed to the ocean over a period of time that is short relative to its half-life. Details of the $^{14}$C long-term dispersion model used in this assessment are available in an Oak Ridge National Laboratory report (Killough, 1977). It was conservatively assumed that no other environmental removal mechanisms were operating for $^3$H and $^{85}$Kr (such as losses to deep ocean water), only radioactive decay. In the special case of $^{222}$Rn emissions from uranium mining and milling, the models used were developed for the USNRC by Argonne National Laboratory (USNRC, 1980b) for populations within 80 km of a model facility, and the National Oceanic and Atmospheric Administration (Heffter and Ferber, 1975) for populations beyond 80 km of a model facility.

In the case of gaseous radioactive releases from light-water-cooled reactor accidents, the atmospheric dispersion as described by the Reactor Safety Study (USNRC, 1975) was assumed. These dispersion estimates are based on a modified Gaussian dispersion model (with vertical dispersion limited by the seasonal mixing depths). Stability, precipitation, wind speeds and directions are based on actual meteorology measured at several different types of U.S. nuclear power station sites (i.e., valley, river, lake, ocean and plains) over extended periods of time. For details on the models, see the Reactor Safety Study, Appendix VI, Section 4 (USNRC, 1975).

### Radiation Dose Models

The radiation dose models used in this assessment are those which permit estimation of collective population dose commitments.[6] Such doses are collective in that they represent the summation of all the individual doses in an exposed population. These doses are also a commitment, since they represent the total collective dose over extended periods of time from all radionuclides released per GW(e)-yr. Two types of commitments are considered in this assessment. For each individual in the exposed population, a 50-year dose commitment is first calculated for each radionuclide that is taken into the body from inhalation and food pathways during the year a modern nuclear power plant and its supporting fuel cycle operates, as well as external exposures from airborne radioactivity, and radioactivity deposited on the ground (and resuspended) during that year. The second type of dose commitment results from similar population exposures to these same radioactive releases for the subsequent years. The summation of the 50-year dose commitments for each of these years is called the environmental dose commitment (EDC). In practice, the EDC estimates are usually limited to periods of time for which reasonable estimates of population doses can be made. In this assessment, a 100- to 1,000-year EDC has been used to estimate the potential health effects one GW(e)-yr might cause among people living now and those living in the distant future.

The EDCs consider, within the limits of the present state of knowledge, collective radiation doses from external exposure to radioactivity suspended in air and water, deposited on the ground and in sediments, and taken up through

Table 1.  Radioactive effluents from the nuclear fuel cycle
per reference reactor year [0.8 GW(e)-yr][a]

| Source of the release | Radionuclide released | Curies |
|---|---|---|
| | **Gaseous** | |
| Uranium mines | $^{222}$Rn | 5,300-19,000[b] |
| Uranium mills and mill tailings (Note: essentially all of the radiological impact is from $^{222}$Rn) | $^{226}$Ra | 0.020 |
| | $^{230}$Th | 0.020 |
| | $^{234}$U | 0.0044 |
| | $^{235}$U | 0.000030 |
| | $^{238}$U | 0.030 |
| | $^{222}$Rn | 1,500-22,000[b] |
| UF$_6$ conversion plants | Uranium | 0.0015 |
| Uranium enrichment plants | Uranium | 0.002 |
| | $^{99}$Tc | 0.046[c] |
| Fuel fabrication plants | Uranium | 0.0002 |
| Light-water-cooled nuclear power plants (Note: over 90% of the total radiological impact is from $^3$H, $^{14}$C, $^{85}$Kr, and $^{133}$Xe) | $^3$H | 1,200 |
| | $^{14}$C | 8.0 |
| | $^{58}$Co | 0.015 |
| | $^{60}$Co | 0.06 |
| | $^{85}$Kr | 470 |
| | $^{90}$Sr | 0.0010 |
| | $^{133m}$Xe | 120 |
| | $^{133}$Xe | 12,000 |
| | $^{135}$Xe | 1,100 |
| | $^{131}$I | 0.33 |
| | $^{134}$Cs | 0.005 |
| | $^{137}$Cs | 0.010 |
| Fuel reprocessing plant (Note: over 90% of the radiological impact is from $^3$H, $^{14}$C, and $^{85}$Kr) | $^3$H | 18,100 |
| | $^{14}$C | 24 |
| | $^{85}$Kr | 400,000 |
| | $^{90}$Sr | 0.016 |
| | $^{99}$Tc | 0.11[c] |
| | $^{106}$Ru | 0.14 |
| | $^{131}$I | 0.83 |
| | $^{134}$Cs | 0.109 |
| | $^{137}$Cs | 0.055 |
| | $^{234}$U | 0.000015 |
| | $^{235}$U | 0.000004 |
| | $^{238}$U | 0.000020 |
| | $^{238}$Pu, $^{239}$Pu | 0.00088 |
| | $^{241}$Pu | 0.020 |

Table 1.   (cont'd)

| Source of the release | Radionuclide released | Curies released |
|---|---|---|
| | **Gaseous** *(cont'd)* | |
| | $^{241}$Am | 0.000014 |
| | $^{243}$Am | 0.0000011 |
| | $^{242}$Cm | 0.0015 |
| | $^{244}$Cm | 0.00011 |
| Geologic repository | $^{129}$I | 1.3 |
| | **Liquids** | |
| Uranium mill tailings | Uranium and daughters | 2.0 (released to ground) |
| UF$_6$ conversion plants | $^{226}$Ra | 0.0034 |
| | $^{230}$Th | 0.0015 |
| | Uranium and daughters | 0.044 |
| Uranium enrichment plants | Uranium and daughters | 0.02 |
| Fuel fabrication plants | $^{234}$Th | 0.010 |
| | Uranium and daughters | 0.02 |
| Light-water-cooled nuclear power plants (Note: most of the radiological impact is from $^{134}$Cs and $^{137}$Cs) | $^3$H | 240 |
| | $^{54}$Mn | 0.0015 |
| | $^{60}$Co | 0.0089 |
| | $^{131}$I | 0.28 |
| | $^{134}$Cs | 0.02 |
| | $^{137}$Cs | 0.034 |
| Shallow land burial | $^{99}$Tc | 1.2[c] |

[a]Only the major releases, in terms of quantity and potential radiological impact, are included.  Multiply all releases by 1.25 to convert to GW(e)-yr releases.

[b]100- to 1,000-year period; includes long-term emanation from tailings piles (see USNRC 1981a for further details).

[c]No $^{99}$Tc source terms are specified in Table S-3 (10 CFR 51) at this time.  The values for $^{99}$Tc shown here are based on current but conservative NRC staff estimates, and are subject to future revisions (see USNRC 1981c for further details).

all potential food pathways (milk, drinking water, red meat, fish, invertebrates, vegetables, and grains) following initial deposition and redistribution in the environment. In general, dose commitments are determined by the concentrations of the radionuclides in air and water. For the U.S. population, most of each 50-year dose commitment is determined by the "first pass" of those radionuclides. Only for a few very long-lived radionuclides, such as $^{14}$C and $^{129}$I, can the subsequent passes contribute significantly to the total EDC. The special case for $^{222}$Rn emissions from uranium mines and mills will be discussed below in some detail since those potential impacts could dominate the impacts of the fuel cycle. Details of the models are presented in USNRC, 1974, 1976a, 1976b, 1977a, but due to space limitations cannot be discussed further here.

In the case of $^{222}$Rn releases, even though $^{222}$Rn is a short-lived radionuclide (3.8-day half-life), its predecessors have very long half-lives. As a result, while $^{222}$Rn impacts are primarily to the U.S. population from the first pass of the $^{222}$Rn over the country, such impacts may continue to accumulate over long timespans depending on certain factors which may increase or decrease $^{222}$Rn emissions with time. In the GESMO Hearing, the $^{222}$Rn impacts were incorrectly overestimated due to a factor-of-10 error in the total-body dose factor for $^{210}$Pb in The International Commission on Radiological Protection (ICRP) Publication 2 (1959). The estimates were subsequently corrected by the USNRC staff in a memorandum to the GESMO Hearing Board (USNRC, 1977c). As a result, the GESMO population dose commitments [Table IVJ(E)-1 in USNRC, 1976a] for uranium mining and milling were reduced by factors of 7.7 for uranium mining and 6.1 for uranium milling (no recycle), and similar factors for the other recycle options.

In addition, the staff subsequently concluded the ICRP lung model (ICRP, 1959) was inappropriate for $^{222}$Rn and its short-lived progeny, since it calculates an averaged dose for the entire lung while the critical tissue is the bronchial epithelium. This assessment, therefore, used the recommended dose conversion factors from USNRC (1981a) for $^{222}$Rn and daughters, based on more appropriate models for dose to the bronchial epithelium, as well as total body and bone.

## Health Effects Models

The area of health effects modeling for radiogenic health effects is one which has undergone considerable

Table 2.  Latent cancer mortality/$10^6$ person-rem[a]

| Dose/dose rate | Male | Female | Both[b] |
|---|---|---|---|
| **Acute exposure** | | | |
| ≦25 rems | 144 | 158 | 151 |
| | | | |
| **Continuous exposure** | | | |
| ≦12 rems/year | | | |
| (1)  General public | 107 | 123 | 115 |
| (2)  Occupational workers | | | |
| (20-65 years) | 81.8 | 113 | 97.6 |

[a]Based on Tables V-16 and V-19; BEIR III (National Research Council — National Academy of Sciences, 1980a). All estimates of cancer risk should be rounded to two significant figures to avoid the unwarranted impression of great precision.

[b]"Both" assumes equal numbers of both sexes (usually not so for occupational workers).

growth during the last decade.  Strangely enough, although more is known about the effects of radiation exposure than most other agents of biological stress, there is considerable controversy about the effects of low-level ionizing radiation.  That controversy continues in spite of the fact that no reliable studies have been able to show a statistically significant increase in latent cancer risk at low doses and low dose rates.  The reader is referred to the 1980 report of the National Academy of Sciences (National Research Council — National Academy of Sciences, 1980a) Committee on the Biological Effects of Ionizing Radiation (BEIR III), for the most up-to-date and authoritative information on this subject.  The risk estimators derived from the BEIR III report concerning exposure to low-level, low linear-energy-transfer (LET) radiation are summarized in Tables 2 and 3 and are the basis for the estimates of latent cancer risk from low-LET radiation in this analysis. Estimates of the risk from high-LET exposure (e.g., the progeny of $^{222}$Rn) are also based on guidance in BEIR III. The risk estimators used for lung and bone cancer resulting from $^{222}$Rn emissions from uranium mines and mills were 70 and 4 deaths per $10^6$ person-rem, respectively, and were derived using the BEIR III linear model.

Table 3. Organ-specific cancer mortality/10⁶ person-rem

| Type of Cancer | Acute exposure (≤25 rem) | | | Continuous exposure (≤12 rem/year)[a] | | | | | |
|---|---|---|---|---|---|---|---|---|---|
| | | | | General population | | | Occupational workers | | |
| | Male | Female | Both[b] | Male | Female | Both | Male | Female | Both |
| Thyroid | 5.2 | 13.0 | 9.1 | 3.7 | 10.0 | 6.9 | 2.7 | 9.1 | 5.9 |
| Lung | 39.7 | 33.1 | 36.4 | 28.6 | 25.4 | 27 | 20.7 | 23.2 | 22.0 |
| Breast | ~0 | 25.4 | 12.7 | ~0 | 19.5 | 9.8 | ~0 | 17.8 | 8.9 |
| Esophageal | 3.4 | 3.1 | 3.3 | 2.5 | 2.4 | 2.5 | 1.8 | 2.2 | 2.1 |
| Stomach | 15.1 | 14.6 | 14.9 | 10.9 | 11.3 | 11.1 | 7.9 | 10.3 | 9.1 |
| Intestinal | 7.0 | 6.9 | 7.0 | 5.0 | 5.3 | 5.2 | 3.6 | 4.8 | 4.2 |
| Liver | 9.2 | 7.8 | 8.5 | 6.6 | 6.0 | 6.3 | 4.8 | 5.5 | 5.2 |
| Pancreatic | 10.8 | 10.0 | 10.4 | 7.7 | 7.7 | 7.7 | 5.6 | 7.0 | 6.3 |
| Urinary | 3.9 | 4.5 | 4.2 | 2.8 | 3.5 | 3.2 | 2.1 | 3.2 | 2.6 |
| Lymphoma | 2.5 | 2.3 | 2.5 | 1.9 | 1.7 | 1.8 | 1.3 | 1.6 | 1.5 |
| Leukemia and bone[c] | 27.4 | 18.6 | 23.0 | 22.7 | 16.1 | 19.4 | 20.9 | 15.7 | 18.3 |
| Others | 20.0 | 18.3 | 19.2 | 14.3 | 14.1 | 14.2 | 10.4 | 12.9 | 11.7 |
| Total | 144 | 158 | 151 | 107 | 123 | 115 | 81.8 | 113 | 97.6 |

[a] Lifetime exposure for general population; 20-65 years of age for occupational exposure.

[b] "Both" assumes equal numbers of both sexes (usually not so for occupational workers).

[c] Bone represents ~2.2% of total for leukemia and bone cancer combined.

It must be stressed that all such estimates are potential, since the actual risks may be much smaller, and for low LET radiation could include zero risk.[7]

To identify possible counterpoint to the current health effects models used in this assessment, it is noted that a recent monograph (Luckey, 1980) has concluded that exposure to radiation up to certain levels may act as a stimulant to biological systems and result in increased life expectancy, greater reproduction, reduced mortality, and so forth. This hypothesis, called radiation hormesis, is supported by over 1,000 documented studies with plants and animals. The studies with mammals indicate that radiation doses of about 10 rem per year represent an optimum for maximum benefit. If radiation exposures did in fact increase life expectancy, then the observed increased risk of cancer could be consistent with such a hypothesis, since cancer rates increase exponentially in old age. Although the radiation biology community has not yet carefully examined this hypothesis, this new information will be reviewed in the years ahead. *If proven*, this hypothesis will radically alter the health effects estimates presented here and elsewhere, because low-level radiation doses would result in positive benefits in terms of a long healthy life perhaps at the cost of a greater lifetime risk of death from cancer resulting from all causes.

As yet no human data are available that clearly define the genetic risks of low-level radiation exposure. Such data are still not available even from the large group of survivors in Hiroshima and Nagasaki who were exposed to very high levels of radiation. As a result, the BEIR III authors found it necessary to rely primarily on animal data, which now span many consecutive generations of exposed animals. The genetic risk estimators derived from the BEIR III report are summarized in Table 4, and were used in this analysis. Such estimates represent all expected genetic risk from exposure of one generation of parents over subsequent generations of offspring (total time of several hundred years).

## Uncertainties in Radiation Risk Assessment

The uncertainties in analyses such as presented here can be quite large or fairly small, depending on their source. For example, extrapolation of health effects into the dim and distant future, by necessity, results in very large uncertainties (one or more orders of magnitude, depending on how distant the upper limit of the integral). All such estimates are only semiquantitative in nature, and include considerable professional judgment. On the

Table 4.  Genetic risk/$10^6$ liveborn[a]

| Genetic effect | Range | Geometric mean |
|---|---|---|
| Autosomal dominant and X-linked disorders | 40-200 | 89 (factor of ±2.2) |
| Irregularly inherited disorders | 20-900 | 130 (factor of ±6.7) |
| Overall risk | 60-1100 | $\Sigma$ = 220 |

[a]Assuming one live birth per person per generation surviving to reproduce (i.e., zero population growth) the risks are approximately the same per $10^6$ person-rem (high- or low-LET radiation).

other hand, estimates of deaths (both radiological and accidental) among uranium miners can be based on recent experience and are probably accurate to within a factor of 2 or 3.

Large uncertainties in predictions of future risk come from several sources, of which the following are of major importance:

1.  It is now, and always will be, impossible to accurately estimate future population dose commitments because it is impossible to accurately project the size of the populations at risk.

2.  The health risks associated with radiation exposure (i.e., cancer and genetic effects) change with time as societies change. Such changes cannot be predicted over long periods of time.

Let us now examine some of the reasons for these statements. Consider, for example, that the U.S. Bureau of the Census claims about ± 25% accuracy on its best population projections over the next 50 years *provided* "there will be no large-scale war, widespread epidemic, or other major catastrophe" (U. S. Bureau of Census, 1977). Clearly, if any one or more of such events befall man, estimates of future populations are left in limbo. Even if mankind avoids large-scale wars and epidemics, other major catastrophes may yet claim earth. One such catastrophe that man may now be abetting is the so-called "greenhouse effect." What the exact outcome might be is very uncertain, but the potential disasters are numerous.  To demonstrate how such an occurrence might affect estimates of future populations, consider, for example, the following fictional scenario which is, nevertheless, consistent with several expert evaluations (Norwine, 1977; Baes et al., 1977; Mitchell, 1977; Mercer, 1978; and Schneider and Chen, 1980):

Year 1995 — The "greenhouse effect" is confirmed, but due to the $CO_2$ already released, there is no way of preventing further heating of the earth's atmosphere, even if *all* future man-made $CO_2$ releases cease.

Year 2000 — The increasing atmospheric temperature has caused a world-wide change in the atmospheric steering winds and ocean currents.  The climate in the United States, U.S.S.R., China, and Europe is becoming warmer and drier, much of Africa and Central America is becoming desert.  Hundreds of millions of people are on the verge of starving due to huge crop failures in the United States, Asia, and Europe.  There are no more surplus grains anywhere in the world, and the outlook is grim.

Year 2020 — Grain production in the United States, Europe, and Asia has stabilized due to breakthroughs in drought resistant grains, and new land in Scandinavia, Siberia, Canada, and other areas coming under cultivation due to warmer weather in these latitudes.  However, over 100 million people are already dead or dying of starvation as a result of grain shortages.

Year 2025 — The West Antartic ice cap is now melting rapidly, and the world's oceans are rising a few feet a year.  There is evidence the main Antartic ice cap and the glaciers in Greenland are also beginning to melt.

Year 2080 — The oceans have now risen over 100 feet, inundating lowlands and all the ocean cities of the world, forcing over 3 billion people to flee to higher ground (see Figure 2).  Territorial wars over the remaining productive farm lands have broken out all over the world — billions have been killed or have starved.  The world population has dropped from 8 billion in 1995 to 2 billion, and is still slowly declining.  The U.S. population has declined to 80 million and is stabilizing.

That scenario is frightening, but may be as probable as the "China Syndrome," and all in the next 100 years.

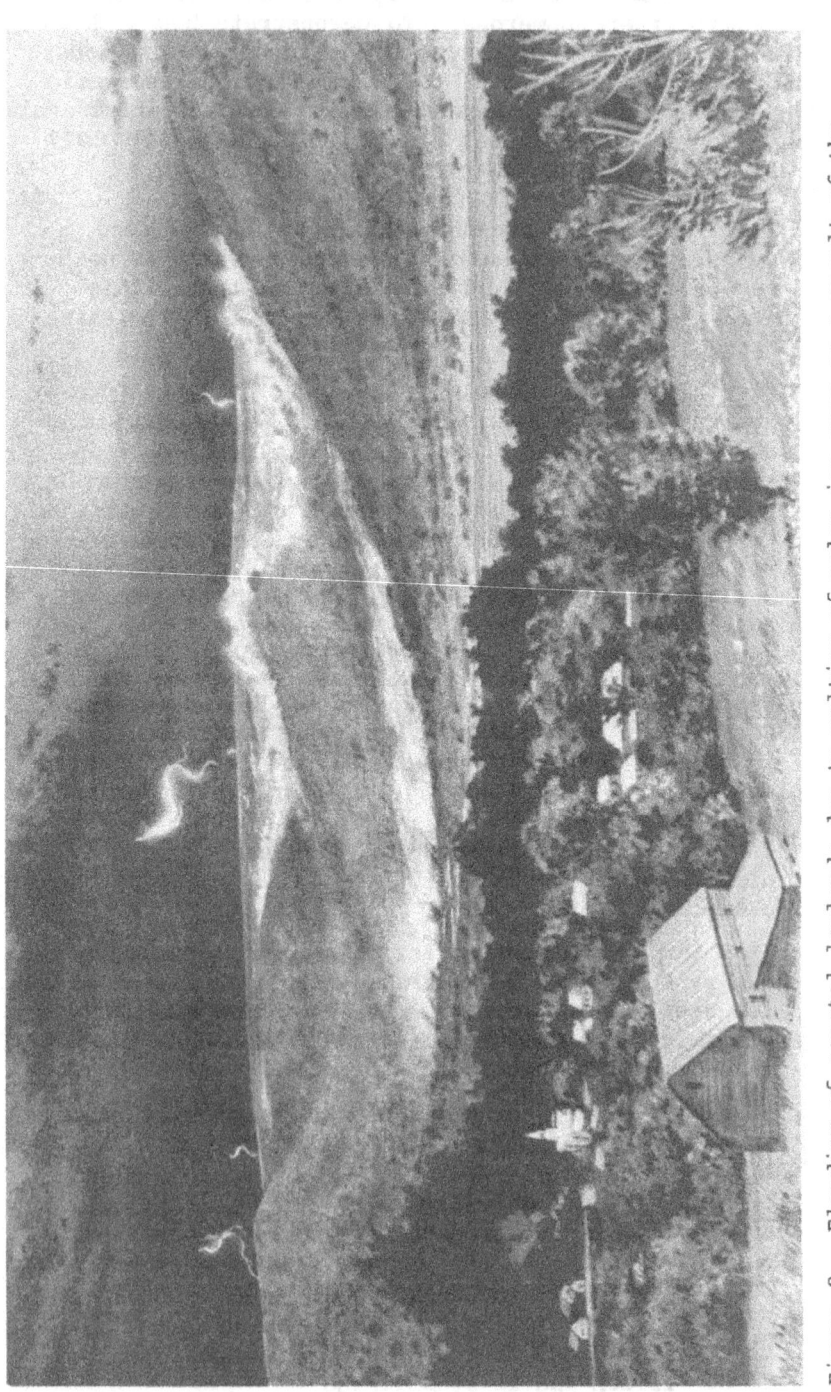

Figure 2. Flooding of coastal lowlands due to melting of polar ice caps as a result of the "greenhouse" effect. Courtesy of *Smithsonian* and the artist, Mr. R. Miller, Woodbridge, Virginia.

How about the next millennium and beyond?  The uncertainties are staggering!

The bottom line, of course, is that just defining the size of a future population at risk has large uncertainties. The easiest course is to assume that everything will stay basically the same as it is today, allowing the U.S. population to grow to 300 million over the next 50 years, and remain stable for the best for the rest of this millennium. While experience has proven beyond any reasonable doubt that the only thing that is constant is change, if one is willing to pretend a little, *perhaps* it is possible to estimate the U.S. population to within a factor of 3 or 4 during the next 100 years.  By really pretending hard, it may be possible to estimate the U.S. population over the next 1,000 years to within a factor of 5 or 10.

Beyond that time, the uncertainties balloon to one or more orders of magnitude.  Why?  After frying for a few thousand years in a warm and extended interglacial period, it now appears probable that the earth will once again slide into another glacial period to freeze for several thousand years before the next interglacial period about 15,000 to 20,000 years from now (see Figures 3 and 4) (Norwine, 1977; Mitchell, 1977; Ponte, 1976; Calder, 1978; and Lamb, 1977). The possibilities for further population changes appear almost limitless.

Recognizing that these uncertainties are almost certainties, what does a reasonable risk assessor do?  Of course he pretends, but within the bounds of reason.  For this analysis, the population dose commitments will be limited to periods of 100 to 1,000 years, recognizing that somewhere during that period we may step "through the looking-glass."[8]

The second major source of uncertainty comes from the recognition that the *potential* risks from low-level radiation are strongly dependent on the characteristics of the exposed population and the capabilities of future medical practice.  Consider, if you will, the differences between the 1900 and 1970 U.S. populations in terms of mortality risks.  As shown in Table 5, cancer and cardiovascular disease were not as important in 1900 as they are today. As a result, it is probable that the somatic risks from radiation exposure were also less per person-rem than they are today because, whatever its causes, cancer is primarily a disease of old age.  In 1900, life expectancy at birth was on the order of 45 years; by 1970, it had increased to over 70 years.  With more people surviving diseases which previously would have killed them before they were 40, the

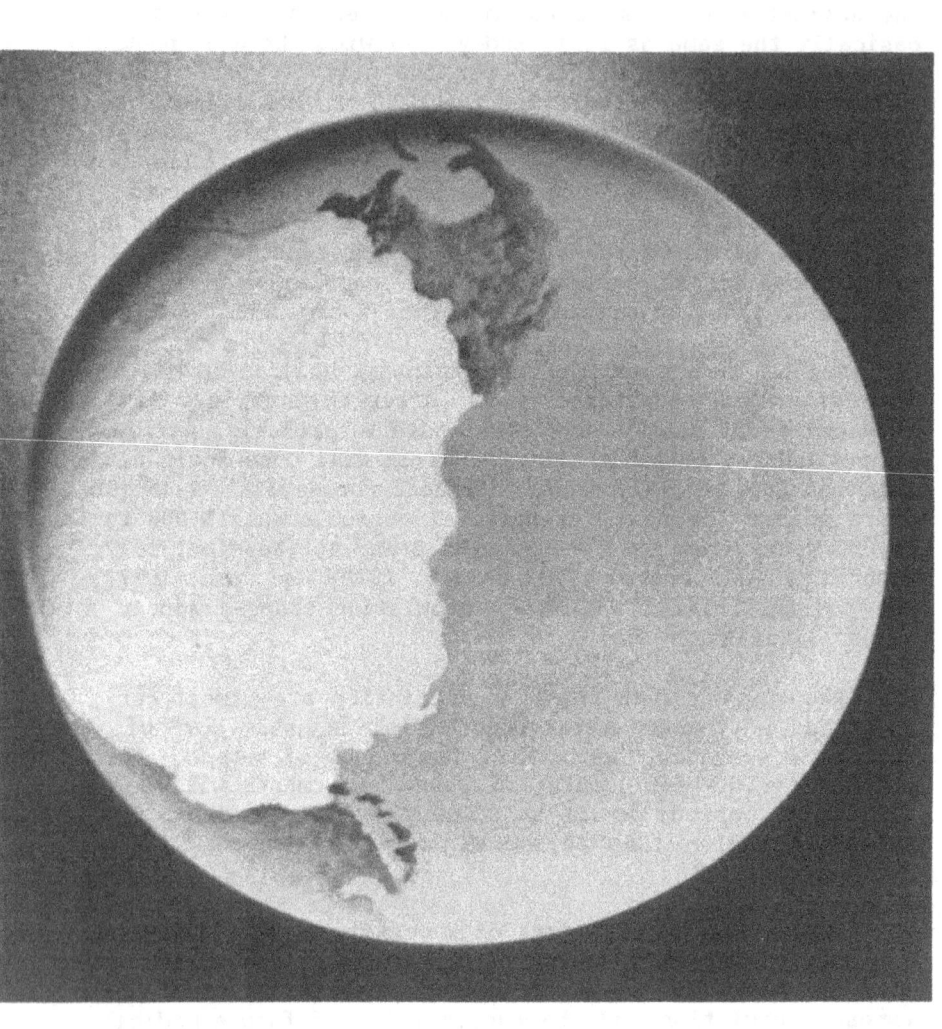

Figure 3. Our next ice age? Photograph courtesy of *Smithsonian* and the artist, Mr. R. Miller, Woodbridge, Virginia.

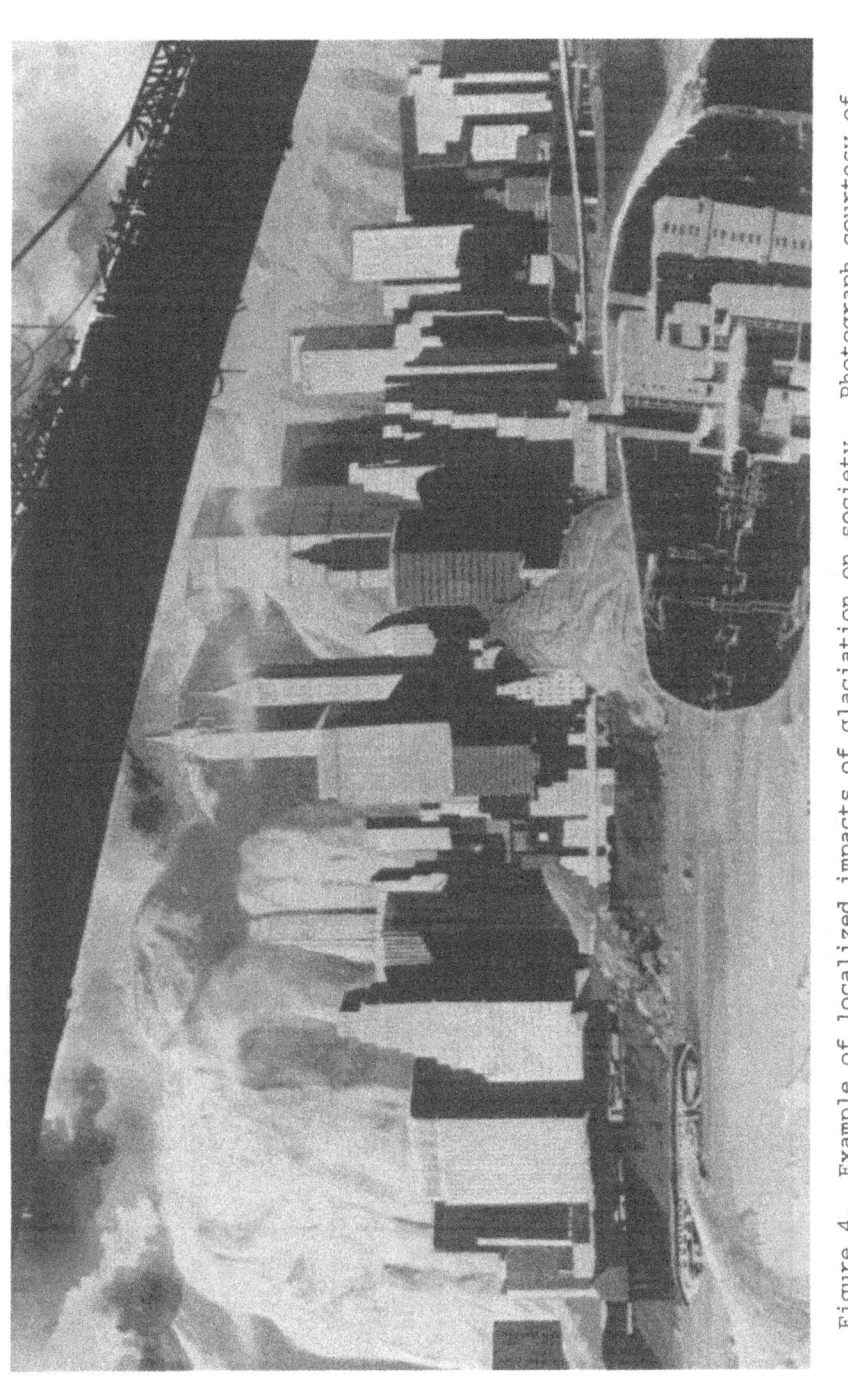

Figure 4. Example of localized impacts of glaciation on society. Photograph courtesy of *Smithsonian* and the artist, Mr. R. Miller, Woodbridge, Virginia.

Table 5. Comparison of causes of mortality in 1900 and 1970 U.S. populations[a]

| Cause of death | Deaths/100,000 population | | Change in risk of mortality by 1970 |
|---|---|---|---|
| | 1900 | 1970 | |
| Tuberculosis | 194.4 | 2.6 | Factor of 75 lower |
| Typhoid and paratyphoid fever | 31.3 | 0.05 | Factor of 600 lower |
| Diptheria | 40.3 | 0.05 | Factor of 800 lower |
| Cancer | 64.0 | 162.8 | Factor of 2.5 higher |
| Major cardiovascular and renal diseases | 345.2 | 496.0 | Factor of 1.4 higher |
| Influenza and pneumonia | 202.2 | 30.9 | Factor of 6.5 lower |
| Gastritis, duodenitis, enteritis and colitis | 142.7 | 0.6 | Factor of 240 lower |
| Accidents (including motor vehicle) | 72.3 | 56.4 | Factor of 1.3 lower |
| Other major diseases | 58.4 | 35.1 | Factor of 1.7 lower |
| Overall | 1150.8 | 784.4 | Factor of 1.5 lower |

[a]U.S. Bureau of the Census (1976).

lifetime risk of radiogenic cancer has gradually increased
since 1900 and may continue to do so until some means is
found to prevent it or cure it (Weiss, 1977; Nagata et al.,
1980; Bloom, 1980; Bram et al., 1980; Sporn, 1980; Derynck
et al., 1980; Goeddel et al., 1980; Avery et al., 1980;
and Zielinski et al., 1980). If that occurs, the risk of
radiogenic cancer will decline until the remaining risk
becomes small relative to other health risks. At that time,
societal resources are likely to be diverted to meet the
next great health risk, which has every indication of being
epidemic senility as a result of more people living long
enough to experience it (Plum, 1979).

In all of this, it is difficult to remember that
Pasteur only demonstrated the existence of pathogenic bacte-
ria about a century ago. What will the future bring? We
can hope it will be change for the better, but in this
analysis, it will be assumed things will remain pretty much
as they are today for the next century. Beyond that it is
probable that the risks from radiogenic cancer and genetic
effects will be much less than they are today because of
medical and technological advances. The uncertainties in
health effects modeling today are probably about a factor
of 5 or 10, but may increase with the time integral to one
or more orders of magnitude during the next millennium.
The competing risks associated with future catastrophic
events like an uncontrolled "greenhouse effect" would be
an added source of uncertainty in estimating the risks of
low-level radiation exposure. Those uncertainties can only
be imagined and will not be considered in this analysis.
Additional discussions of these problems can be found in
other work (USNRC, 1978, 1981b; Gotchy, 1978, 1979).

## Collective Population Dose Commitments and Potential Health Impacts

The detailed results of the calculations using the
various source terms and models just discussed are presented
in Tables 6 and 7. In general, only those radionuclides
which could result in dose commitments in excess of 1 person-
rem are identified in the tables. All others are summed
under the category "Others." The combined potential health
impacts of radionuclides in both gaseous and liquid
effluents are summarized in Table 8.

Tritium, carbon-14, krypton-85, and iodine-129 also
contribute to exposure of populations outside the United
States. However, most of the world population dose commitments during the next 1,000 years from $^3$H, $^{129}$I, and $^{222}$Rn
would be due to the first-pass exposure of the U.S. population, and the population dose would not significantly

Table 6. Collective U. S. general population dose commitments and potential health impacts due to the release of gaseous radioactive effluents from normal operations of the nuclear fuel cycle per GW(e)-yr[a]

| Source of the dose commitment | Nuclide | Dose commitments (person-rem) | | | | Total body risk equivalent | Potential health impacts | |
|---|---|---|---|---|---|---|---|---|
| | | Total body | Bone | Lung | Thyroid | | Potential latent cancer mortality | Potential genetic effects |
| Uranium mines | $^{222}$Rn | 53–190 | 720–2,600 | 520–1,900 | | 210–740 | 0.063–0.22 | 0.012–0.042 |
| Uranium mills and tailings | $^{222}$Rn | 15–120 | 200–1,600 | 150–1,200 | | 58–460 | 0.033–0.15 | 0.013–0.036 |
| | $^{226}$Ra | 42 | 45 | <1 | | 42 | | |
| | Others | 0.83 | 28 | 31 | | 9.3 | | |
| Light-water-cooled nuclear power plants | $^{3}$H | 16 | | | | 16 | 0.011–0.013 | 0.021–0.024 |
| | $^{14}$C | 54–71 | | | | 54–71 | | |
| | $^{60}$Co | 11 | | | | 11 | | |
| | $^{85}$Kr | <1 | | | | <1 | | |
| | $^{133}$Xe | 4.8 | | | | 4.8 | | |
| | $^{131}$I | <1 | <1 | <1 | 61[b] | <1 | | |
| | Others | 6.4 | 13 | ~1 | ~1 | 6.8 | | |

Table 6. (continued)

| Source of the dose commitment | Nuclide | Dose commitments (person-rem) | | | | | Potential health impacts | |
|---|---|---|---|---|---|---|---|---|
| | | Total body | Bone | Lung | Thyroid | Total body risk equivalent | Potential latent cancer mortality | Potential genetic effects |
| Fuel reprocessing plants | $^3$H | 230 | | | | 230 | 0.050-0.055 | 0.092-0.10 |
| | $^{14}$C | 130-170 | | | | 130-170 | | |
| | $^{85}$Kr | 28 | | | | 28 | | |
| | $^{131}$I | <1 | <1 | <1 | 120[b] | <1 | | |
| | $^{134}$Cs | 9.9 | | | | 9.9 | | |
| | $^{137}$Cs | 15 | | | | 15 | | |
| | Others | 2.8 | 39 | 1.4 | <1 | ~3.3 | | |
| Geologic repository | $^{129}$I | 5.5 | | | 440 | 33 | 0.0040 | 0.0012 |
| 100- to 1,000-year totals: | | | | | | 0.16-0.44 | | 0.14-0.20 |

[a]Totals are for time periods of 100 and 1,000 years into the future when ranges are given. The impacts of all other fuel cycle facilities are insignificant by comparison, and result in population dose commitments of less than 1 person-rem each.

[b]A dose effectiveness factor of 1/10 is applied in computing thyroid cancer risk from exposure to $^{131}$I, since $^{131}$I is only about 10% as effective as x-rays, gamma rays, or other shorter-lived iodine isotopes.

Table 7. Collective U. S. general population dose commitments and potential health impacts due to the release of liquid radioactive effluents from normal operations of the nuclear fuel cycle per GW(e)-yr[a]

| Source of the dose commitment | Nuclide | Dose commitments (person-rem) | | | | | Potential health impacts | |
|---|---|---|---|---|---|---|---|---|
| | | Total body | Bone | Lung | Thyroid | Total body risk equivalent | Potential latent cancer mortality | Potential genetic effects |
| UF$_6$ conversion plants | $^{226}$Ra | 120 | 130 | <1 | <1 | 125 | 0.038 | 0.026 |
| Light-water-cooled nuclear power plants | $^3$H | 5.3 | | | | 5.3 | 0.0008 | 0.0014 |
| | $^{131}$I | <1 | <1 | <1 | 19[b] | <1 | | |
| | $^{137}$Cs | ~1 | | | | ~1 | | |
| Totals: | | | | | | | 0.039 | 0.027 |

[a]The impacts of all other fuel cycle facilities are insignificant by comparison and result in population dose commitments of less than 1 person-rem each.

[b]A dose effectiveness factor of 1/10 is applied in computing thyroid cancer risk from exposure to $^{131}$I, since $^{131}$I is only about 10% as effective as X rays, gamma rays, or other shorter-lived iodine isotopes.

Table 8. Summary of potential health impacts among the U.S. general population from normal operations of the nuclear fuel cycle per GW(e)-yr.[a,b]

| Source | Potential latent cancer mortality | Potential genetic effects |
|---|---|---|
| Uranium mines | 0.063-0.22 | 0.012-0.042 |
| Uranium mills and tailings | 0.033-0.15 | 0.013-0.036 |
| $UF_6$ conversion plants | 0.038 | 0.026 |
| Light-water-cooled nuclear power plants | 0.012-0.014 | 0.021-0.025 |
| Fuel reprocessing plants | 0.050-0.055 | 0.092-0.10 |
| Geologic repository | 0.0040 | 0.0012 |
| Totals: | 0.20-0.48 | 0.17-0.23 |

[a] The impacts of all other fuel cycle facilities are insignificant by comparison and result in population dose commitments of less than 1 person-rem each.

[b] Where ranges are given, the values represent impacts for 100- and 1000-year environmental dose commitments.

change if the world were considered.  In the case of $^{14}C$, however, the world population dose would be about five times greater than that for the United States for the next 100 years, and about 10 times greater than that to the United States over the next 1,000 years.  Similarly, the $^{85}Kr$ population dose to the world would be about 20 times greater than to the U. S. population.  Examination of Tables 6 and 7, however, show that such increases would result in about 60-70% increases in the total cancer risk and 140-230% increases in the genetic risks shown in Table 8.  Given the much larger uncertainties in projecting health impacts on other populations in the world (e.g., due to differences in life expectancies, spontaneous cancer mortality and competing risks), the relatively conservative estimates presented for the United States could be considered to reasonably reflect the cancer risk to the entire world from the U. S. nuclear fuel cycle.

The risk of developing cancer is, in general, greater than the cancer mortality because some cancers (e.g., thyroid) have a relatively small risk of mortality.  The BEIR III report (National Research Council — National Academy of Sciences, 1980a) indicates overall cancer incidence for external or whole body exposure is about 1.5 to 2 times higher than mortality.  However, since a large fraction of the fuel cycle cancer mortality is from bone and lung cancer (from $^{222}Rn$ releases) which have an assumed 100% mortality in the BEIR III models, the overall fuel cycle cancer incidence should not be much greater than the mortality.  In this assessment it was assumed the incidence would be 1.5 times the mortality risk.

Finally, lest it be forgotten, there is a radiological risk associated with almost any human activity, including tilling the soil ($^{222}Rn$ releases and resuspension of $^{40}K$ to the air where it can be inhaled), congregating for scientific conferences ($^{40}K$ gamma rays from internal depositions in attendees), building tight energy-efficient homes, particularly with brick and stone ($^{40}K$ and $^{222}Rn$ from the building materials), or generating electricity by coal combustion (principally $^{238}U$, $^{235}U$, $^{230}Th$, $^{226}Ra$, $^{222}Rn$, and $^{40}K$ emitted with the fly ash).  Such releases may have public radiological risks that are comparable to those from normal operation of the nuclear fuel cycle (Chapter 3 of this volume; Travis et al., 1979; McBride et al., 1978; USEPA, 1979; Camplin, 1980; NCRP, 1975; 1977; UNSCEAR, 1977).

Further, Cohen (1981) has calculated that over geologic times, the nuclear fuel cycle may even save hundreds of human lives, giving a negative health risk per GW(e)-yr. This original idea, which surely deserves a special title (e.g., the Cohen Effect; analogous to the Suess Effect for coal combustion), comes from the fact that the uranium fuel cycle removes $^{235}U$ and $^{238}U$ from uranium ore for use as fuel, leaving the balance of the chain now headed by $^{230}Th$. Since $^{230}Th$ has a half-life that is only about 0.002% that of $^{238}U$, the emanation of $^{222}Rn$ from uranium mill tailings is greatly reduced over billions of years relative to undisturbed ore, since erosion of the continent will continually bring these radionuclides to the surface of the earth. Such calculations over billions of years into the future must be considered with caution, because of the uncertainties in populations and cancer risk over long periods of time. However, they should give second thoughts to those who would calculate health risks over billions of years in order to condemn uranium mill tailings and the nuclear fuel cycle as being unacceptable.

## Occupational Radiation Risks

With regard to occupational radiation risks from the nuclear fuel cycle, the Table S-3 (10 CFR Part 51) analysis provides a detailed current assessment of occupational dose commitments (USNRC, 1976b; 1977a; 1977b). These estimates and the potential health risks are summarized in Table 9. Since most of the occupational dose commitments are from whole body exposures to external radiation sources, no breakdown by radionuclide is practical. Only in the case of uranium miners do the risks from internally deposited radioactivity (short-lived $^{222}Rn$ progeny in the bronchi of the lungs) become of great importance. The major source of genetic risk among workers in the nuclear fuel cycle comes from nuclear power plant exposures. The total cancer and genetic risk over the next century for the nuclear fuel cycle per GW(e)-yr is about equally divided between workers (0.25 and 0.17) (see Table 9) and the general public (0.20 and 0.17) (see Table 8), respectively. However, due to the much smaller numbers of nuclear workers, the average individual risks to occupational workers or their descendants are much higher than for the general public, although still small compared to the normal risk of cancer to non-nuclear workers, or cancers associated with exposures to other non-radiological agents (e.g., vinyl chloride, arsenic compounds, asbestos, benzene, etc.).

A recent report to the President indicates that occupational exposure to such carcinogens is believed to be a factor in more than 20% of all cases of cancer, while an unknown number of persons are at risk because of the seepage of carcinogenic chemicals into domestic water supplies from waste dumps and other types of exposure (CEQ, 1980).

Table 9. Collective occupational dose commitments and potential health impacts of the nuclear fuel cycle per GW(e)-yr[a]

| Source of the dose commitment | Dose commitments (person-rem) | | | | | Potential health impacts[a] | |
|---|---|---|---|---|---|---|---|
| | Total body | Bone | Lung | Thyroid | Total body risk equivalent | Potential latent cancer mortality | Potential genetic effects |
| Uranium mines | 88 | 360 | 1,400 | 250 | 470 | 0.096 | 0.019 |
| Uranium mills | 88 | 440 | 1,000 | 40 | 370 | 0.076 | 0.019 |
| UF$_6$ conversion plants | <1 | 10 | 6.9 | <1 | 2.3 | 0.0005 | ~0 |
| Enrichment plants | <1 | 5.9 | 14 | <1 | 6.2 | 0.0013 | ~0 |
| UO$_2$ fuel fabrication plants | 12 | 4.4 | 450 | <1 | 130 | 0.027 | 0.0026 |
| Light-water-cooled nuclear power plants | 560 | | | | 560 | 0.046 | 0.12 |
| Irradiated fuel storage | 3.6 | | | | 3.6 | 0.0003 | 0.0008 |
| Reprocessing | 28 | | | | 28 | 0.0023 | 0.0062 |
| Transportation | 1.8 | | | | 1.8 | 0.0001 | 0.0004 |
| Waste management | <1 | | | | <1 | ~0 | ~0 |
| Totals | | | | | | 0.25 | 0.17 |

[a]Based on an essentially all-male population of workers.

## Radiological Health Risks from Accidents

The potential health risks resulting from catastrophic accidents in the nuclear fuel cycle appear to be dominated by the risks associated with low probability, high consequence accidents in nuclear power plants (Erdman et al., 1979). In particular, the Reactor Safety Study found most of the risk of all potentially serious nuclear power plant accidents depends on only a few types of accidents in either pressurized or boiling water reactors (PWRs and BWRs). Even though the probabilities of occurrence are estimated to be vanishingly small, the potential health consequences could be very large in the event of an actual accident, approaching in total numbers the annual death rate on U.S. highways.

The Reactor Safety Study (USNRC, 1975) estimated that the potential risk of cancer mortality from nuclear power plant accidents was 0.02 deaths per year of operation for a 1,000 MW(e) plant. However, that risk estimate included the application of so-called dose and dose-rate effectiveness factors which reduced the "upper bound" risk by a factor of 2. In the absence of BEIR III guidance on that matter, it is felt that, while there are sound radiobiological reasons for such factors (e.g., biological repair mechanisms), it is prudent to raise the WASH-1400 (USNRC, 1975) risk estimate to 0.04 deaths per GW(e)-yr. It is important to note that although the uncertainties may be larger then originally believed, even if the catastrophic risks of nuclear power are as much as 100 times greater than estimated by the Reactor Safety Study, such accidents could result in about two deaths (acute fatalities and latent cancers) per GW(e)-yr. Such an increase, combined with those from normal operations, would make the risks from the nuclear fuel cycle approximately equal to the low end of the range of mortality risk from the coal fuel cycle. Furthermore, as will be shown later, such risks are small in relation to everyday risks people are more familiar with (e.g., cigarette smoking, travel, and recreation.)

## Non-radiological Health Risks from Accidents

Some additional risks (other than cancer and genetic effects) involved in occupational activities (largely mining, etc.) come from estimates in the latest National Academy of Sciences Report by the Committee on Nuclear and Alternative Energy Systems (CONAES) (National Research Council – National Academy of Sciences, 1980b, pp. 427-432). That analysis indicates the following mortality risks per GW(e)-yr: (1) mining, 0.2 deaths; (2) processing, 0.001 deaths; (3) transport, 0.01 deaths; and (4) power generation, 0.01 deaths, for a total of about 0.22 accidental

Table 10. Comparisons of the potential health risks among the U.S. general population from the nuclear fuel cycle per GW(e)-yr with similar risks from other sources of radiation exposure

| Population at risk | Population total-body dose commitments (person-rem) | Potential health risks | |
|---|---|---|---|
| | | Potential latent cancer deaths | Potential genetic effects |
| Average for U.S. from the nuclear fuel cycle for 100 years per GW(e)-yr | 1,700[a] | 0.20 | 0.17 |
| Average for U.S. from natural background radiation (∼102 mrem/year) (Oakley, 1972) | 22,000,000 | 2,500 | 4,800 |
| Average for Denver, CO, from natural background radiation (∼180 mrem/year) (Oakley, 1972; NCRP, 1975) | 180,000 | 21 | 40 |
| Average for U. S. from television viewing (∼1 mrem/year from low-energy X-rays) (NCRP, 1977) | 220,000 | 25 | 48 |
| Average for U.S. for diagnostic X-rays (∼72 mrem/year) (National Research Council-National Academy of Sciences, 1972) | 16,000,000 | 1,800 | 3,500 |

[a]Includes both external total body doses and specific organ doses from internally deposited radionuclides. The genetically significant dose is about 750 person-rems.

deaths per GW(e)-yr. A similar CONAES estimate for total accidental injuries per GW(e)-yr for the entire nuclear fuel cycle is 20 injuries per GW(e)-yr. Although no details are provided, the draft report of the CONAES Risk Impact Panel (which is referenced by the main report of the CONAES) indicates a range of about 7 to 20 injuries per GW(e)-yr. Further, most of those injuries are associated with accidents in uranium mines (i.e., it follows the same pattern as accidental deaths). The value of 7 comes from Table A-1 of the Council on Environmental Quality (CEQ) report (1973), but no reference is provided in the Risk Impact Panel report for the value of 20 per GW(e)-yr. The CEQ report gives the following breakdown on accidental injuries per GW(e)-yr: (1) mining, 4.6; (2) processing ($UF_6$, enrichment, fabrication, reprocessing, waste management), 0.76; (3) transportation, 0.06; and (4) light-water reactors, 1.7.

## Perspectives

Having calculated the potential health impacts of the nuclear fuel cycle (remembering that the lower bound radiological risks, particularly those among the public, may actually be zero for low doses and dose rates of low-LET radiation), it lends perspective by comparing these estimates with other commonplace risks, even though many of these risks result from voluntary individual activities (see Tables 10 and 11). The following comparisons are not intended to be all inclusive, and other comparisons are possible. The calculated health risks among the general public associated with these exposures are for the general U.S. population. No attempts were made to quantify equities, distribution of risks, etc., since, as noted earlier by Dr. Fischoff and his colleagues in Chapter 1, that is presently beyond the state of the art. (See Gotchy, 1982, for additional discussion.)

The first comparison in Table 10 is with naturally occurring background radiation. The major sources for such doses are from cosmic rays and terrestrial radioactivity, which result in both external and internal exposures.

Another comparison in Table 10 is with similar risks from other common sources of radiation exposure, such as from medical X-rays and color television-viewing.

A third comparison is of the naturally occurring annual risks of health impacts to the U.S. population as shown in Table 11.

Finally comparisons of the radiological mortality risks to occupational workers with other mortality risks people

Table 11.   Normal annual risk of mortality among the U.S.
            general population

| Source of risk | Risk of mortality |
|---|---|
| All causes of death (NCHS, 1976) | 2,100,000 |
| Major cardiovascular diseases (NCHS, 1976) | 1,100,000 |
| Total cancers (ACSI, 1980) | 400,000 |
| Smoking cigarettes (ACSI, 1980) | 330,000 |
| All accidents (NCHS, 1976) | 120,000 |
| Automobile driving (NSC, 1979) | 57,000 |
| Falls (NCHS, 1976) | 17,000 |
| Fires and hot substances (NCHS, 1976) | 7,000 |
| Drowning (NCHS, 1976) | 6,200 |
| Accidental poisoning by drugs and medicaments (NCHS, 1976) | 2,400 |
| Air travel (NCHS, 1976) | 1,500 |
| Accidental electrocution (NCHS, 1976) (regardless of how it is generated) | 1,100 |
| Railway travel (NCHS, 1976) | 660 |
| Lightning (NCHS, 1976) | 88 |
| Nuclear fuel cycle per GW(e)-yr | 0.2[a] |
| Substitution of a coal-fired plant for a nuclear plant per GW(e)-yr of plant operation (based on estimates by Dr. Morris in Chapter 3) | 10-21 |

[a]This would approximately double if occupational risk
is included.

are more familiar with (generally from other causes which lead to larger losses of life expectancy than would radiogenic cancer) are presented in Table 12. These comparisons clearly demonstrate that the lifetime risks associated with the nuclear fuel cycle are extraordinarily small when compared with other everyday risks people face with relatively mild trepidation.

## Risks Associated with
## Proliferation and Terrorism

Although this assessment does not address the potential health risks associated with proliferation of nuclear weapons and terrorism, these concerns have been evaluated by the NAS Committee on Nuclear and Alternative Energy Systems (CONAES) (National Research Council – National Academy of Sciences, 1980b). CONAES itself is split on the issue of proliferation, and no one can yet reasonably quantify such risks.

CONAES carefully examined the sociopolitical question of linkage between commercial nuclear power and the risk of proliferation of nuclear weapons.[9] It was concluded that even stopping commercial nuclear power could not stop proliferation, since other less expensive alternatives for producing weapon materials (e.g., such as that used by India) are readily available. However, CONAES argued for the use of political barriers to reduce the *rate* of proliferation, with the belief that slower proliferation would allow institutions to evolve to the point where the risk of nuclear war will be comparable to or less than it is today. These barriers would include strengthening of the Non-Proliferation Treaty and placing fuel cycle operations involving weapons-usable material under international control. CONAES concluded that a potential linkage may exist between expansion of commercial nuclear power in the world and the risk of nuclear war, but it is at most a weak linkage. Thus, in time, other sociopolitical controls must be developed or proliferation could occur with or without commercial nuclear power programs.

With regard to terrorism, CONAES wisely noted that many energy sources face the terrorist threat. Examples are dams and fuel storage facilities (oil, natural gas, liquefied fuels, etc.). However, the risk of terrorist attacks on nuclear facilities (or diversion of nuclear materials) are easier to control than these other sources since the areas and number of personnel involved are smaller, making security tighter and facilities more defensible.

Table 12. Lifetime mortality risks numerically equivalent to the potential risks of mortality associated with occupational radiation exposures [based on estimates by Pochin (1975)]

| Type of activity | 1 rem | 25 rem (emergency) | 45 rem/lifetime[a] |
|---|---|---|---|
| Smoking cigarettes | 1 carton | 25 cartons | 0.5 cigarettes/day[b] |
| Drinking wine | 66 bottles | 33 bottles/year[b] | 1 liter/week[b] |
| Automobile driving | 6,600 miles | 3,300 miles/year[b] | 5,900 miles/year[b] |
| Commercial flying | 33,000 miles | 17,000 miles/year[b] | 30,000 miles/year[b] |
| Rockclimbing[c] | 3.3 hours | 10 days | 18 days |
| Canoeing[c] | 1.6 days | 1.3 months | 2.4 months |
| Being a man aged 60 | 1.8 days | 1.5 months | 2.7 months |

[a] 1 rem/year for 45 years (ages 20 to 65).

[b] 50 years of use (ages 20 to 70).

[c] 8 hours/day activity.

Levels of security now required for nuclear facilities are not greatly different from those involved in high security projects such as the Manhattan Project, or in the protection of the gold in Fort Knox, which have succeeded in their objectives. Historically, personnel clearance for employment has been routinely used in the past without a significant compromise of civil liberties. Thus it is reasonable to believe the same can be accomplished for the commercial nuclear fuel cycle. Furthermore, CONAES concluded that high security would add little to the cost of nuclear power.

## Summary and Conclusions

The estimated health impacts of the nuclear fuel cycle per GW(e)-yr from this assessment are summarized in Table 13. While any breakdown of potential health impacts represents a somewhat indigestable mixture of apples, oranges, and other assorted fruits and nuts, it is clear that the potential impacts on the general public and occupational workers for the entire nuclear fuel cycle are small in absolute numbers, and in relation to other everyday risks. While one may argue that cancer risks to occupational workers are accepted voluntarily and the public's cancer risks are involuntary in nature, this distinction does not change the pain and economic distress suffered, or the cost to society in the loss of one of its members because of a premature death. Furthermore, occupational risks, which must be borne by any worker regardless of occupation, may be dictated by forces outside the control of most workers (e.g., economics, chance, and tradition) obscuring the distinction between the voluntary or involuntary nature of the risks. In that respect, the total cancer risks may be additive. In addition, there are other potentially greater occupational cancer risks which have not been included here (for example, those resulting from exposure to industrial solvents and dusts), since such data are not readily available. However, the 1980 Report to the President by the Toxic Substances Strategy Committee indicates that occupational exposure to carcinogens (primarily nonradiological) may be a factor in more than 20% of all cancers (CEQ, 1980).

It is also interesting to note how much the coal fuel cycle impacts on the nuclear fuel cycle if (using the estimates by Dr. Morris in Chapter 3) it is assumed the 0.056 GW(e)-yr of electric power needed to operate the nuclear fuel cycle [per GW(e)-yr] comes entirely from coal power. Since most of that energy is currently used for uranium enrichment, and much of that power is in fact derived from coal combustion, such additions are probably not unreasonable.

Table 13. Summary of potential health risks among the total U. S. population per GW(e)-yr for the nuclear fuel cycle[a]

| Source of the risk | Potential latent cancer mortality | | Potential latent cancer incidence | |
|---|---|---|---|---|
| | Occupational | General public | Occupational | General public |
| Uranium mining | 0.096 | 0.063-0.22 | ∿0.1 | ∿0.07-0.25 |
| Processing[b] | 0.10 | 0.071-0.19 | ∿0.1 | ∿0.08-0.21 |
| Power generation | 0.046 | 0.012-0.014 | 0.071 | 0.020-0.023 |
| Transportation | 0.0001 | NA[c] | 0.0002 | NA |
| Reprocessing | 0.0023 | 0.050-0.055 | 0.0035 | 0.097-0.11 |
| Waste management | NA | 0.0040 | NA | 0.006 |
| Catastrophic accidents | NA | 0.04 | NA | ∿0.06 |
| Subtotals | 0.25 | 0.24-0.52 | ∿0.3 | ∿0.33-0.66 |
| Coal combustion to operate the nuclear fuel cycle[d] | NA | 0.017[e] | NA | 0.025[f] |
| Totals: | ≧0.25 | 0.26-0.54[e] fatal cancers | ≧0.3 | 0.36-0.69[f] cancer cases |

[a]Where ranges are given, the values represent impacts for 100- and 1000-year environmental dose commitments.

[b]Includes uranium milling, $UF_6$ conversion, enrichment, and fuel fabrication.

[c]These values are expected to be small but are presently not available (NA).

Table 13. (continued)

| Occupational accidents and diseases | | Potential genetic effects in future generations | |
|---|---|---|---|
| Mortality | Nonfatal cases | Occupa-tional | General |
| 0.2 | 4.6-14 | 0.019 | 0.012-0.042 |
| 0.001 | 0.76-2.3 | 0.021 | 0.039-0.062 |
| 0.01 | 1.7-5.1 | 0.12 | 0.021-0.025 |
| 0.01 | 0.06-0.18 | 0.0004 | NA |
| | | 0.0062 | 0.092-0.10 |
| NA | NA | NA | 0.0012 |
| NA | NA | NA | 0.08 |
| 0.22 | 7-20 | 0.17 | 0.25-0.31 |
| 0.069-0.074 | 5.3-5.5 | NA | ~0-0.035 |
| 0.29 | 12-26 | ≧0.17 | 0.25-0.35 |

[d]Production of 56 MW(e)-yr of power by coal combustion to operate the nuclear fuel cycle [per GW(e)-yr] from estimates by Dr. Morris, Chapter 3.

[e]An additional 0.56-1.2 deaths are estimated from sulfate pollution.

[f]An additional 0.15 nonfatal injuries among public are estimated from transport accidents.

In closing, it should now be obvious that it is not possible to live without being at risk (except prior to conception and perhaps after death; theologians have been hotly debating the latter for centuries). Yet needless risk can and should be avoided *if* the incremental reduction in risk can justify the expenditure of public resources. This important criterion for making such decisions was clearly stated by the NAS-BEIR Committee (National Research Council – National Academy of Science, 1972):

> "The public must be protected from radiation but not to the extent that the degree of protection results in substitution of a worse hazard for the radiation avoided. Additionally, there should not be attempted the reduction of small risks even further at the cost of large sums of money that, spent otherwise, would clearly produce greater benefit" (p.2).

It is hoped that this assessment and attendant perspectives will assist decision makers as well as scientists and citizens in making the difficult decisions on America's future energy course with understanding and reason.

## Notes

[1]This chapter was prepared by an employee of the U. S. Nuclear Regulatory Commission which has neither approved nor disapproved its technical content.

[2]See, for example, transcript of the environmental hearings for the Perkins Nuclear Power Station, following page 2369, and following page 2425, (USNRC, 1978).

[3]Evidentiary Hearing before an Appeal Board on the Radon Release Issue, (USNRC, 1980a). Atomic Safety Licensing Appeal Board, see decision of May 13, 1981 (ALAB-640).

[4]See, for example, USNRC, 1976a, pp. IV E-23–E-28.

[5]See in particular Section IVJ of NUREG-0002 (USNRC, 1976a).

[6]For example, the annual radiation dose to the total body of an average American is about 0.1 rem (1.0 milliSievert) from natural background radiation. Most of the dose occurs during the year from external radiation (cosmic rays and terrestrial gamma radiation). However, some of the doses from internally deposited primordial radionuclides (uranium, thorium, and the actinium series) continue to give doses to certain specific organs (e.g., lung and bone) for many subsequent years (i.e., a committed dose). The collective annual total body dose commitment from natural back-

ground radiation in the United States is about 0.1 rem/yr × 220-million persons, or 22-million person-rem (0.22 million person-Sieverts).

[7]National Research Council — National Academy of Sciences, 1980a, p. 139).

[8]A reference to Lewis Carrol's fantasies, *Alice's Adventures in Wonderland* (1865) and *Through the Looking-Glass and What Alice found There* (1872).

[9]See especially pp. 326-337 and 483-488 of the CONAES report.

## References

American Cancer Society, Inc. (ACSI). 1980. *Cancer Facts and Figures: 1981.* p. 19. New York, N. Y.

Avery, R. J. et al. 1980. Interferon inhibits transformation by murine sarcoma viruses before integration of provirus. *Nature* 288:93-95.

Baes, C. F. et al. 1977. Carbon dioxide and climate: the uncontrolled experiment. *Am. Scientist* 65:310-320.

Bloom, B. R. 1980. Interferons and the immune system. *Nature* 284:593-595.

Bram, S. et al. 1980. Vitamin-C preferential toxicity for malignant melanoma cell. *Nature* 284:629-630.

Calder, N. 1978. Head south with all deliberate speed: ice may return in a few thousand years. *Smithsonian* 8(10).

Camplin, W. C. 1980. *Coal-Fired Power Stations — The Radiological Impact of Effluent Discharges to Atmosphere*, Report NRPB-R-107, National Radiological Protection Board, UK.

*Code of Federal Regulations* (CFR). 1981. Title 10. Energy. Part 51. Licensing and Regulatory Policy and Procedures for Environmental Protection.

Cohen, B. L. 1981. The role of radon in comparisons of effects of radioactivity releases from nuclear power, coal burning, and phosphate mines. *Health Phys.* 40(1):19-25.

Council on Environmental Quality (CEQ). 1973. Energy and the Environment: Electric Power. Table A-11. Washington, D. C.

Council on Environmental Quality (CEQ). 1980. *Toxic Chemicals and Public Protection*, A Report to the President by the Toxic Substances Strategy Committee, Washington, D.C.

Derynck, R. et al. 1980. Expression of human fibroblast interferon gene in escherichia coli. *Nature* 287: 193-197.

Erdmann, R. C. et al. 1979. *Status Report on the EPRI Fuel Cycle Accident Risk Assessment.* NP-1128. Electric Power Research Institute. Palo Alto, California.

Goeddel, D. V. et al. 1980. Human leukocyte interferon produced by E. coli is biologically active. *Nature* 287:411-415.

Gotchy, R. L. 1982. *Potential Health and Environmental Impacts Attributable to the Nuclear and Coal Fuel Cycles.* NRC report NUREG-0332. U. S. Nuclear Regulatory Commission, Washington, D. C.

Gotchy, R. L. 1979. NRC Estimates of Health Risks Associated with Low-Level Radiation Exposure, *Proceedings of the 10th Annual National Conference on Radiation Control, Harrisburg, Pennsylvania, April 30-May 4, 1978,* HEW Publication (FDA). June 1979. 79-8054, USHEW/ USPHS/FDA, Bureau of Radiation Health, Rockville, Maryland 20857.

Gotchy, R. L. 1978. Comparison of long-term environmental impacts; more questions than answers. 1978 Annual Meeting of the American Nuclear Society, San Diego, California, June 18-27, 1978. TANSAO 28 1-804.

Heffter, J. L. and G. J. Ferber. 1975. A regional-continental scale transport, diffusion, and deposition model. NOAA Technical Memorandum ERL ARL-50. Air Resources Laboratories, Silver Spring, Maryland.

International Commission on Radiological Protection (ICRP). 1959. *Report of Committee II on Permissible Doses for Internal Radiation.* ICRP Publication 2. Pergamon Press. Oxford.

Killough, G. G. 1977. *A Diffusion-Type Model of the Global Carbon Cycle for the Estimation of Dose to the World Population from Releases of Carbon-14 to the Atmosphere.* ORNL-5269. Oak Ridge National Laboratory, Oak Ridge, Tennessee.

Lamb, H. H. 1977. *Climate: Present, Past and Future,* Vol. 2. Methuen: London; Barnes and Noble: New York.

Luckey, T. D. 1980. *Hormesis with Ionizing Radiation.* CRC Press, Boca Raton, Florida.

McBride, J. P., R. E. Moore, J. P. Witherspoon, and R. E. Blanco. 1978. Radiological impact of airborne effluents of coal and nuclear plants. *Science* 202(4372): 1045-1050.

Mercer, J. H.  1978.  West Antarctic ice sheet and $CO_2$ greenhouse effect: a threat of disaster.  *Nature* 271:321-325.

Mitchell, J. M. Jr.  1977.  *Carbon Dioxide and Future
Climate.*  EDS.  National Oceanic and Atmospheric Administration, U. S. Department of Commerce.

Nagata, S.  et al.  1980.  Synthesis in E. coli of a poly-
peptide with human lencocyte interferon activity.
*Nature* 284:316-318.

National Center for Health Statistics (NCHS).  *Vital Statistics of the United States:  1972; 1976, Vol. II –
Mortality, Part A.*  U. S. Department of Health, Education and Welfare, Washington, D. C.

National Council on Radiation Protection and Measurements
(NCRP).  1975.  *Natural Background Radiation in the
United States.*  Report NCRP-45.

National Council on Radiation Protection and Measurements
(NCRP).  1977.  *Radiation Exposure from Consumer Products and Miscellaneous Sources.*  Report NCRP-56.

National Research Council, National Academy of Sciences.
1972.  *The Effects on Populations of Exposure to Low
Levels of Ionizing Radiation.*  NAS Committee on the
Biological Effects of Ionizing Radiation (BEIR I).
Washington, D. C.

National Research Council, National Academy of Sciences.
1980a.  *The Effects on Populations of Exposure to Low
Levels of Ionizing Radiation.*  NAS Committee on the
Biological Effects of Ionizing Radiation (BEIR III).
Washington, D. C.

National Research Council, National Academy of Sciences
1980b.  *Energy in Transition:  1985-2010.*  Committee on
Nuclear and Alternative Energy Systems (CONAES).  Washington, D. C.

National Safety Council (NSC).  1979.  *Accident Facts – 1979
Edition.*  Chicago, Illinois.

Norwine, J.  1977.  A question of climate.  *Environment*
19(8):6.

Oakley, D. T.  1972.  *Natural Radiation Exposure in the
United States.*  USEPA Report ORP/SID/2-1, Washington,
D. C.

Plum, F.  1979.  Dementia:  an approaching epidemic.  *Nature*
279:372-73.

Pochin, Sir Edward.  1975.  The acceptance of risk.  *Brit.
Med. Bull.* 31(3):184-190.

Ponte, L. 1976. *The Cooling.* Prentice-Hall, Englewood Cliffs, New Jersey.

Schneider, S. H. and R. S. Chen. 1980. Carbon dioxide warming and coastline flooding: physical factors and climatic impact. *Annual Rev. of Energy* 5:107-140.

Sporn, M. B. 1980. Combination Chemoprevention of Cancer. *Nature* 287:107-108.

Travis, C. C. et al. 1979. *A Radiological Assessment of Rn-222 Released from Uranium Mills and Other Natural and Technogically Enhanced Sources.* USNRC Report NUREG/CR-0573 (ORNL/NUREG-55), Oak Ridge National Laboratory, Oak Ridge, Tennessee.

U. N. Scientific Committee on the Effects of Atomic Radiation (UNSCEAR). 1977. *Sources and Effects of Ionizing Radiation.* Report to the General Assembly. United Nations, New York.

U. S. Department of Commerce, Bureau of Census. 1976. *Bicentennial Edition — Historical Statistics of the United States: Colonial Times to 1970, Part 1,* Series B149-166. 93rd Congress, 1st Session. House Document No. 93-78 (pt. 1).

U. S. Department of Commerce, Bureau of Census. 1977. *Projections of the Population of the United States: 1977 to 2050.* Series P-25, No. 704. Washington, D. C.

U. S. Environmental Protection Agency (USEPA). 1979. *Radiological Impact Caused by Emissions of Radionuclides into the Air in the United States.* Prelim. Report EPA 520/7-79-006. Washington, D. C.

U. S. Nuclear Regulatory Commission (USNRC). 1974. *Environmental Survey of the Uranium Fuel Cycle.* WASH-1248.

U. S. Nuclear Regulatory Commission (USNRC). 1975. *The Reactor Safety Study, An Assessment of Accident Risks in U. S. Commercial Nuclear Power Plants.* WASH-1400 (NUREG-75/014).

U. S. Nuclear Regulatory Commission (USNRC). 1976a. *The Final Generic Environmental Statement on the Use of Recyle Plutonium in Mixed Oxide Fuel in Light Water Cooled Reactors (GESMO).* NUREG-0002.

U. S. Nuclear Regulatory Commission (USNRC). 1976b. *Environmental Survey of the Reprocessing and Waste Management Portion of the LWR Fuel Cycle.* NUREG-0116 (Supp. 1 to WASH-1248).

U. S. Nuclear Regulatory Commission (USNRC). 1977a. *Public Comments and Task Force Responses Regarding the Environmental Survey of the Reprocessing and Waste Management Portions of the LWR Fuel Cycle.* NUREG-0216 (Supp. 2 to WASH-1248).

U. S. Nuclear Regulatory Commission (USNRC). 1977b. Docket RM-50-3. *Hearing Record for the Final Rule Making for Uranium Fuel Cycle Impacts from Spent Fuel Reprocessing and Radioactive Waste Management.* Washington, D. C.

U. S. Nuclear Regulatory Commission (USNRC). 1977c. Memorandum to the GESMO Hearing Board. Docket No. RM-50-5.

U. S. Nuclear Regulatory Commission (USNRC). 1978. *Environmental Hearings for the Perkins Nuclear Power Station.* Docket No. 50-488, -489, and -490.

U. S. Nuclear Regulatory Commission (USNRC). 1980a. *Evidentiary Hearing, Appeal Board on the Radon Release Issue, (ALAB-640).* Harrisburg, Pennsylvania. Docket No. 50-277, -278; 50-320; 50-354, -355; and 50-485.

U. S. Nuclear Regulatory Commission (USNRC). 1980b. *Generic Environmental Impact Statement on Uranium Milling.* NUREG-0706. Argonne National Laboratory.

U. S. Nuclear Regulatory Commission (USNRC). 1981a. *Radon Releases from Uranium Mining and Milling and Their Calculated Health Effects.* NUREG-0757.

U. S. Nuclear Regulatory Commission. 1981b. Proposed Narrative Explanation of Table S-3, Uranium Fuel Cycle Environmental Data, 10 CFR 51, *Federal Register 46*, No. 42, pp. 15129-15255, March 4.

U. S. Nuclear Regulatory Commission. 1981c. *Testimony of E. F. Branagan and R. K. Struckmeyer on the Potential Radiological Health Effects of Technetium-99 Releases from the Fuel Cycle, Susquehanna Steam Electric Station,* Docket No. 50-387 and 50-388, October 14.

Weiss, R. 1977. Vaccination against virus induced tumors. *Nature* 267:205-206.

Zielinski, C. C. et al. 1980. Surface phenotypes in T-cell leukemia are determined by oncogenic retroviruses. *Nature* 288:489-491.

# 3. Health Risks of Coal Energy Technology

## Introduction

Everyone is familiar with Hubbert's graph of fossil
fuel use in human history (Figure 1).  The early rise in
this curve in the 19th and early 20th century was based on
coal.  Increasing use of coal was a cornerstone in the
development of world industrial power.  Coal has been re-
placed largely by oil and natural gas and now contributes
<30% of world energy supplies.  The rapid increase in the
price of oil over the past decade and the uncertainty of an
adequate supply at any price have dictated a shift away from
oil.  Eventually this shift must be away from all fossil
fuels, and growth in that direction is essential.  But
neither nuclear nor renewable sources are able to fill in
the gap as rapidly as coal.  In the United States, coal is
available domestically and in large supply – but not without
risk.  Societal memory of the time when coal was our primary
energy source reflects heavy smog, dirt, and grime in the
cities and disasters in the mines.  It is not a picture to
which one wishes to return.  But neither is today's coal
technology the technology of the 1920's and 30's.  Moreover,
the spector of January 1974 haunts us every time the Organi-
zation of Petroleum Exporting Countries (OPEC) meets.
Finally, we are beginning to discover that no energy source
– not even conservation – is without risk.  There must be a
full and careful assessment of the risks of coal.  These
risks can then be compared with those from other energy
sources to help decide overall energy policy and to determine the appropriateness of coal in individual cases.
It seems almost certain that in the face of a comparison of
the risks of coal against the risks of doing without, use of
coal will increase over the remainder of this century.  In
that case it will be important to compare the risks of
various ways of using coal (e.g., large and small electric

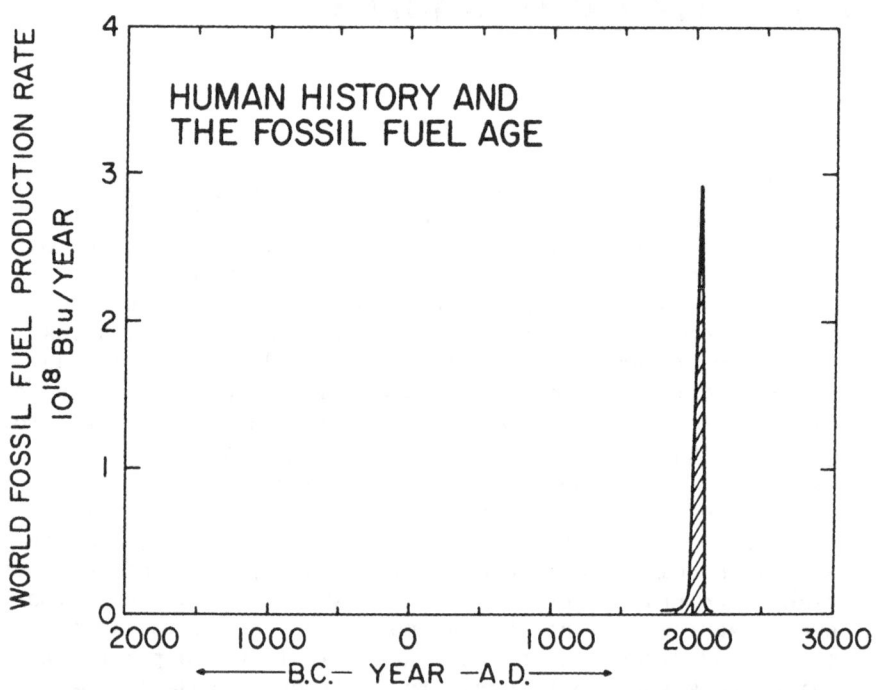

Figure 1.  Epoch of fossil fuels.  After Hubbert (1962).

generating plants, industrial and residential heating and cogeneration plants, residential stoves and furnaces, and coal-derived fuels - liquids, gases, and solids).

The general public and workers in a wide variety of trades are subjected to risks from coal production and use. These risks include accidental injury, respiratory disease, and cancer. In addition, there are more long-term, indirect risks stemming from environmental change from acid rain and $CO_2$ induced climate change.

Despite over a century of study of the health effects of coal, there are still great uncertainties. Risk assessments will reflect these uncertainties and thus will not lead to clear-cut or noncontroversial answers. But decisions must be made in the face of this uncertainty. The analytical assessment of risks imposes a discipline which hopefully will facilitate the use of what information does exist.

The health risks of coal through the complete fuel-cycle including mining, cleaning, transport, combustion and conversion to synthetic fuels are systematically examined below. Risks are quantified where possible in terms of both individual risk (risk per person-year) and per unit energy [per ton of coal or GW(e)-yr of electricity].

## Coal Mining and Cleaning

The principle and most well-documented health effects of coal mining are occupational. With the exception of individual disasters involving flooding or landslides associated with coal mining and cleaning wastes that are difficult to extrapolate to a general situation, risks to the general public are ill-defined. There are a number of potential sources of such risk. In some cases, surface mining on steep slopes may threaten homes below with rock slides. Current regulations presumably prevent this. Near-by populations are exposed to noise and fugitive dusts from surface mines, although this may be more of a nuisance than a health problem. Changing local hydrology may affect water supplies, causing contamination, interference with treatment, or use of less safe sources of water. Acid mine drainage, primarily from coal waste piles and underground mines, can affect water supplies, increasing the concentration of trace elements. Water pollution control requirements on new facilities result in most emissions originating in abandoned facilities (National Research Council, 1980). Coal cleaning wastes have been shown to have considerable

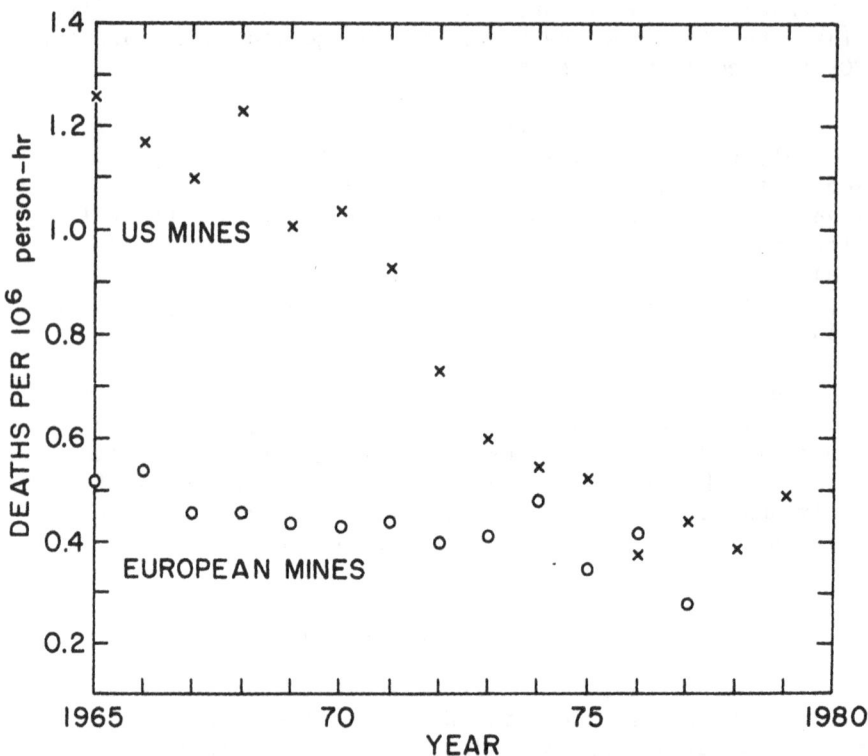

Figure 2.  Fatal injuries per million person-hours in underground bituminous coal mining.  U.S. Data from Mine Safety
and Health Administration (1976-1979) and Mining Enforcement
and Safety Administration (1971-75).  Adjusted to remove
large accidents (see text).  European data from Amoudru
(1980).

potential for producing highly acid leachates that dissolve
toxic trace elements (e.g., cadmium) concentrated in the
wastes (Chiu et al., 1980). Air emissions from diesel
equipment at surface mines may pose a public health risk.
Subsidence can pose direct risk as well as more subtle
effects on ground water flows. Burning mines and waste
piles can release large quantities of air pollutants, particularly $H_2S$. This was at one time a major problem but has
been brought largely under control.

## Accidental Injuries and Fatalities in Coal Mines and Coal Cleaning Plants

Coal mines have always been subject to a high occupational accident rate. The Coal Mine Health and Safety Act
of 1969 (CMHSA) introduced changes affecting this risk. An
analysis was carried out of the time trend of accident risk
with the aim of estimating future accident rates. The
trends reflect a complex mix of influences: changes in
safety methods and attitudes, government regulation, mining
technology, and work force characteristics. The individual
influence of each factor could not be determined. Since
risk is proportional to time exposed in the mine, injury
rates were taken as deaths and injuries per person-hour, a
measure of risk to the individual miner. The effects of
changes in productivity rate or tons produced per person-
hour are discussed later. The combination of the two give
the aggregate risk per unit energy produced.

The analysis is based on data from 1965 through 1979.
Although there do not appear to be important discrepancies,
changes in record keeping and reporting of the data were
made in 1972 and 1978. Changes in the degree of regulatory
supervision of reporting and record keeping may also intro-
duce artifacts into the data. Data from 1979 are preliminary. The 1965-75 data were obtained from the Mining
Enforcement and Safety Administration. Data for 1976-79
were obtained from the Mine Safety and Health Agency (MSHA).

Fatal accidents in underground bituminous coal mining.
Recent years have averaged about 0.4 deaths per $10^6$ person-
hour in U.S. underground bituminous coal mines. There is a
long-term decline in these fatality rates however, most
notable after the passage of CMHSA in 1969 (Figure 2). This
trend is presumably due to changing mining technology and
safety methods and standards. Current rates are now comparable to coal mine fatality rates in the European community
(Figure 2).

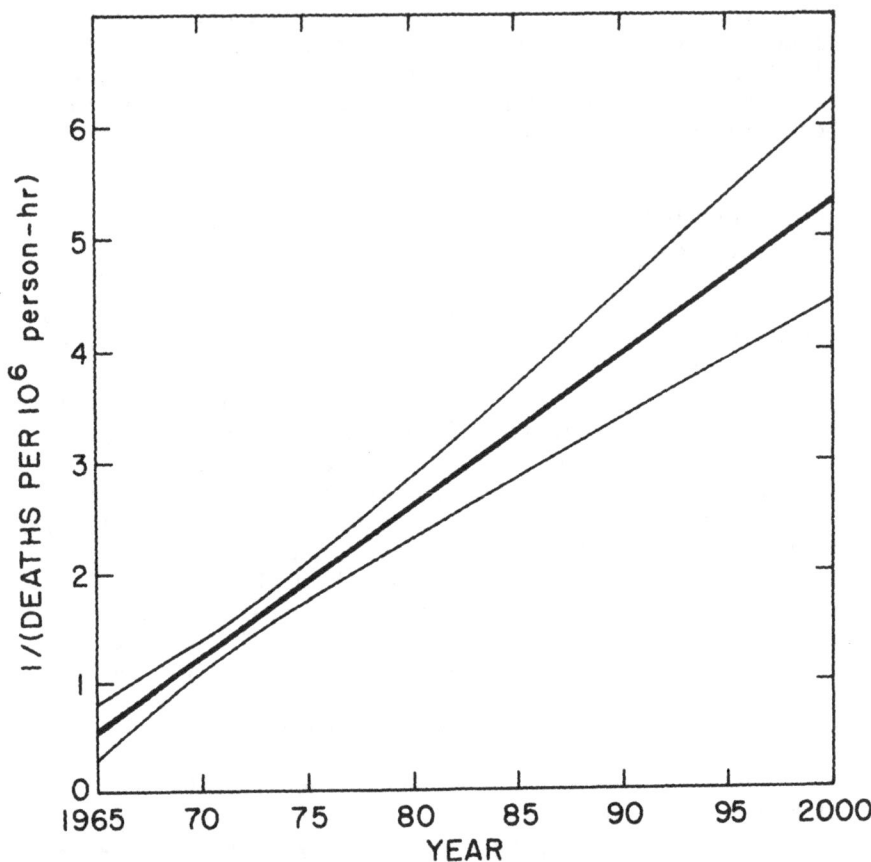

Figure 3.  Fatal injuries in U.S. underground bituminous
coal mining, reexpressed from Fig. 2 as the reciprocal of
fatality rate per million person-hourly adjusted to remove
large accidents.  Regression line, $Y = 0.419 + 0.136 X$,
where $X$ = year with 1965 = 1, extended to year 2000 with 95%
statistical confidence interval.

The analysis is limited to an extrapolation of the 1965-79 trend. To aid in analysis, the trend was linearized by reexpressing the parameter as the reciprocal of fatality rate or person-hours per fatality (compare Figures 2 and 3). The curve was smoothed by distributing the effects of large mine catastrophes, defined as more than 10 miners killed in a single event. Most mine fatalities occur singly, and the large accidents distort the effect. These disasters are sufficiently infrequent that the 15-year study period was inadequate to detect a trend in large accidents. The cases distributed are listed in Table 1. Deaths in these disasters were subtracted from the figures for the year they occurred, and the 142 total deaths were distributed evenly over all 15 years to yield adjusted annual rates. The regression on these adjusted and reexpressed rates was highly significant ($R^2 = 0.85$; $F_{1,13} = 76$; $p < 0.01$).

Table 1.    Underground bituminous mine disasters killing over 10 miners, 1965-79

| Date | Place | Deaths |
|------|-------|--------|
| 7 Nov. 1968 | Farmington, W.Va. | 78 |
| 20 Dec. 1970 | Hyden, Ky. | 38 |
| 11 Apr. 1976 | Partridge, Ky. | 26 |
| Total | | 142 |

Source:  *World Almanac,* 1977, p. 748.

The derived relationship was $Y = 0.419 + 0.136X$, where Y is the inverse of mortality rate in deaths per $10^6$ person-hour and X is the year, 1965 = 1. Typical 1980 rate is 0.4 deaths per $10^6$ person-hour with a 95% confidence interval 0.34-0.43. The extrapolated confidence interval of Figure 3 is shown as predicted deaths per person-hour in Figure 4.

The analysis predicts fatality rates will be reduced to one-half current levels by the end of the century. Despite the lack of sophistication in this approach, given the long-term, continuing emphasis on mine safety, the result seems reasonable. One must take care in using such predictions, of course. Changes in underlying factors may change the trend; in such a case, the confidence interval given would be too narrow. The prediction is for the trend line (e.g., the confidence interval of the 1990 level does not

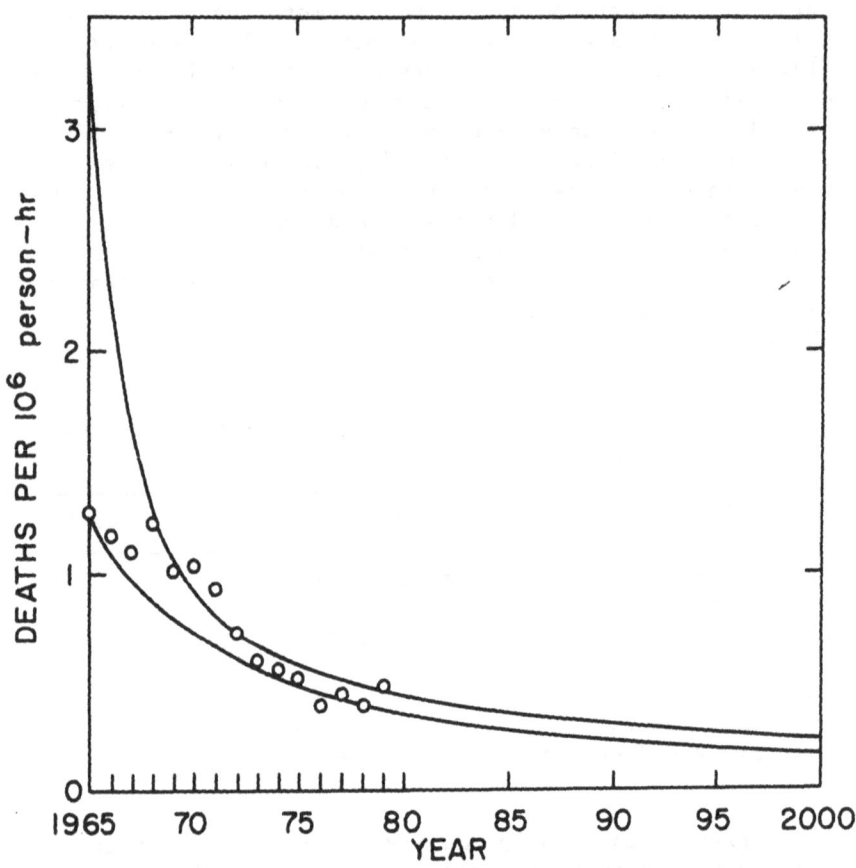

Figure 4. Fatal injuries in U.S. underground bituminous
coal mining, 95% confidence interval reexpressed from Fig. 3
extended to year 2000. Effects of large accidents removed.

refer to where the 1990 rate per se will fall, but what a typical rate will be around 1990).

While any one year might fall beyond these confidence limits, the statistically derived confidence limits provide a means of estimating the likely bounds of future effects. Examination of Figure 3 shows that the data become more erratic during the last four years. This also might indicate a widening confidence interval. There is no indication of a break from the long-term trend, however. While there is some evidence that rates are correlated with worker age and experience (Theodore Barry and Associates, 1971), with younger less-experienced miners demonstrating a higher accident rate, this does not show up in the trend despite the increase in younger miners.

Trends in the national rate may reflect shifts among mining regions or among coal firms. In addition, the variation by region and firm provide some perspective to the factor of 2 reduction in the trend prediction over the 1980-2000 period. Mortality rates by region differ by more than a factor of 2 (1971-79 geometric mean by Federal Region: Region III, 0.42; Region IV, 0.68; Region V, 0.29). The President's Commission on Coal (1980) found a sevenfold difference in injury rates among coal firms (15 to 105 injuries per $10^6$ person-hour).

Nonfatal disabling accidents in underground coal mines. Disabling work injuries are injuries that arise in the course of employment resulting in permanent or temporary disability. The latter renders the worker unable to work for one or more days subsequent to the date of injury. Unlike fatalities, there is no discernable long-term trend in nonfatal disabling accidents (Figure 5). The long-term geometric mean is 48 injuries per $10^6$ person-hours, with a geometric standard deviation of 1.15. Over the past 6 years there has been a sharp upward trend in injury rates. Given the opposite trend in fatalities and the strong regulatory trend it does not seem reasonable yet to base future rates on this short-term trend. A similar trend in 1969-71 was not continued.

Divergent trends in fatality and injury rates do not seem likely to continue. Possible explanations of the difference are: (1) Increased regulation and other factors have increased the number of people underground who are exposed to accidental injury but have not increased the number of miners in the most hazardous positions where accidents are likely to be fatal. (2) Regulation and safety

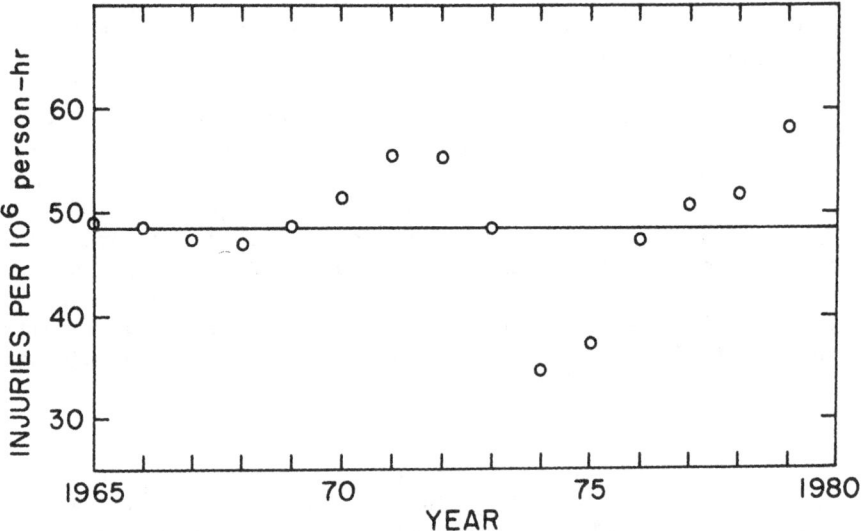

Figure 5. Nonfatal disabling injuries per million person-hours in U.S. underground bituminous coal mining, 1965–79, geometric mean 48.4, geometric standard deviation 1.15. See Fig. 2 for data sources.

programs have been concentrated and effective on conditions likely to lead to fatal accidents but have not been effective for nonfatal accidents. (3) Injury data are more subject to reporting bias than fatality data, and the nonfatal accident rate trend may be merely a reflection of this bias. Of interest, both underground and surface (after removal of downward trend) nonfatal accidents seem cyclical with maximum at 1971 and minimum at 1974. This may well indicate a reporting effect or a problem with the denominator.

### Fatalities and nonfatal disabling injuries in surface coal mining.
Surface mining fatalities and disabling injury trends are shown in Figure 6. The reexpressed trends are shown in Figures 7 and 8. Both trends are statistically significant.

An analysis of the residuals in the linear regression for surface mine fatalities suggests a nonlinear relationship. Both linear and nonlinear regression lines are shown in Figure 7. The better fit ($R^2 = 0.91$) is provided by:

$$Y = 0.01396X^2 - 0.12806X + 1.6102.$$

This results in a substantially lower estimate in the year 2000 (0.004 deaths per $10^6$ person-hour) than would be predicted from a linear extrapolation (0.05 deaths per $10^6$ person-hour). Results of extrapolating the trend to future years are shown in Figure 9.

The surface mine disabling nonfatal injury regression was $Y = 3.478 + 0.1659X$, where $Y = 100$ cases per $10^6$ person-hour ($R^2 = 0.72$; $F_{1,13} = 33.5$; $p < 0.01$). Typical 1980 rate is 16.3 cases per $10^6$ person-hour with 95% confidence interval 15.0–17.8. This rate compares favorably with a U.S. average for the private sector (Bureau of Labor Statistics, 1979). Predictions for future years are shown in Figure 10. Injury rates are predicted to decrease to 2/3 of the current levels by the year 2000, a much slower rate of decrease than fatality rates. This is a pattern similar to underground mining in which the nonfatal injuries are predicted not to decrease at all.

### Coal cleaning plants.
There is no trend in either fatality or nonfatal disabling injury rates in coal cleaning plants (Figure 11). The long-term geometric mean for injury rate is 26 cases per $10^6$ person-hour with a geometric standard deviation of 1.3. The long-term geometric mean for

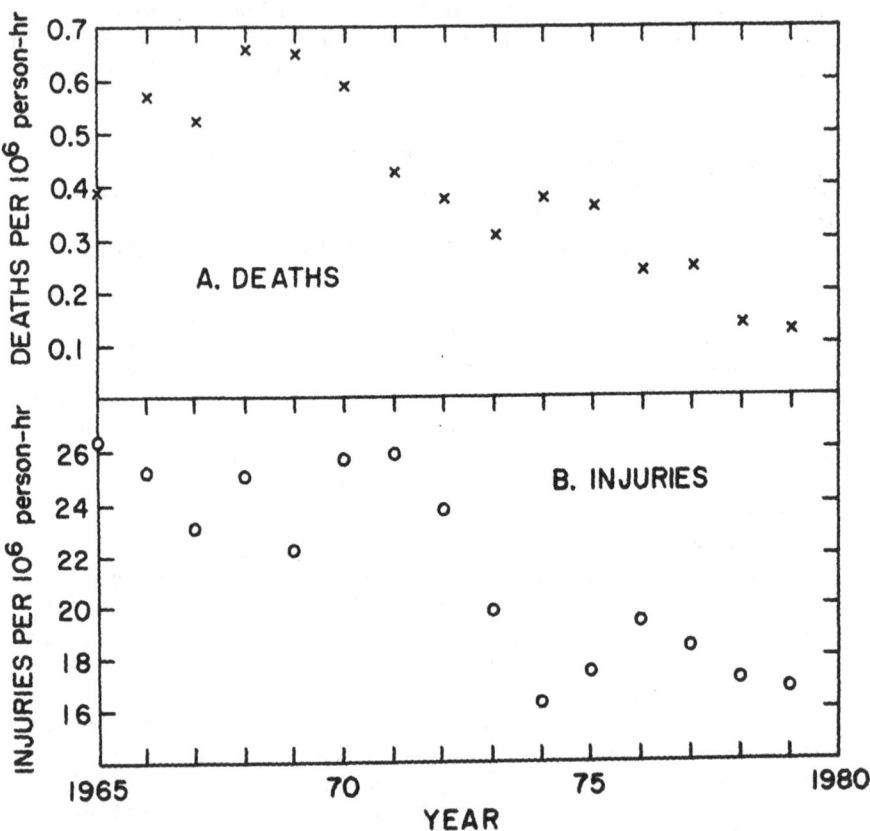

Figure 6.  Fatal (A) and nonfatal disabling injuries (B) in
U.S. surface bituminous coal mining per million person-
hours.  See Fig. 2 for data sources.

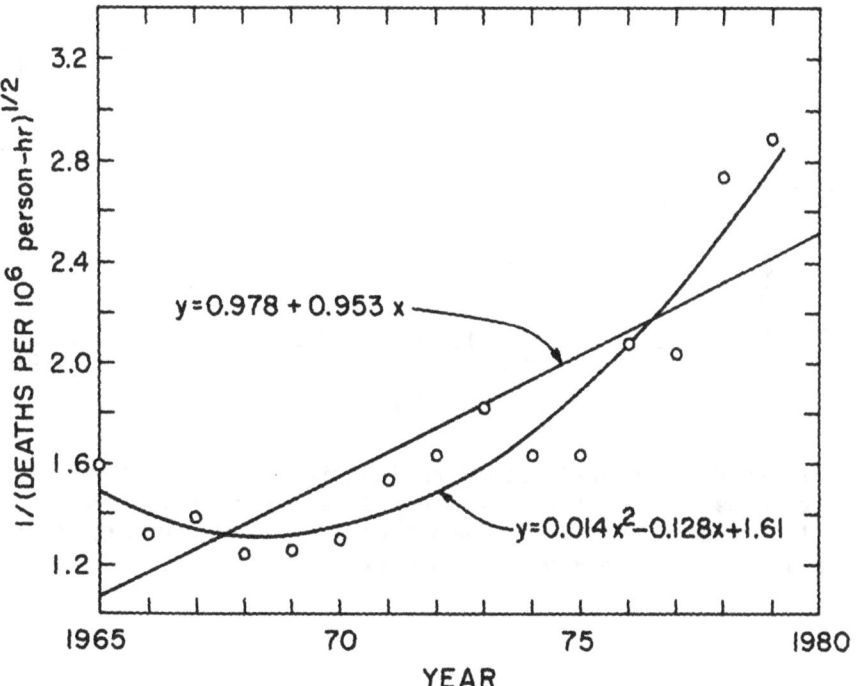

Figure 7. Fatal injuries in U.S. Surface bituminous coal mining, reexpressed from Fig. 6 as $1/$(deaths per million person-hours) $^{1/2}$ = Y. Both linear (Y = 0.978 + 0.953 X) and non-linear (Y = 0.014 X$^2$ - 0.128 X + 1.61) regression results are shown.

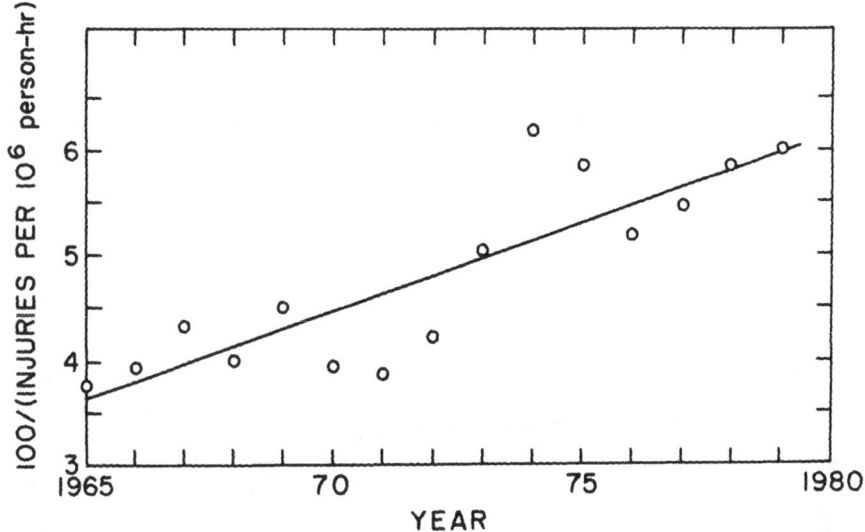

Figure 8.   Nonfatal disabling injuries in U.S. Surface bituminous coal mining, reexpressed from Fig. 6 as 100/
(injuries per million person-hours) = Y.   Linear regression
result, Y = 3.48 + 0.166 X shown.

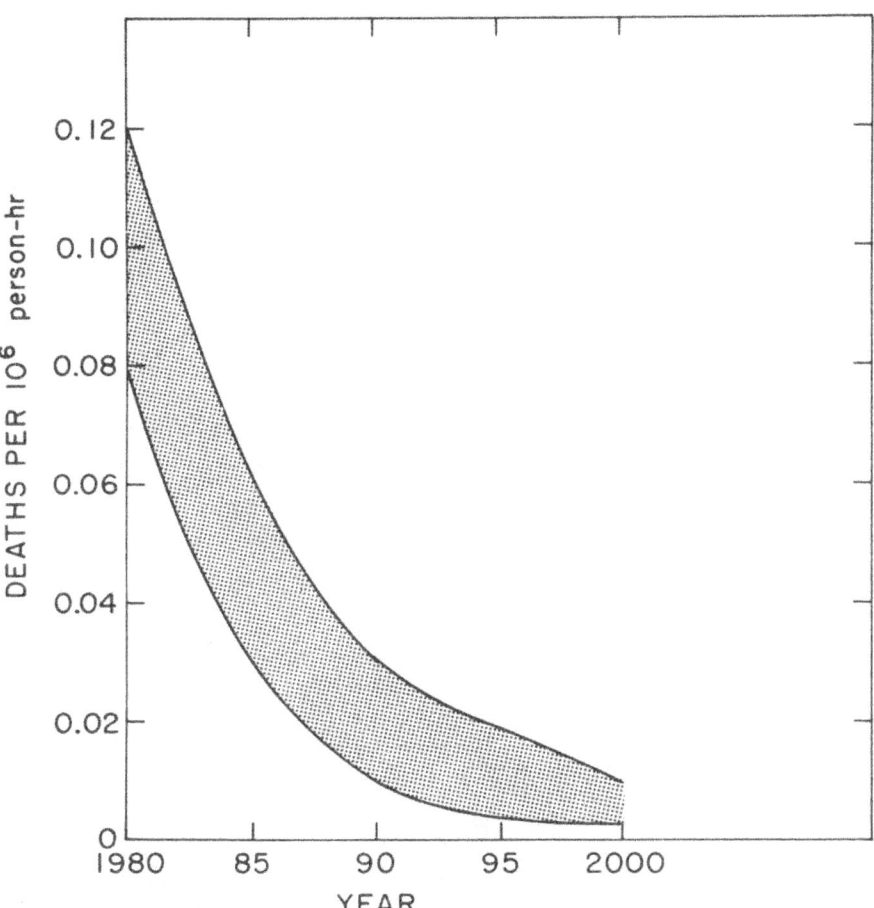

Figure 9. Fatal injuries in U.S. Surface bituminous coal mining. Extension of 95% confidence in interval of trend from Fig. 7 to year 2000.

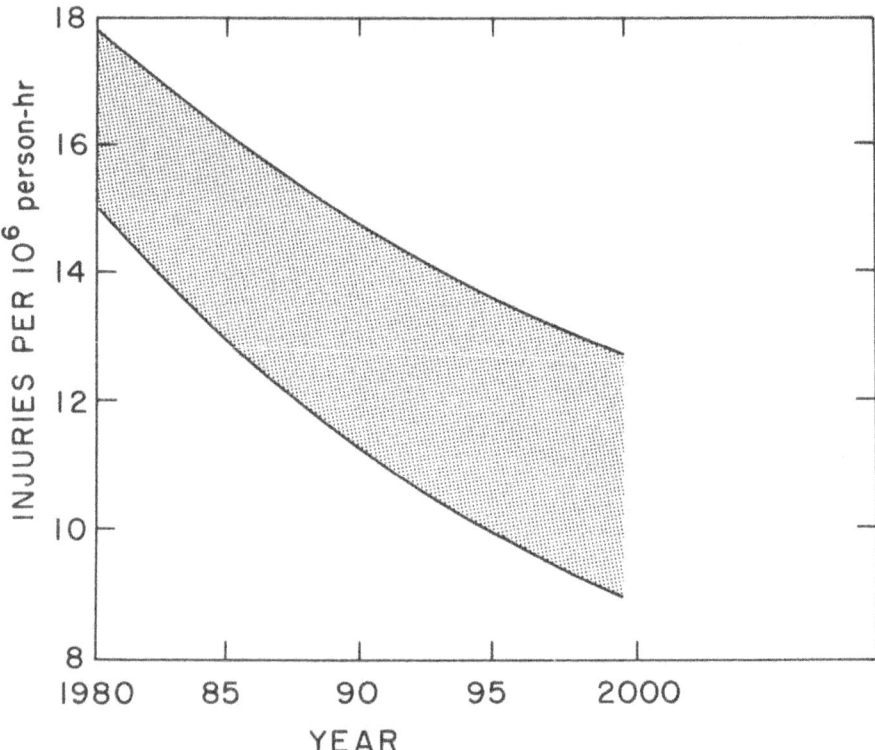

Figure 10.    Nonfatal disabling injuries in U.S. Surface
bituminous coal mining; extension of 95% confidence interval
of trend from Fig. 8 to year 2000.

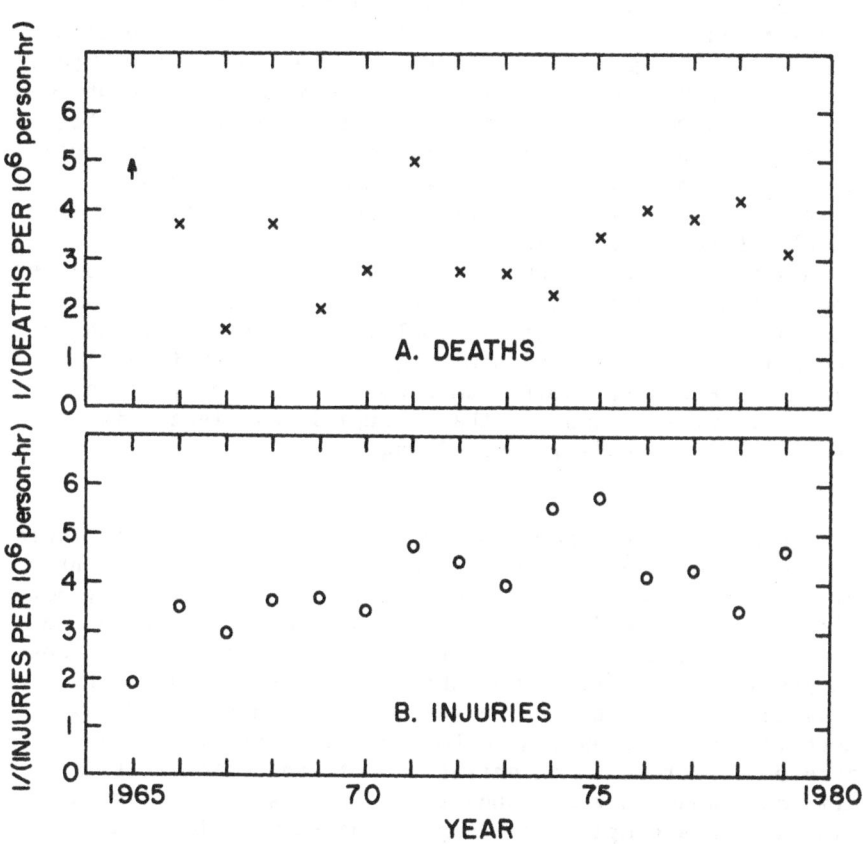

Figure 11. Fatal (A) and nonfatal disabling injuries (B) in U.S. coal cleaning plants, reexpressed as reciprocal of rate per million person-hours. See Fig. 2 for data sources.

fatality rate is 0.29 deaths per $10^6$ person-hour with a
geometric standard deviation of 1.8.


## Occupational Disease in Underground Coal Mining

Continuing dust exposure in underground coal mining
leads to coal workers' pneumoconiosis (CWP) and industrial
bronchitis (Morgan, 1980). Despite extensive research (cf.
Selikoff, Key, and Lee, 1972), the specific etiology of both
diseases is unknown, and it is thus impossible to predict
with any assurance the health impact of current dust exposure in the mines. Estimates are made below, however, based
on results of earlier exposures considering changes in dust
level. Although not detracting from the seriousness of
occupational respiratory disease in coal miners, it provides
some perspective to realize that its effect is less than
that of cigarette smoking in coal miners who smoke. While
there may be exposure in some surface mines sufficiently
high to yield CWP, studies have not produced support for
this. It will be assumed that occupational disease is
associated with underground mining only.


Coal workers' pneumoconiosis (CWP). This disease takes
two forms, simple and complicated, the latter known as progressive massive fibrosis (PMF). Simple CWP is usually not
disabling in itself. It is a response to deposition of coal
dust in the lung, but there are marked regional differences
in prevalence of simple CWP which cannot be explained by
measurements of mass dust exposure alone (Morgan, 1980).
Certain trace elements have been hypothesized to act as factors or cofactors. Concentrations of iron, nickel, titanium, and vanadium were found to be increased markedly in
miners' lungs compared to lungs of non-miner, long-term
residents of the same county (Sweet et al., 1974). Cause
and effect are difficult to determine, however. The differ-
ential trace element enrichment may be a result of differen-
tial retention caused by the disease, rather than a cofactor
in the disease (Davis, Ohery, and LeRoux, 1977; National
Research Council, 1980.) Morgan (1980) indicates that probably more important than chemical composition is the propen-
sity for some coals to fragment into particles of 0.5-2 µm,
whereas others fragment into a higher proportion of 4-6 µm-
size particles. The small size particles are more important
in the development of CWP. Individual susceptibility is
also important in CWP. Not all miners similarly exposed
develop the disease.

Table 2. Prevalence of CWP by years underground, percent[a,b]

| Years under-ground | Appalachia | | Midwest | | West | |
|---|---|---|---|---|---|---|
| | Round 1 | Round 2 | Round 1 | Round 2 | Round 1 | Round 2 |
| 0-9 | 10 (193) | 1 (34) | 10 (43) | 0.3 (2) | 3 (11) | 0.5(3) |
| 10-19 | 26 (231) | 4 (40) | 27 (53) | 3 (4) | 8 (9) | 7 (8) |
| 20-29 | 42 (717) | 16 (222) | 30 (89) | 10 (18) | 16 (40) | 8 (15) |
| 30-39 | 54 (170) | 22 (211) | 42 (57) | 8 (8) | 25 (30) | 5 (5) |
| 40+ | 57 (189) | 31 (89) | 65 (43) | 22 (7) | 30 (11) | 15 (5) |

[a]Number of cases shown in parentheses;
[b]Data from Appalachian Laboratory for Occupational Safety and Health; round 1 from Morgan et al., 1973, round 2 from Attfield and Hudak, 1980.

Progressive massive fibrosis (PMF) is a much more serious form of CWP. It develops only following an advanced simple CWP. It does not require continued exposure to coal dust, as advancing grades of simple CWP do, but depends on other factors. In a British study of coal mine-face workers, while total dust exposure was the most significant factor in determining probability of progression to PMF, progression appeared to fall with increasing mineral content (Walton et al., 1977). This might also be interpreted as a diminishing effect of decreasing coal rank (Naeye, Mahon, and Dellinger, 1971; Walton et al., 1977). Progression might also be related to immunologic factors. Relative risk of PMF was found to be markedly greater in miners lacking antigen W18 (Heise et al., 1977).

The Appalachian Laboratory for Occupational Safety and Health has completed two rounds and begun a third of a national study of CWP prevalence (Morgan et al., 1973; Attfield and Hudak, 1980). The overall prevalence of CWP in the second round (1972-75) was 8% compared to 30% in the first round (1969-71). In part, the decreased prevalence represented an influx of younger miners between rounds, who would not have had time to develop the disease. Prevalence generally decreased by factors of 2-3, however, between groups with the same work experience (Table 2). The decrease in prevalence was believed to be partly an artifact introduced through differences in interpretation of x rays rather than a real decrease. An increasing prevalence in CWP by years underground was found in both rounds (Table 2). Prevalence rates, of course, do not account for miners

who have taken ill and left the mines.  Petersen and
Attfield (1980) indicate a bias of about 70% for PMF but
only about 5% for CWP from this cause.  Nonetheless, taking
the rates of round 2 (Table 2) on their face yields an
essentially uniform annual incidence in CWP after a ten-year
latent period.  Allocating the prevalence of CWP in miners
with 25 to 45 years underground to each year gives an incremental risk of CWP of about 0.6% per miner-year or 600 per
$10^5$ miner-year.  If 10-20% of CWP progresses to PMF
(Cochrane, 1962), the risk of disabling disease is 0.006  x
(0.1-0.2) = 60-120 per $10^5$ miner-year.  Round 1 rates do not
fit this model as well and give a risk 2.5 times higher.

Coal miner diseases develop over decades.  Conditions
in the mines have changed considerably over that time; these
changes cannot be completely taken into account.  Dust concentrations in coal mines have decreased by a factor of 3 to
4 in recent years, and the character of exposure may have
changed as well.  The effect of this dust exposure change is
likely to be nonlinear.  Rae (1971) established a concave
upward exposure-response function that suggested CWP might
be virtually eliminated below 2 mg/m$^3$.  Thus, the lower
limit on effects at current levels might be zero.  An upper
limit might be taken as a linear extrapolation of the above
estimates downward by a factor of 3.5.  Taking the upper end
of the range, 0.0012/3.5 = 3.4 x $10^{-4}$ PMF cases per miner-
year.  Using round 1 rates yields 3.4 x $10^{-4}$ x 2.5 = 8.6 x
$10^{-4}$ PMF cases per year.

Based on British and German data, Morgan (1980) estimates that at dust levels below 3.5 mg/m$^3$ fewer than 4% of
miners will develop CWP over 35 years.  This is a rate of
0.0011 per year.  Assuming 20% progression yields a PMF rate
of 2.3 x $10^{-4}$ per year.  This is well within the range defined by the upper limit calculated above.

Bronchitis.  Morgan (1980) makes a case that coal miners develop an obstructive airway disease related to dust
exposure but different from CWP and from the bronchitis
induced by cigarette smoking.  There is often a poor relationship between the symptoms of this bronchitis and CWP.
This may be because the larger, 5-100 μm particles produce
this effect in the upper airways and these larger particles
are removed by the mucociliary escalator leaving no radio-
graphic evidence (Morgan, 1980).  In a 1977-78 survey of 242
Utah miners, a 25% prevalence of CWP and a 57% prevalence of
chronic bronchitis was found.  The chronic bronchitis prevalence was similar among smokers and nonsmokers.  Only 7% of
the miners surveyed were diagnosed as having both CWP and
chronic bronchitis (Rom et al., 1980).  Based on review of

five studies of pulmonary function and respiratory symptoms,
Reger and Hancock (1980) concluded that the prevalence of
chronic obstructive airways disease is roughly equivalent to
CWP in coal miners.  Like CWP, chronic bronchitis is disabling only in its more advanced form.  It seems clear that
even if estimates of simple CWP are used instead of the disabling PMF, and an equal incidence of occupational chronic
bronchitis is included, the incidence of occupational
disease in underground mining is much lower than the accidental injury rate.  It must be realized, however, that the
disease is chronic; once having gotten it the miner
continues to have it for the remainder of his life.


   Disease mortality.  Comparing deaths in 1950 for which
"usual occupation" was designated coal mining with 1950
U.S. census count of coal miners ("present or most recent
occupation"), Enterline (1964) reported coal miners to have
twice the risk of mortality as other employed U.S. males
(SMR = 195)[1].  Liddell (1973) in a similar study of British
coal miners for 1961 found their overall mortality risk to
be lower than the population of working and retired males
(SMR for face workers, 60; other underground workers, 76;
surface workers, 108).  This might be explained on the basis
that only those with exceptionally strong constitutions were
able to work in the mines, and of them only the fittest at
the mine face.  Liddell's control group included retired
workers while Enterline's control included only actively
employed males, which may be one reason why Enterline got a
high SMR.  The mortality rate for occupational pneumoconiosis, however, was several times that of the control in the
Liddell study.  The mortality rate for occupational pneumoconiosis in the control population was 212 deaths x $10^{-5}$.  In
the groups of miners it was 1.9-5.6 times higher, indicating
an occupationally induced increase of 4.2-12.2 deaths x
$10^{-5}$.

   With full information and steady-state conditions,
studies such as these should yield reasonable occupation-
specific mortality rates; however, some people die years
after leaving the mines and may have worked in other jobs in
the interval.  Thus, reporting of usual occupation on the
death certificate may not fully reflect mining experience.

   More reliable information comes from studies that follow groups of miners over long periods to evaluate their
risk.  Hollingsworth (1970), Enterline (1972), Ortmeyer et
al. (1973, 1974) and Rockette (1977a,b) conducted such studies.  Hollingsworth (1970) and Enterline (1972) reported a
statistically significant increased mortality rate in a

Table 3.  Mortality in coal miners for selected causes
          of death[a]

| Cause | Observed number of deaths | SMR[b] | Excess rate deaths x $10^{-5c}$ |
|---|---|---|---|
| Stomach cancer | 127 | 138.2 | 4.3 |
| Lung cancer | 352 | 113.7 | 2.6 |
| Nonmalignant respiratory disease | 741 | 157.1 | 37.9 |
| Asthma | 32 | 166.0 | 1.8 |
| Tuberculosis | 63 | 148.0 | 2.4 |
| Total excess rate | | | 49.0 |

[a]Data from H. E. Rockette 1977a.  Based on mortality
experience 1959 through 1971 of a 10% sample of those men
covered by UMWA Health and Retirement Funds on January 1,
1959.

[b]SMR = (observed deaths/expected deaths) x 100.
Expected deaths based on 1965 U.S. white male mortality
rates.  All SMR's are significant at the 5% level.

[c]Excess rate calculated as [(SMR - 100)/100 x 1965
U.S. white male rate].

cohort of 553 West Virginia miners followed from 1938 to 1971 (SMR = 158). This was a small group, but a much longer than usual follow-up period.

Ortmeyer et al. (1974) followed 3,726 miners that had been selected randomly in 1962-3 for a CWP study. No significant overall excess mortality rate was found for the group as a whole (SMR = 104) compared to the total U.S. male population, but miners previously diagnosed with PMF in the earlier study showed a markedly higher mortality rate than those with simple or no CWP. In an earlier study (Ortmeyer, Baier, and Crawford, 1973), Pennsylvania coal miners who had been compensated for disability had a significant overall excess mortality rate (SMR = 119) compared to white Pennsylvania males. Rockette (1977a,b) analyzed mortality in a cohort of 23,000 coal miners covered by the International Union, United Mine Workers of America (UMWA) Health and Retirement Funds between 1959 and 1971. No significant excess was found in overall mortality rate (SMR for all causes = 101.6). Significantly increased mortality rates were reported for lung and stomach cancer, nonmalignant respiratory diseases, asthma, tuberculosis, accidents, and ill-defined causes (Table 3). The total excess rate for these causes was $49 \times 10^{-5}$.

Rockette (1980) summarizes the current understanding of mortality studies as follows: (1) The doubling of coal miner mortality risk based on the 1950 census data is not supported by the studies as a group, but there is a consistent excess (SMR slightly over 100). Because of the "healthy worker effect," this excess is probably larger than the studies indicate; (2) Results for lung cancer show great variability and are well within the range that might be explained by differences in smoking habits; (3) Stomach cancer shows a consistent excess. This may be related to nonoccupational factors such as socioeconomic status, diet, and ethnic background, but the consistency among studies of different coal mining populations strengthens the possiblity of an occupational factor. (4) Nonmalignant respiratory diseases are consistantly high. (5) Cardiovascular disease deaths are generally lower than in the control populations.

If one takes the small overall increase in mortality rate (SMR = 102-104) with a standard mortality rate of about $9 \times 10^{-3}$, the excess mortality rate for coal miners is $18-36 \times 10^{-5}$. The Liddell (1973) study gives no excess on this basis but includes an excess of $4-12 \times 10^{-5}$ in the mining-related diseases alone. The Rockette (1977a) study gives $49 \times 10^{-5}$ in the mining-related diseases alone (higher than an excess of the overall since it is balanced against a

decreased cardiovascular mortality rate). Since the
Rockette study is the most recent and most extensive, the
latter value will be taken as the best estimate.

As with morbidity, improved conditions may reduce or
eliminate excess mortality. An upper limit might be taken
as a linear extrapolation by a factor of 3.5 (based on the
3-4 times decrease in dust level). This reduces the
Rockette estimate to $49 \times 10^{-5} \times (1/3.5) = 14 \times 10^{-5}$ excess
deaths per person-year. Two other factors come into play.
First, the "healthy worker effect" could increase the overall disease mortality excess by 10-40%. Second, the risk of
excess disease mortality follows the miner even after he has
left the mines. If the period at risk is actually 50-70
years while the period in the mines is 20-35 years, this
would increase the disease mortality estimate by 2-3 times.
An increase in disease mortality risk of 3-4 times to $50 \times 10^{-5}$ is more consistent with the PMF rates calculated above
of $34-86 \times 10^{-5}$. Since accidental death rates are about 0.4
per $10^6$ person-hour or about $80 \times 10^{-5}$ deaths per person
year, accidental and disease fatalities are much closer than
is the case for nonfatal incidents.


## Estimating Health Risk in Coal Mining on a Unit Energy Basis

The effectiveness of CMHSA must ultimately be measured
in terms of total health damage. Effects per person-hour
describe risk to the individual miner, but the overall societal effect depends also on how many miners are exposed
(i.e., on impact per unit of coal produced). Overall, the
decrease in individual risk has in fact been largely offset
by an increase in numbers exposed: since CMHSA, there has
been a sharp drop in underground productivity and - beginning later - an indication of a lesser drop in surface productivity. Baker (1979) demonstrates convincingly that
CMHSA and its enforcement procedures have been the principal
contributors to this change. Thus, on balance it would
appear that to date, regulation has not substantially improved health effects of coal mining in terms of effects per
ton produced.

Before 1969 there was evidence of a trade-off between
safety and productivity. States with high accident rates
generally had high productivity (Baker, 1979). The CMHSA
required an influx of "nonproductive" labor and tended to
slow down the production process (Wool and Ostbo, 1980). In
addition, the enforcement process itself affected productivity: mines that essentially met the standards before 1969
subsequently suffered sharp productivity losses attributable

to the enforcement procedures themselves, since no significant improvement in operation would have been required
(Baker, 1979).

Other factors contributing to the decline in productivity were labor unrest during the period and new UMWA contract work rules (Wool and Ostbo, 1980). The influx of
inexperienced workers has been cited as a source of decreased productivity, but Baker found the increase in miners
under 25 had a small but positive impact on productivity.
Turnover in employment, on the other hand, was shown to
affect productivity adversely. Age distribution and experience presumably affect accident rates directly, but evidence as to their net result is contradictory. If inexperienced miners have higher accident rates, the expected
increase of younger miners to meet increasing production
needs would thus lead to higher risk. Samples from Social
Security records indicate, however, that the fraction of
miners under 25 increased from 11.1 to 20.9% between 1969-70
and 1975, and the fraction between 25 and 34 increased from
19 to 30% (Wool and Ostbo, 1980), during a period of improvement in the accident rate. In this same period, miners
with less than 1 year of experience increased from 11% of
the workforce to 20%, and those with 1 to 4 years of experience increased from 19 to 28% (Wool and Ostbo, 1980). It
may be, however, that the effect of CMHSA overwhelmed a
reverse tendency to increase accident rates. If this is
true, future rates might increase as the proportion of
younger, less experienced miners continues to grow.

Technological change (the cause of productivity increases between 1950 and 1969) would be expected to counter-
act the declining productivity trend after 1969, but Baker
found little influence. In fact, an unexpected negative
relationship was shown to be associated with introduction of
longwall mining (Wool and Ostbo, 1980). The judgment of
Wool and Ostbo was that in the near term (to 1985) there
will be a slight improvement in productivity in eastern underground mines and a substantial increase in western surface mines, but continued decline elsewhere. After 1985,
eastern underground mines would again decline. Due to regional shifts in coal production, they expect an overall
national reversal in the downward productivity trend.

For mine accidents, continued low productivity in underground mines will be important. For example, within the
range of expected variation, for the worst case (1980 individual risk, declining productivity) a tripling of underground coal production by the year 2000 could be expected to
lead to perhaps 720 fatalities, 6 times the 1980 estimate.

Table 4.  Occupational injury risks per GW(e)-yr in surface
and underground coal mining under varying
productivity and individual risk levels

| | Productivity (man-hr/ ton) | Individual risk per $10^6$ man-hr | | Effect per GW(e)-yr ($3.4 \times 10^6$ ton) | |
|---|---|---|---|---|---|
| | | Deaths | Injuries | Deaths | Injuries |
| **Underground accidents** | | | | | |
| c. 1980 estimate | 1.05 | 0.39 | 48 | 1.4 | 170 |
| Alternative | 1.05 | 0.19 | 48 | 0.67 | 170 |
| 2000 estimates | 2.06 | 0.19 | 48 | 1.3 | 340 |
| | 2.06 | 0.39 | 48 | 2.7 | 340 |
| **Underground disease (PMF)** | | | | | |
| c. 1980 estimate | 1.05 | 0.07[a] | 0.17 | 0.25 | 0.6 |
| Alternative | 1.05 | 0.07[a] | 0.17 | 0.25 | 0.6 |
| 2000 estimates | 2.06 | 0.07[a] | 0.17 | 0.49 | 1.2 |
| **Underground disease (CWP & occupational bronchitis)** | | | | | |
| c. 1980 estimate | 1.05 | | 6 | | 21 |
| Alternative | 1.05 | | 6 | | 21 |
| 2000 estimates | 2.06 | | 6 | | 42 |
| **Surface mine accidents** | | | | | |
| c. 1980 estimate | 0.297 | 0.12 | 16 | 0.12 | 16 |
| Alternative | 0.297 | 0.05 | 11 | 0.05 | 11 |
| 2000 estimates | 0.297 | 0.12 | 16 | 0.12 | 16 |

[a]Does not include possible 3-4 times increase discussed
in text.

For the best case (declining risk, 1980 productivity), a tripling of underground coal production by 2000 would lead to some 180 accidental fatalities, 1.5 times the 1980 estimates. The effect of a variety of possibilities of productivity levels and accident and disease rates are summarized on a GW(e)-yr basis in Table 4.

## Coal Transport

Accustomed as we are to the carnage on the highways, it should be no surprise that the transport of over 600 million tons of coal annually over an average of hundreds of miles leads to a significant number of accidental deaths and injuries. The level of individual risk is generally very low compared to coal mining, since a large fraction of the effect is spread over the general public.

Coal is transported by rail, water (rivers, Great Lakes, and intercoastal waterways), truck, and/or conveyor belt. One slurry pipeline is in operation and pipelines are a potentially significant mode of coal transport in the future.

## Railroad Transportation

Most coal moves by rail. Coal constitutes 29% of all rail freight in the U.S. and 13% of all freight revenue. By comparison, coal transport makes up 20% of all rail freight in the U.S.S.R. Coal is moved in hopper cars, which are unloaded by turning the car itself over, by opening bottom hoppers, or, more rarely, by unloading from the top. The cars are generally loaded at mine sidings or tipples that collect from several mines. The average hopper car carries 75 tons of coal; older cars, 55 tons; and newer ones, 100 tons. Size of hopper car used depends on the condition of the track. Modern unloading facilities are frequently trestles running over storage piles into which coal is dumped from moving cars. Many have loading and unloading rates of thousands of tons per hour (Congressional Research Service, 1977).

Because railroad transportation statistics for accidental deaths and injury are not maintained by type of freight carried, it is not possible to determine directly the mortality effects of transporting coal by rail. There are, however, several ways to estimate this value. The simplest is to assign a proportionate share of all railroad deaths to coal transport. This apportionment may be on the basis of total weight or bulk of material transported, train-miles traveled, or ton-miles traveled.

Over 60% of accidental deaths associated with freight traffic result from rail-highway grade crossing accidents, primarily due to collisions between trains and motor vehicles (Federal Railroad Administration, 1966-1972). The number of intersections crossed and the characteristics of each crossing (e.g., highway vehicle and train traffic density, type of crossing protection) are crucial parameters. Several models have been developed to predict the accident risk at grade crossings based on such factors (Coleman and Stewart, 1976). Rogozen et al. (1977) use such a model to estimate the impact of specific unit train routes compared to coal slurry pipelines. They conclude that train impacts are nonlinearly related to statistics such as train-miles or ton-miles. In a typical example, as the average number of trains per day increased by 70%, the predicted number of accidents increased by only 30%.

While there are many factors which cannot be considered in these models, it seems clear they offer the best approach to quantifying impacts for particular cases. A great deal of information is required, however. The routes to be followed must be specified, and for each grade crossing the average daily highway traffic, average daily train traffic, type of crossing protection, location (urban or rural), and single or multiple tracks.

For broad assessment purposes - in which specific routes are unknown - a simpler approach is required. Train-mile apportionment gives results much closer to the detailed model results than ton-mile. Estimates below are based on ton-mile and a train-mile apportionment of total freight but are reported on a ton-mile basis. Since the detailed models indicate a nonlinear response, these are average estimates, rather than marginal. Examples cited by Rogozen et al. (1977) suggest the marginal estimates may vary downward from the average by as much as a factor of 5. Since coal represents a substantial share of all rail transport, and an even greater share in areas with heavy coal traffic, the average figure may be more reasonable when estimating effects of total U.S. coal transport. When estimating the incremental effect of a single plant or a perturbed scenario, a marginal estimate would be desired. All grade crossing accidents involving trains have been charged against coal transport in calculations made below. One might argue that since the fault frequently lies with the motor vehicle, only a portion (and perhaps a small portion) should actually be charged to coal transport.

There is some reason to believe that unit coal trains –
in which coal is the only cargo – may create different exposure situations than the average freight train. Coal has
a greater density than average freight; coal cars are generally bigger and heavier; and coal trains are longer than
average. Train velocity may be different. Unit trains generally operate on well-used and maintained lines, and it has
been suggested that they may be less likely than average
freight trains to pass signal-less crossings. Concerning
the 40% of accidents not at grade crossings, unit trains
generally can avoid hazardous switching and yard operations.
While one might suspect that unit trains are less likely to
be involved in fatal accidents than are average freight
trains, there are no data on which to base an adjustment.
Occupational accidents associated with unit trains seem
likely to be concentrated at on- and off-loading facilities.

Schoppert and Hoyt (1968), in a sample of grade crossing accident reports from six states, found that grade
crossings have a turbulent effect on motor vehicle traffic,
resulting in accidents not involving trains: one third of
the accidents occurred when a train was present but not
involved and one third when a train was not even present.
Based on detailed data from 16,000 crossings in Illinois, it
was found that the fatality rate was much higher in accidents involving trains but the nonfatal injury rate was
higher in non-train crossing accidents. Accidents not
involving trains have not been included in calculations
below.

In unit trains, and for the most part in non-unit
trains also, the cars must return to the mine empty. Thus,
train-mileage refers to the round-trip distance per trip
times the number of trips, while ton-mileage is calculated
as tonnage hauled per trip times one-way distance (no ton-
miles are incurred on the empty return trip) times the
number of trips.

There were $6.78 \times 10^{12}$ ton-miles of freight movement on
U.S. railroads during the period examined, 1966-74. Freight
trains logged $3.97 \times 10^9$ train-miles (Association of
American Railroads, 1977). Statistics for deaths and injuries among employees and the public are given in Table 5 per
ton-mile and per train-mile for the years 1966 to 1974 and
for the nine years averaged. The annual statistics show a
slight down-trend in public deaths and injuries. Given that
both railroad and automobile traffic is increasing, this
must reflect the effort of the railroads, state highway
departments, and Federal Department of Transportation (DOT)
to reduce accidents, particularly at grade crossings.

Table 5. Deaths and injuries associated with railroad freight operations per ton-mile and train-mile[a]

| Year | Public deaths | | Public injuries | | Employee deaths | | Employee injuries | |
|---|---|---|---|---|---|---|---|---|
| | Per $10^9$ ton-mi | Per $10^6$ train-mi | Per $10^9$ ton-mi | Per $10^6$ train-mi | Per $10^9$ ton-mi | Per $10^6$ train-mi | Per $10^9$ ton-mi | Per $10^6$ train-mi |
| 1966 | 2.16 | 3.65 | 4.30 | 7.25 | 0.050 | 0.085 | 5.33 | 9.00 |
| 67 | 2.08 | 3.55 | 4.47 | 7.65 | 0.060 | 0.102 | 4.41 | 7.55 |
| 68 | 1.98 | 3.43 | 4.26 | 7.38 | 0.059 | 0.103 | 5.13 | 8.88 |
| 69 | 1.95 | 3.45 | 4.50 | 7.97 | 0.072 | 0.127 | 4.94 | 8.75 |
| 70 | 1.95 | 3.50 | 3.86 | 6.90 | 0.077 | 0.138 | 4.50 | 8.06 |
| 71 | 1.94 | 3.33 | 4.05 | 6.97 | 0.041 | 0.070 | 3.89 | 6.69 |
| 72 | 1.82 | 3.14 | 3.99 | 6.87 | 0.048 | 0.082 | 3.56 | 6.14 |
| 73 | 0.38 | 0.68 | 0.45 | 0.81 | 0.068 | 0.124 | 3.54 | 6.44 |
| 74 | 1.62 | 2.95 | 3.56 | 6.45 | 0.055 | 0.100 | 4.02 | 7.28 |
| 66-74 | 1.74 | 3.05 | 3.66 | 6.42 | 0.059 | 0.103 | 4.44 | 7.78 |

[a]Ton-mile and train-mile data from Association of American Railroads (1977). Injury and death data from Federal Railroad Administration (1966-74). Data for 1975 and later years are not available in this form. Grade crossing accidents were not included in the 1973 record.

Statistics were not calculated later than 1974, since accident data were no longer reported separately for freight traffic by DOT after that year.

The average haul length for the industry as a whole is over 500 miles, (Association of American Railroads, 1977), but coal shipments are reported to have an average haul length of 300 miles (National Coal Association, 1976). Assuming a 300-mile haul and using average figures over the 1966-74 interval, production of 1 GW(e)-year of electricity (requiring $3.4 \times 10^6$ tons of coal) would correspond to $1.02 \times 10^9$ ton-miles. Assuming an optimum unit train size of 15,000 net tons (Bailey and Waring, 1967), then 227 train trips would be required, which at 600 miles per round trip yields $1.36 \times 10^5$ train-miles per GW(e)-year. Non-unit train movement would involve more train-miles to deliver the same amount of coal, but only a share of the effort can be charged to coal transport. If one takes the results of these two methods of calculation as the range of effects for a 300-mile haul, the resulting estimates are given in Table 6.

Table 6.  Health damage from coal transport by rail

|  | Cases per GW(e)-year[a] | $10^{-10}$ cases per ton-mile[b] |
|---|---|---|
| Public deaths | 0.41 –1.8 | 4.1 |
| Public injuries | 0.87 –3.7 | 8.6 |
| Employee deaths | 0.014–0.06 | 0.14 |
| Employee injuries | 1.06 –4.4 | 10. |

[a]Lower value based on train-mile, upper value on apportionment.
[b]Derived from train-mile apportionment.

The higher estimates correspond to data per ton-mile. For haul distances other than 300 miles, the estimates are linearly proportional to changes in haul distance. The lower estimates, from the train-mile approach, give a closer fit with the results of the more detailed approach of Rogozen et al. (1977) when compared in actual cases. Since ton-miles are easier to use, a more valid approach to calculating coefficients in terms of ton-miles is to derive them from the train-mile apportionment statistics. Assuming a load of 15,000 tons gives an average trip load of 7,500 tons (to account for the empty return trip). Note that accidents involving the public (mostly collisions between motor vehicles and trains), have a high death-to-injury ratio, whereas occupational accidents involve many more injuries than deaths.

Railroad accident rates vary by region. Since the bulk of such accidents involve collision with automobiles, the rate presumably depends on the density of automobile traffic and on driving patterns. The difference in deaths per train-mile among regions is less than a factor of 2 and in injuries less than 10%.

Additional health risk, not quantified here, results from the air pollution contribution of diesel exhaust from coal train locomotives and to the possible impairment of emergency medical service in communities where major streets are frequently blocked by unit trains.

## Truck Transportation

Truck transport has been the most rapidly growing mode of coal transport. Twelve percent of total coal production, about $8 \times 10^7$ tons, is delivered by truck. Haul distance averages 50 to 75 miles (Congressional Research Service, 1977). This does not include truck-haul of coal to tipples for loading on rail or barges. We assume a 30-ton load of coal per trip, giving an average trip load of 15 tons, including the empty return trip. Common carrier truck fleets average 7 accidents per $10^6$ vehicle-miles (National Safety Council, 1978). Assuming 0.03 deaths and 0.5 injuries per $10^6$ accidents results in 0.21 deaths and 3.5 injuries per $10^6$ vehicle-mile, with the following coefficients for deaths and injuries in terms of ton-miles:

$$\text{Deaths} = (0.2 \times 10^{-6}) = 1.4 \times 10^{-8} \text{ deaths/ton-mile.}$$

$$\text{Injuries} = (3.5 \times 10^{-6}) = 2.3 \times 10^{-7} \text{ injuries/ton-mile.}$$

It is assumed that these are split equally between employees and the public. The production of 1 GW(e)-year of electricity production, requiring $3.4 \times 10^6$ tons of coal, results in $(3.4 \times 10^6 \text{ tons})/(30 \text{ tons/truck}) = 1.13 \times 10^5$ trips per GW(e)-year. Assuming an average round trip of 100 miles, there are $1.13 \times 10^7$ vehicle-miles per GW(e)-year. This yields 2.4 deaths and 40 injuries per GW(e)-year. Again, these are assumed to be split equally between employees and the public.

## Barge Transportation

Deaths in barge transportation of coal are calculated on a ton-mile basis, based on accident data obtained from the Coast Guard and tonnage data from the Department of Commerce.

Coast Guard data for 1970-72 (excluding deaths or injuries due to natural causes, homicide, suicide and fights) indicate 76% of reported deaths and 92% of reported injuries among longshoremen and crew (occupational) as opposed to passengers and others (314/415 total deaths and 1,177/1,281 total injuries). Table 7 shows calculations of deaths in water transport. Occupational injuries overall are 3.7 times occupational deaths.

Table 7. Calculations of occupational deaths attributable to coal in water transport

| | Total[a] (ton-miles x $10^9$) | Coal[b] (ton-miles x $10^9$) | Ratio | Total annual deaths[c] | Deaths assigned to coal[d] |
|---|---|---|---|---|---|
| Coastal | 62.5 | 2.4 | 0.0384 | 174 | 6.68 |
| Gt. Lks. | 115.2 | 10.1 | 0.0877 | 8 | 0.70 |
| Rivers | 125.2 | 35.5 | 0.284 | 36 | 10.22 |
| Total | 302.9 | 48.0 | 0.158 | 218 | 17.60 |

[a]U.S. Department of Commerce, 1975:598.
[b]Assuming 480-mile average trip (Congressional Research Service, 1977).
[c]1969-72 U.S. Coast Guard data.
[d]Total deaths x coal transport ratio.

Using the coal totals from Table 7 yields 3.6 x $10^{-10}$ deaths per ton-mile, which is apportioned according to the above percentages to yield 2.8 employee deaths and 0.88 public deaths per $10^{10}$ ton-mile of coal transported. Employee injuries, at 3.7 times occupational deaths, are therefore 1.0 x $10^{-9}$ per ton-mile. Since occupational injuries represent 92% of the total, there are 9.0 x $10^{-11}$ public injuries/ton-mile. For one GW(e)-yr, 3.4 x $10^6$ tons of coal need to be delivered, with an average barge haul distance of 480 miles, yielding 1.632 x $10^9$ ton-miles/GW(e)-yr. The above rates can then be recast as follows:

|  | Cases per GW(e)-yr from barge transport |
|---|---|
| Public deaths | 0.14 |
| Public injuries | 0.15 |
| Employee deaths | 0.46 |
| Employee injuries | 1.6 |

## Pipeline Transportation

Slurry pipeline accident rates have been estimated to occur at a rate of 0.0019 fatalities and 0.0032 nonfatal injuries per $10^{12}$ Btu transported (EPA, Environmental Protection Agency, 1977). Health damage is entirely occupational.

Converting 1 GW(e)-yr to $8.16 \times 10^{13}$ Btu, assuming $2.4 \times 10^7$ Btu per ton of coal and $3.4 \times 10^6$ tons of coal per GW(e)-yr, allows conversion of the above rates to 0.16 deaths and 0.26 injuries per GW(e)-yr. The average length of proposed slurry pipelines is 700 miles; thus, one GW(e)-yr is equivalent to $700 \times 3.4 \times 10^6 = 2.38 \times 10^9$ ton-miles. Using this factor for renormalization yields $6.7 \times 10^{-11}$ deaths and $1.1 \times 10^{-10}$ injuries per ton-mile.

Table 8 summarizes the health effects of coal transport via rail, truck, barge, and slurry pipeline in terms of deaths and injuries per ton-mile and GW(e)-yr. The highest accident rate, not surprisingly, is for truck transport, with accident levels one and two orders of magnitude higher than for other transportation modes. Only for rail is the death rate very much greater for the public than for employees.

Although the numbers of accidental deaths per unit energy in coal transport can approach that in mining, the level of individual risk is much lower due to greater numbers of exposed individuals.

## Coal Combustion

### Air Pollution

Health risks of air pollution from coal combustion have the greatest uncertainty in the coal fuel cycle. A wide range of air pollutants, including particulates, $SO_2$, $NO_x$, CO, polycyclic organic matter (POM) and trace metals such as

Table 8.  Summary of deaths and injuries from coal
transportation

|  | Public death | Public injury | Employee death | Employee injury |
|---|---|---|---|---|
| Accidents per ton-mile | | | | |
| Rail | $4.1 \times 10^{-10}$ | $8.6 \times 10^{-10}$ | $1.4 \times 10^{-11}$ | $1.0 \times 10^{-9}$ |
| Truck | $7.0 \times 10^{-9}$ | $1.2 \times 10^{-7}$ | $7.0 \times 10^{-9}$ | $1.2 \times 10^{-7}$ |
| Barge | $8.8 \times 10^{-11}$ | $9.0 \times 10^{-11}$ | $2.8 \times 10^{-10}$ | $1.0 \times 10^{-9}$ |
| Pipeline | 0 | 0 | $6.7 \times 10^{-11}$ | $1.1 \times 10^{-10}$ |
| Accidents per GW(e)-yr | | | | |
| Rail | 0.41 | 0.87 | 0.014 | 1.1 |
| Truck | 1.2 | 20.0 | 1.2 | 20.0 |
| Barge | 0.14 | 0.15 | 0.46 | 1.6 |
| Pipeline | 0 | 0 | 0.16 | 0.26 |

iron, mercury, and cadmium are produced. All the well-documented air pollution episodes were associated with the sulfur-particulate mix in coal combustion products. Shifts to oil and gas for home heating and air pollution control measures have essentially eliminated such episodes. Current concern is for exposures to comparatively low levels of pollutants, frequently spread over large areas. Long-range transport of fine particles can expose populations thousands of miles distant from the pollution source. Any single plant contributes a negligible amount at such distances, of course, but the combined contribution of hundreds of remote sources can be a significant part of the total exposure to particles. The $NO_2$ emissions from coal combustion may also contribute significantly to ozone exposures at remote sites. Complicating any assessment is the chemical transformation of coal combustion products in the atmosphere: $SO_2$ to various sulfate and sulfite species, $NO_2$ to nitrates, possibly nitrosamines and ozone. There remain large uncertainties in air chemistry and transport mechanisms and loss rates. The nature of these uncertainties is such that it is difficult to even assess the potential error in exposure estimates. There is considerable controversy over whether long-term exposures to comparatively low concentrations of pollutants can cause chronic effects, or whether there is some threshold below which no effects occur. Even if there were a threshold on an individual level, in a heterogenous population individual thresholds would span a wide range exhibiting a gradient of effects. Recent results of animal experiments have underscored the extent of individual variation in response to sulfate exposures (Wolff et al., 1979).

Four years ago an air pollution-health damage function based on sulfates was developed at Brookhaven (Morgan et al., 1978). At that time animal toxicology (Amdur, 1976), epidemiology (Environmental Protection Agency, 1974), and correlational analyses (Lave and Seskin, 1978) all seemed to point to sulfate as the harmful agent in the sulfur-particulate mix of air pollution. Even at that time, however the Brookhaven assessment of the evidence was that, if the usual statistical requirements of "proof" used in science were applied, the conclusion was "not proved". For questions of public policy that must be decided on the basis of existing evidence, however, "not proved" does not mean the best estimate is zero. On the contrary, adverse effect on health of sulfate exposures was likely. This effect was expressed in terms of a linear, no-threshold relation between sulfate exposure and increased mortality rate. The underlying hypothesis was that chronic exposure increased the incidence of acute respiratory infection in children and eventually lead to increased incidence of chronic heart and respiratory disease in adults. This is then reflected in an increased mortality rate. Because of the long latent periods involved, deaths attributable to a given years' air pollution exposure do not occur that year, but are distributed over the lifetime of the exposed population. Reasonable estimates of the age distribution of deaths lead to the conclusion that 5-15 years lost per attributable death are likely.

Under steady-state conditions, the number of deaths occurring over future years attributable to a pollution exposure this year equals the number of deaths occurring this year due to the summated pollution exposure of all previous years. Based partly on this, a linear health-damage function was drawn from cross-sectional studies as a simplified way to estimate effects of alternative energy strategies. By this simplified, linear damage function, incremental sulfate exposure this year inevitably leads to an increment of health damage and a given number of premature deaths. The incremental health damage is proportional to the incremental sulfate exposure and is independent of the total sulfate exposure. Use of a linear function to estimate effects of small changes in sulfate levels in areas with high-background levels seems reasonable. Estimates of the effects of substantial changes in background levels, or of small changes in areas with low initial background levels, increase the uncertainty in the estimation of damage.

The function was described as a probability distribution with a 14% probability of zero effect and a 10% probability of greater than 8 attributable deaths per $10^5$ person-$\mu g/m^3$ sulfate (Figure 12). Because of a wide focus in the United States on sulfates, considerably more toxicological and clinical work has become available since this function was developed, much of which fails to support effects at existing exposure levels (Avol et al., 1979; Schlesinger, Lippman, and Albert, 1978; Wolff et al., 1979). In addition, much of the epidemiology linking health damage with sulfate has come into question (Committee on Science and Technology, 1976). Recent work in air chemistry has shown that, while free $H_2SO_4$ aerosol does exist in the atmosphere, most sulfate is in the form of $(NH_4)_2SO_4$ which airway resistance studies in animals show is of lower potency than $H_2SO_4$ or some metallic sulfates but still higher than $SO_2$ gas (Amdur, 1971). A Brookhaven-Carnegie Mellon University effort is currently reevaluating the sulfate damage function. There is still a probability of an effect. In a recent review, Leikauf and Lippmann (1980) conclude that "...there is no clear evidence that the United States

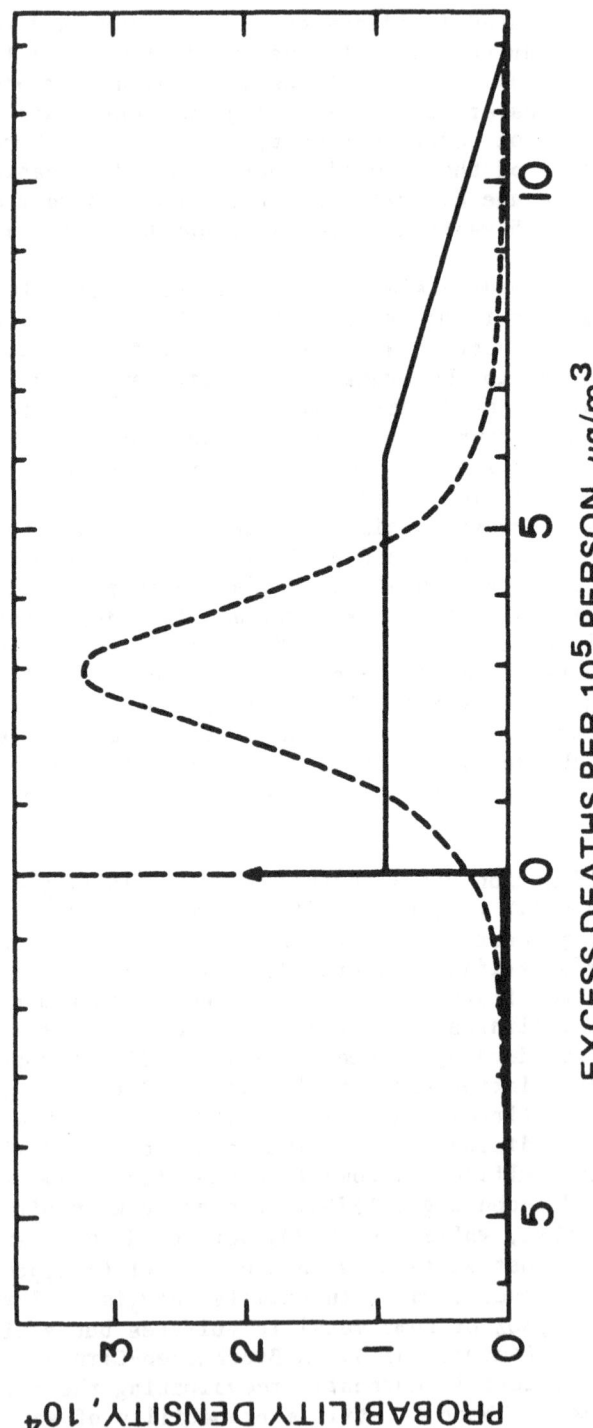

Figure 12. Probability density functions representing uncertainty in the slope of assumed linear sulfate health damage function. From Morgan et al. (1978).

population is currently suffering any direct health effects from the inhalation of various sulfur oxide compounds [but] our current knowledge on mechanisms of action, dose-response, and possible interactions with other pollutants is so poor, however, that we clearly have no basis for complacency either." Much current research identifies the sub-micrometer sulfate aerosol, particularly the acidic species, to be of special concern. There may be a practical threshold. In addition, concern must be expanded to include fine particles as a class, rather than just sulfates.

Working from the existing damage function, however, provides a reference point. Figure 13 is based on a concept developed by Rowe (1980) to estimate total population expo-sure to sulfate from a unit $SO_2$ emission. The figure is based on results from computer simulation of meteorological and chemical processes using a long-range pollution trans-port model developed by Meyers and Cederwall of the Atmospheric Sciences Division at Brookhaven National Laboratory (Meyers and Cederwall, 1975; Meyers, Cederwall, and Ohmstede, 1979). In the Ohio Valley, for example, $SO_2$ emissions yield 30 to 40 person-$\mu g/m^3$ sulfate exposure across the United States annual emission. The average for the United States is 24 person-$\mu g/m^3$ sulfate exposure per ton of $SO_2$ annual emission. Taking an Ohio Valley figure of 35 person-$\mu g/m^3$ per ton $SO_2$ emission with an $SO_2$ emission rate of 0.4 pounds $SO_2$ per Btu thermal coal (0.24% sulfur, 12,000 Btu/lb. coal or equivalent flue gas desulfurization) with the existing damage function yields 0 to 60 attrib-utable deaths annually across the United States (90% confi-dence interval, median 21). Some notion of the effect of a potential threshold for sulfates can be gained from Figure 14, which shows the fraction of the total population expo-sure to sulfate above given concentrations. Since the mon-itoring network does not have sufficient density to describe accurately the full distribution of exposure, this figure is also based on the results of the Brookhaven long-range transport model. The model tends to over estimate at higher concentrations so the true curve probably comes down some-what steeper than that shown in Figure 14. A population threshold of about 10 $\mu g/m^3$ would reduce the health damaging population exposures to about 1/5 to 1/4 of the total expo-sure. This would reduce the effect of an Ohio Valley plant to ~5 attributable deaths per year. Sulfur-particulate pollution at existing levels does not lead to any unique effects but aggrevates or adds to a background of existing disease making the identification of effects at existing pollution levels an almost impossible task. Five attrib-utable deaths annually nationwide is about a 0.0025% increase in mortality rate. Thus, even the effect of 100

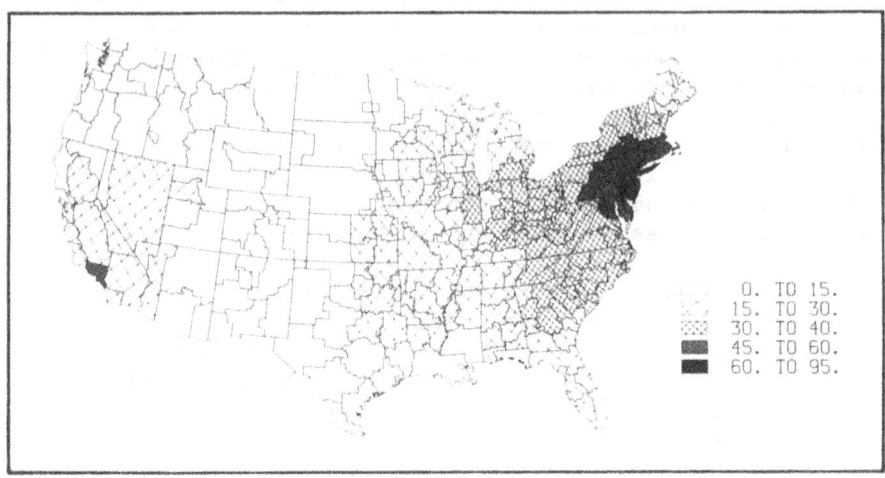

Figure 13. Annual average sulfate exposure per unit $SO_2$ emission, person–$\mu g/m^3$ per ton annual $SO_2$ emission, by air quality control region.  From M. D. Rowe (work in progress).

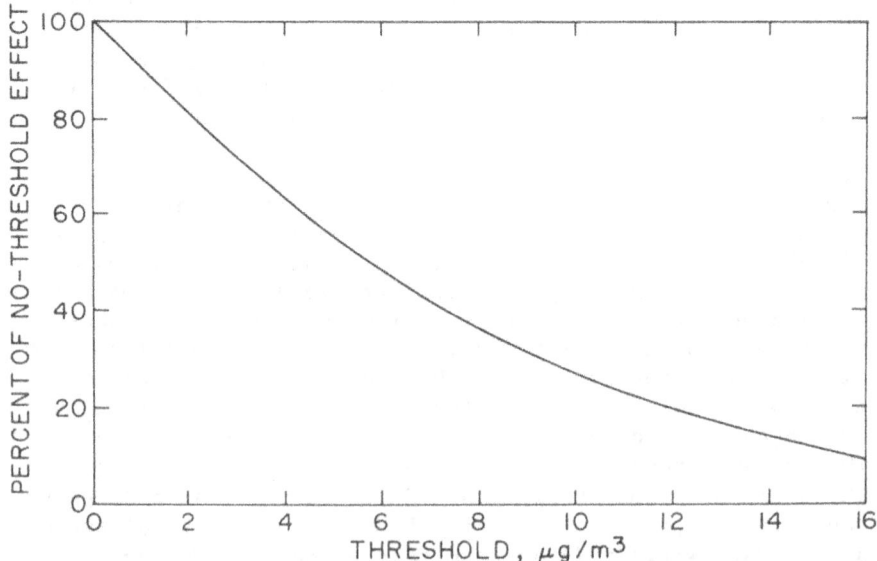

Figure 14.  Fraction of U.S. population exposed to sulfate air pollution above given concentrations.  Indicates fraction of health effect calculated with linear, no threshold model which would occur given a threshold model with the same damage function slope and exposure pattern similar to total sulfate exposure.

plants would be difficult to detect. Exposure to the various components of the sulfur-particulate mix are so well correlated that it is difficult to assign effects to a particular pollutant. Pollutant classes that are receiving considerable attention are polycyclic organic material (POM), trace metals and radionuclides. In addition to direct effects of pollutants, global $CO_2$ emissions pose the potential for significant health risks through climatic change. These risks are discussed in more detail elsewhere in this volume (Von Hippel, 1981).

## Polycyclic Organic Matter (POM)

Coal combustion products contain a number of polynuclear aromatic hydrocarbons including polycyclic and heterocyclic compounds with nitrogen, oxygen, or sulfur in the ring systems. Many of these polycyclic organics have been proven to be mutagenic in bacterial tests and carcinogenic in animals. For some, such as benzo(a)pyrene, there is strong direct evidence of such effects from occupational studies of carcinogenesis in man. Most of these organics normally exist in the particulate phase.

Fine particles present a greater surface area per unit weight than large particles for absorbing organic compounds. Those with dimensions <2 μm may then carry organics into the lung. That elution of POM takes place in the lung has been demonstrated by the observation that carbon deposits recovered from lungs at autopsy are depleted in POM (Falk, Kotin, and Markul, 1958); however, the amount of elution is decreased for very fine particles (<80 nm) (Falk and Jurgelski, 1979).

A synergistic effect between benzo(a)pyrene and $SO_2$ has been demonstrated in animals (Laskin, Kuschner, and Drew, 1970), and the presence of such irritants as $SO_2$ may explain the much higher carcinogenic activity of POM in coke oven workers (Redmond et al., 1972; Redmond, 1976) compared with roofers (Hammond et al., 1976).

There are large differences in POM levels between urban and rural areas, among cities and even within single cities, but drawing dose-response information from such situations through studies of the exposed populations presents a number of difficulties. One is the overwhelming effect of cigarette smoking. The relationship between smoking and cancer has been firmly established, and the corresponding cancer rate is at least several times greater than the cancer potential of air pollution. Thus, differences in

hard-to-measure smoking habits among different populations
could account for much of the observed differences in lung
cancer rates. Another difficulty is in the measurement of
POM exposure level. There are many potentially carcinogenic
chemical species, and the relative amounts of each vary
significantly with combustion source and atmospheric conditions. Moreover, the net activity of such mixtures has been
shown in bacterial mutagenesis tests to depend on interactions among the compounds and is not simply additive. The
use of index measures such as benzo(a)pyrene or total
benzene- or cyclohexene-soluble extract leaves considerable
uncertainty between estimated and actual exposure. This
compounds the more common problem of extrapolating population exposure from fixed outdoor measuring sites.

Some estimates have been made of health damage functions using general population studies. Most prominent is
the estimate by the National Academy of Sciences (NAS) that
an increase in urban air pollution corresponding to an average benzo(a)pyrene increase of 1 ng/m$^3$ may result in an
increase of 5% in the lung cancer death rate (NAS, 1972).
For the reasons stated above, this estimate appears highly
speculative.

Better epidemiological results are available from occupational studies. Perhaps the best is from the Pittsburgh
long-term mortality study of steelworkers. A tenfold increase in lung cancer was observed for men employed >5 years
full-time topside at coke ovens (Lloyd, 1971; Redmond et
al., 1972), to typical exposures of about 10$^4$ ng/m$^3$ (NAS,
1972). Increased cancer has been related directly to estimates of exposure to coal tar pitch volatiles (Mazumdar et
al., 1975).

Extrapolations required in applying such results to estimate effects of low-level general population exposures to
POM differ from those required in animal studies or direct
observations of vital rates in large populations. For coke
oven workers, although both exposure and specific relationship with disease are well characterized, exposures are
higher than for the general population; the chemical character of the POM is different; the age and health status of
the population are very restricted (healthy adult males);
and the lifetime distribution of exposure differs. Nevertheless, these factors can all be taken into account to some
degree, and - despite uncertainties in extrapolation - the
data can provide an important approach to quantitative estimation of health effects in the general population. Such

studies are currently under analysis by the U.S. Environmental Protection Agency's Carcinogen Assessment Group, with the aim of developing more general health damage functions.

To put the risk from increased POM emissions in some perspective, it is instructive to consider the relative contributions from different sources. Residential furnaces burning bituminous coal have POM emission rates $10^3$ to $10^5$ times higher than other fossil fuel sources (NAS, 1972). An analysis of airborne concentration trends suggests that on a national aggregate basis such residential furnaces dominate other sources despite their relatively small energy production (Faoro, 1975). Emission rates from residential anthracite coal combustion are 50 times lower (DeAngelis and Reznic, 1979). Gas, oil combustion, and coal combustion in large steam power plants have POM emissions 10 to 100 times lower still. While residential coal furnaces are estimated to have emitted about one-third of the anthropogenic benzo(a)pyrene in the United States in 1968, coal steam electric plants emitted only about 0.1% (EPA 1975). When actual exposure is considered rather than emission concentrations, it is significant that sidestream cigarette smoke contributes benzo(a)pyrene concentrations in typical rooms on the same order as that of urban air (1-20 $ng/m^3$). Public areas with heavy smoking can reach concentrations over 100 $ng/m^3$ (NAS, 1972).

There is also a background level of POM produced by natural processes. Polycyclic organic matter with mutagenic and carcinogenic potential is emitted by volcanoes and forest fires and is produced in biosynthesis. The former, like anthropogenic emissions, is released to the atmosphere while the latter remains fixed in the plants and microorganisms in which it is formed (Suess, 1975). Analysis of soils and sediments suggest that preanthropogenic POM concentrations most likely were due to airborne deposition from forest fires occurring over geologic time spans (Blumer and Youngblood, 1975).

Finally, assessment of POM hazards suffers from a more general difficulty: the mechanisms of health damage are complex - too complex to be understood fully and too complex even to permit reduction of all those aspects that are understood to damage functions that may be used for analyzing the health effects of energy technologies. Any quantitative health effects estimate will suffer from uncertainties in estimating model parameters as well as uncertainties in the model itself.

A number of carcinogen models are discussed in detail
by Hoel et al. (1975) and Schneiderman, Decoufle, and Brown
(1979).  Some assume no threshold; others allow the possibility.  While most models are compatible with available
data, they predict effects that vary by several orders of
magnitude in the low dose range, which is usually the region
of most interest and for which good data are not available.
In this region the individual risk is quite low, and effects
become lost in the "noise" of background cancer occurrence.
Models have been used to extrapolate from animal experiments
to man, but in general such extrapolation has not been
accepted widely in a quantitative sense; animal testing has,
however, been accepted for qualitative identification of
carcinogens or potential carcinogens.

The advance of in vitro systems for mutagenesis testing
has led to additional efforts to extrapolate quantitatively
from mutagenesis tests and animal experiments to man (Crouch
and Wilson, 1979; Campbell, 1980).  Such approaches may
prove particularly useful in determining relative rankings
of carcinogens, which can then be calibrated using compounds
for which good studies are available in vitro, in animals
and in man.

Studies by a number of workers (Crisp, Fisher, and
Lamment, 1978; Fisher, Crisp, and Raabe, 1979; Kubitschek
and Venta, 1979) conclude that coal fly ash emitted to the
atmosphere is mutagenic in the Ames Salmonella reversion
assay.  None of the studies, however, report any mutagenic
activity in the collected fly ash.  This has been substan-
tiated by Bonnell, Schilling, and Massey, (1980), who find
no mutagenic activity in fly ash collected in the electro-
static precipitator of a British power plant.  Fisher,
Crisp, and Raabe, (1979) look further into the physical
factors affecting the mutagenicity of fly ash and find that
the greatest mutagenic activity is associated with the
finest particles of the ash.  This leads to a tentative
conclusion that mutagenic effects are caused by compounds
that volatilize during combustion or are formed during or
after combustion.  Condensation presumably takes place after
exhaust gases pass through the precipitator.

In addition to mutagen assay studies there have been
reports of specific mutagenic agents in fly ash.  There is
considerable controversy over these findings.  Lee et al.,
(1980) report finding dimethyl sulfate, a proven mutagen, in
the particles emitted from a stoker-type coal-fired heating
plant and a large coal-fired power plant.  Dow Chemical
Corporation reports 38 ng/g *tetrachlorodibenzo-p-dioxin*
(TCDD) in the stack effluent of an industrial power plant

burning coal and fuel oil (Dow, 1978). These findings are disputed in a report finding no evidence of TCDD in the fly ash emitted from a coal-fired power plant stack (Kimble and Gross, 1980).

## Trace Metals

Coal may contain every naturally occurring element. Most are present in trace amounts with concentrations that vary considerably from seam to seam. Upon combustion, these trace elements are redistributed among the bottom ash and the collected and escaping fly ash. Elements of greatest concern are arsenic, cadmium, lead, and mercury. These commonly occur at concentrations higher than the earth's crust and are highly toxic to most biological systems. Of more moderate concern are chromium, vanadium, copper, zinc, nickel, and fluorine (National Research Council, 1980).

Natusch, Wallace, and Evans (1974) report that concentrations of toxic trace metals increase in fly ash as particle size decreases. The degree of trace element enrichment with decreasing particle size still has to be evaluated satisfactorily. Natusch, Wallace, and Evans, (1974); Ondov, Rugaini, and Biermann, (1978); and Campbell, et al., (1978) all report strong increases with decreasing particle size. The work of Gladney et al., (1976), however, indicates very much lower enrichment factors.

Natusch, Wallace, and Evans, (1974) explain enrichment by a volatilization-condensation mechanism. Their model suggests that when coal is burned, the more volatile elements are vaporized and thus depleted from the slag and bottom ash. As flue gases cool, these elements preferentially condense out on the smaller fly ash particles because of their larger surface area-to-volume ratio. Selective retention of coarser fly ash particles by pollution control devices further enhances the concentration in escaping fly ash. Such elements thus pose a greater hazard than simple chemical analysis would indicate.

Smaller particles are deposited more efficiently in the pulmonary region of the lung where long residence times enhance absorption rates of trace metals (Natusch, Wallace, and Evans, 1974). Concentration of volatile toxic trace elements on particle surfaces would enhance the toxicity of small particles. Finally, the chemical form of elements deposited in the lung requires evaluation, as this is an important factor in determining solubility and hence uptake into the pulmonary bloodstream.

The large quantities of coal burned for production of
electricity result in large annual emissions, even of trace
contaminants.  Little is known about the fate of metals
emitted from tall stacks, although it is clear they travel
long distances.  Less than 10% of the metal emissions can be
accounted for within 50 km of the source (National Research
Council, 1980).  Vaughn et al., (1975) modeled the behavior
and accumulation of trace metals in soil, water, biota, and
man around a large power plant.  They concluded that the
food chain was the only pathway of potential consequence to
man and that, in general, excessive bioaccumulation was not
expected.


## Radionuclides

Coal contains trace amounts of three naturally occurring radioactive decay series headed by uranium-238,
uranium-235, and thorium-232.  Radionuclides from these
series are present in the particles emitted during coal combustion.  In addition, radon isotopes appear in each of the
three decay series, and radon gas is released during coal
combustion and from ash piles.  The risk from radon is considered small compared to that from radionuclides in particle emissions (EPA, 1979).  Coal typically contains about
1-2 ppm uranium and 2-4 ppm thorium (Swanson et al., 1976,
McBride, et al., 1978); on this basis, the uranium-thorium
inventory in the coal cycle is orders of magnitude less than
in the nuclear fuel cycle.  Maximum dose to individuals in
the vicinity of a coal-burning facility may, however, be
comparable to maximum dose from a nuclear facility; and dose
to bone may be higher owing to the differences in the
radionuclides released (McBride et al., 1978; EPA, 1979).

Solubility of the particulate matter influences both
the amount of radionuclide taken up by green plants and the
amount of inhaled or ingested fly ash cleared from the human
lung or digestive tract.  In both cases, solubility - and
therefore potential impact - is believed to be low (Beck et
al., 1980; EPA 1979).

There are many human exposure pathways for radionuclides.  Individuals are exposed to gamma radiation exter-
nally by immersion in an atmosphere containing suspended
radioactive particles and to particles deposited on the
ground.  Individuals are exposed internally via inhalation
or ingestion.  Sources of ingested material include foliar
deposition and radionuclides extracted from the soil by
plants.  Internal exposure involves alpha radiation as well
as beta and gamma radiation.

Beck et al. (1980) surveyed the area around three coal-burning plants and found elevated levels of radionuclides at only one, which had concentrations comparable to what their model predicted. They report a projected human health impact only via the inhalation pathway and only for the maximally exposed individual.

McBride et al. (1978) and EPA (1979) modeled health effects as a function of a number of variables including location, stack height, and consumption of locally produced food. Applying dose-response values (Committee on the Biological Effects of Ionizing Radiation, 1972) to these model results and normalizing to 1 GW(e)-yr. of electricity production yields estimates of 0.0001 to 0.29 latent cancer deaths per GWe-yr.

## Occupational Health at Coal-Fired Power Plants

Workers at coal-fired power plants are exposed to noise, solvents, coal dust and possibly other environmental hazards. The only quantitative estimates of risk are for occupational accidents, however. The Council on Environmental Quality (1973) estimated 0.01 deaths and 1.2 injuries per plant-year. Bertolett and Fox (1974) surveyed the accidental injury rate for four utility companies with over 13,000,000 person-hours of exposure at coal-fired power plants. They found a fatality rate of 0.10 and a nonfatal injury rate of 3.3 per 1000 MW plant year for coal plants. Factoring in a 75% capacity factor gives a fatality rate of 0.13 per GW(e)-yr. and a nonfatal injury rate of 4.4 per GW(e)-yr.

## Coal Conversion

Problems with reliability and cost of foreign oil imports has created a demand for substitute gaseous and liquid fuels in the United States. An enormous research and development program and the beginnings of a potentially large industry have sprung up. However, limited information exists which directly applies to assessing the potential health risks of such an industry. No full scale plants exist in the United States. Town gas plants and German coal hydrogenation plants of the 1930's and 1940's were of a much smaller scale and different in design from those being planned today. More important, no evidence apparently exists from these older plants on which to base health risk assessments. Existing facilities in South Africa, Yugoslavia and

East Germany offer some opportunity to obtain information.
The United States EPA has been carrying out cooperative
research on environmental emissions of the Kosovo plant in
Yugoslavia for several years (Lee and Stara, 1980). There
are a number of pilot plants in the United States, some of
which have been operating for several years. There are
large programs at EPA and DOE conducting chemical analysis
of effluents, mutagenesis testing, and animal toxicology
studies. These pilot plants are not complete facilities nor
are they operated in the same manner as commercial facilities would be, however. The greatest amount of applicable
health risk information is from a Union Carbide pilot coal
hydrogenation plant at Institute, WV which operated 1952-
1956 (Sexton, 1960). Much of the concern for potential
hazards at coal synfuels plants stems from a number of studies of coke oven and coal gas retort workers in which there
was clear evidence of increased cancer (Doll, 1965; Doll,
1972; Lloyd, 1971; Redmond et al., 1972). In addition, it
would seem that certain experiences at petroleum refineries
would be of some inferential use, but suprisingly, very
little information is available on refinery workers (Lloyd,
1980; Hanis, Stauraky, and Fowler, 1979; Schottenfield, et
al., 1980; Thomas, Decoufle, and Moure-Eraso, 1980).

Wiser (1980) presents some useful insights into what
lies behind potential health risks from coal conversion.
Most (60-75%) of the carbon in coal exists in aromatic ring
structures, connected with ether or short aliphatic links.
Thus, breaking up the coal structure would result in many
potentially carcinogenic compounds. Most coal gasification
processes and indirect liquefaction processes which first
gasify the coal (such as the SASOL plant in South Africa)
expose coal to molecular oxygen and steam at temperatures
>900°C. Under these conditions, the carbon structure of the
coal is not just broken up, but is completely destroyed.
Most of the carbon goes to carbon monoxide. The potential
carcinogenic hazard is largely eliminated, but acute risks
of carbon monoxide exposure are created. Because of its
acute hazard and its virtual ubiquitousness in the process
stream, it has been recommended that carbon monoxide serve
as an overall hazard indicator in such plants (National
Institute for Occupational Safety and Health, 1978). In
direct liquefaction plants (such as SRC I, SRC II, and Exxon
Donor Solvent processes) temperatures are generally 450-
500°C. This environment just breaks the connecting links in
the coal structure, releasing the wide variety of aromatic
ring compounds. Refining the product through further hydrogenation opens these rings, yielding 1- or 2-ring compounds
that are unlikely to be carcinogenic but may still be highly
toxic. Thus, the major carcinogenic risk is in the

intermediate product. An important difference between the aromatic compounds derived from coal and those for which a wider exposure experience exists in the petroleum industry is the greater number of oxygen, nitrogen and sulfur heterocyclic compounds and of organometallic compounds (Koppenaal and Manahan, 1976).

The principle health risk of coal conversion plants appears to be to the workers, particularly maintenance workers who are apt to have the greatest exposures. A number of fractions from coal liquefaction processes were found to be mutagenic in microbial test systems, causing neoplastic changes following intramuscular injection into rodents, and producing carcinomas in animals when they remain on the skin for extended periods (Harris et al., 1980). Considerable effort has gone into assessment of industrial hygiene needs to protect these workers (White, 1979). The risk may not be as great as has been feared. A 1950's study of 359 workers at the Institute, West Virginia, plant identified 50 workers with skin abnormalities of which 10 were diagnosed with skin cancer. Forty-nine of the 50 were later followed up in a National Institute for Occupational Safety and Health (NIOSH) study (Palmer, 1979, Harris et al., 1980). Only 5 of the 10 were confirmed as having had skin cancer, and no excess systemic cancers were found. Current pilot plants have greater emphasis on occupational health and industrial hygiene. The occupational health record in these plants is excellent, although basal cell carcinomas reportedly occurred on the lip, ear, and nose of 3 of 190 employees at a plant with 11 years operation. The significance of these cases was considered questionable by NIOSH due to the small number of employees and the lack of adequate reference data available (Harris et al., 1980). Salmon (1980) made a bounding calculation of 0.05 to 0.12 cancers per plant-year for gasification plants and 0.26-0.30 cancers per plant-year for liquefaction plants assuming exposures were similar to coke oven workers; actual expected exposures were estimated to be lower by more than 10 times.

What public exposures to POM, hydrogen sulfide, carbonyl sulfide, carbon disulfide, and other pollutants will be is impossible to judge now, but as the processes are pressurized and contained, they are likely to be nil, certainly much lower than exposures to workers. Fugitive air emissions and leachates from waste tars and sludges are possible sources of public exposure.

In addition to the direct health risk of the conversion plant, coal synfuels introduces changes in demands - and thus health effects - throughout the entire coal fuel

Table 9. Health and safety effects of fuel supply processes per GW(e)-yr[a]

| | Central-station electric | | | | | Direct combustion | | |
|---|---|---|---|---|---|---|---|---|
| | FGD[b] | SRC-II[b] | Low Btu[b] | AFB[b] | High Btu | SRC-II | Natural gas | Petroleum |
| **Extraction** | | | | | | | | |
| Disease death | 0-1.3[c] | 0-1.8 | 0-1.3 | 0-1.2 | 0-1.0 | 0-0.9 | | |
| Nonfatal disease | 7.5-14. | 10.-20. | 7.5-14. | 6.3-13. | 5.6-11. | 5.3-10. | | |
| Accident death | 0.7-1.9 | 1.-2.6 | 0.7-1.9 | 0.5-1.8 | 0.4-1.6 | 0.4-1.5 | 0.006 | 0.003 |
| Accident injury | 81.-91. | 116.-126. | 82.-92. | 71.-79. | 63.-71. | 58.-66. | 0.04-0.8 | 0.1 |
| **Transport[d]** | | | | | | | | |
| Accident death | 0.4-1.8 | | | 0.3-1.5 | | | | |
| Accident injury | 16.-21. | 0.06 | 0.06 | 14.-18. | 0.03 | 0.03 | 0.06-1.3 | 0.03 |
| **Processing** | | | | | | | | |
| Accident death | 0.13 | 0.19 | 0.09 | 0.13 | 0.16 | 0.09 | | 0.009 |
| Accident injury | 8.4-12. | 15.-19. | 7.5-11. | 7.5-11. | 11.-12. | 5.6-8.4 | 0.06 | 0.3-1.5 |

[a]Derived from Morris et al., 1979.

[b]FGD is conventional coal electric with flue gas desulfurization; SRC-II is direct coal liquefaction by the solvent-refined coal process; Low Btu is direct conversion of coal to low BTU gas; High Btu is direct conversion of coal to high Btu gas; AFB is atmospheric fluidized bed combustion of coal.

Notes:

[c]Ranges are 60% confidence intervals based on a normal approximation to the Poisson, with the exception of disease in extraction which represents the range of various published studies. Because of the indirect method of estimation, this method probably results in too narrow a range for transport and distribution.

[d]Transport and distribution effects are highly dependent on assumptions of mine-mouth vs remote operation of coal consumption facilities; SRC-II plants and low-Btu gas plants are assumed to have mine-mouth locations.

cycle. These system-wide effects have been examined in detail (Morris et al., 1979). Introduction of synfuel conversion processes can decrease overall system efficiency (mine-to-ultimate use) resulting in a need for more mining per unit energy delivered. Relative effects in this part of the fuel cycle are shown in Table 9 for synfuels options compared to standard coal steam electric with flue gas desulfurization (FGD) and natural gas and petroleum in direct combustion.

Air pollution exposures are changed considerably; system-wide emission of particles and sulfur oxides are reduced since higher removal efficiencies are possible in the conversion plant. The location of emissions may shift from power plant to conversion plant which is likely to be located nearer the mines. There is the possibility of carry-over of coal pollutants in the product synfuels, leading to exposures at the point of combustion; this may be of concern particularly for fuels to be used in urban areas. The overall system efficiency loss also leads to an increase in $CO_2$ emissions for synfuels. The additional $CO_2$ for a large synfuels industry is substantial in absolute terms, but represents only a small fraction of expected global $CO_2$ growth (Moskowitz, Morris, and Albanese, 1980).

## Conclusion

Any of man's activities involve risk; estimates presented here of the risks of coal must be taken in this context. The effects estimated are those which can reasonably be attributed to the direct operation of the coal fuel cycle. Where possible, these risks have been expressed as effects per GW(e)-yr. Occupational health effects are summarized in Table 10. Underground coal mining is the source of the bulk of the occupational impact; these values are subject to an uncertainty of about a factor of 2 in either direction. Public health risks are much more uncertain. Table 11 shows public health estimates of transport risks and alternative estimates of air pollution risks with and without thresholds. Air pollution poses the largest potential risk. The incremental risk is probably too small to expect it to be detectable in any reasonable epidemiological study, however, both air pollution and coal transport are low-level risks distributed over a large population. On an individual risk basis, the effects are sufficiently low as to be unlikely to cause any health concern except in particularly sensitive populations. On the other hand, the cumulative effect in millions of people exposed to low risk levels may be sufficient to justify control measures.

128    Samuel C. Morris

Table 10.  Coal fuel cycle occupational health effects
           summary[a]

|  | Per GW(e)-yr | |
|---|---|---|
|  | Deaths | Non-fatal cases |
| Coal Mining | | |
| Underground[b] | | |
|   Accidents | 1.7 | 170 |
|   Disease | 0-0.2 | 0.1-5 |
| Surface[b](accidents) | 0.12 | 18 |
| Coal cleaning (accidents) | 0.06 | 3-5 |
| Coal Transport (accidents) | | |
|   Rail[b] | 0.014 | 1.1 |
|   Barge[b] | 0.46 | 1.6 |
|   Truck[b] | 1.2 | 20. |
| Power Plant (accidents) | 0.13 | 5 |
| Total[c] | 1.3 | 96. |

[a]See text for discussion of derivation and levels of
uncertainty.
   [b]Assumes 1 GW(e)-yr from this source alone.
   [c]Assumes a mix of mining: 57% surface, 43% underground;
Transport: 53% rail, 22% barge, 11% truck, 14% mine-mouth,
etc., and middle values where ranges are given.

Table 11.  Coal fuel cycle public health effects summary

|  | Per GW(e)-yr | |
|---|---|---|
|  | Deaths | Non-fatal cases |
| Transport accidents | | |
|   Rail | 0.41 | 0.87 |
|   Barge | 0.14 | 0.15 |
|   Truck | 1.2 | 20. |
| Air pollution | | |
|   Sulfate Surrogate | | |
|   (no threshold) | 21 (0-60) | |
|   Sulfate Surrogate | | |
|   (10 µg/m$^3$ threshold) | 10 (0-30) | |
|   Radionuclides | 0-0.3 | |

Such a balance must include consideration of the uncertainty in effects estimates, valuation of effects and attitudes toward risk.

## Acknowledgements

This work was supported by the Health and Environmental Risk Analysis Program, Office of Health and Environmental Research, U.S. Department of Energy.  Earlier work supported by the DOE Office of Technological Impacts has been incorporated.  Particular acknowledgements are due H. C. Thode, Jr., for assistance with statistical analysis of mine accident data; J. Nagy, from whom calculations of risk from radionuclides were drawn; S. Rosenblatt, for assistance with the sulfate threshold analysis, and A. Link who typed repeated drafts of the manuscript.  I thank M. A. Crowther, B. L. Cohen, S. J. Finch, H. Fischer, L. D. Hamilton, P. D. Moskowitz, K. M. Novak, M. D. Rowe, W. A. Sevian, J. Stebbings, and A. Watson for their help and comments on various stages of this work.

## Notes

[1]The Standardized Mortality Ratio (SMR) is the ratio of observed to  expected deaths during the period of a study multiplied by 100.  Expected  deaths are obtained by applying age-sex-specific mortality rates from a  control population to the number of people in the corresponding groups in the study population and summing the result.

# References

Amoudru, C.  1980.  A study of trends on occupations risks associated with coal mining.  *IAEA Bulletin* 22:80-91.

Amdur, M. O.  1971.  Aerosols formed by oxidation of sulfur dioxide, review of their toxicology.  *Arch. Environ. Health* 23:459-468.

Amdur, M. O.  1976.  Toxicological guidelines for research on sulfur oxides and particulates.  In *Fourth Symposium on Statistics and the Environment*, pp. 48-55.  National Academy of Sciences, Washington, D.C.

Association of American Railroads.  1977.  *Yearbook of Railroad Facts.*  Washington, D.C.

Attfield, M. and J. Hudak.  1980.  Prevalence of coal workers' pneumoconioses:  comparison of first and second rounds.  In *Health Implications of New Energy Technologies*, pp. 203-212.  W. N. Rom and V. E. Archer (Eds.).  Ann Arbor Science Publishers, Inc., Ann Arbor, Michigan.

Avol, E. L., M. P. Jones, R. M. Bailey, N. N. Chang, M. T. Kleinman, W. S. Linn, K. A. Bell and J. D. Hackney.  1979.  Controlled exposures of human volunteers to sulfate aerosols.  *Am. Rev. Respir. Dis.* 120:319-327.

Bailey, A. G. and M. L. Waring.  1967.  *Economics of Unit Trains and Unit Train Operations.*  Railway Systems and Management Association, Chicago, Illinois.

Baker, J. G.  1979.  *Determinants of Coal Mine Labor Productivity Change.*  DOE/IR/0056.  U.S. Government Printing Office, Washington, D.C.

Beck, H. L., C. V. Gogolak, K. M. Miller and W. M. Lowder.  1980.  Perturbations on the natural radiation environment due to the utilization of coal as an energy source.  In *Natural Radiation Environment III*, pp. 1521-1557.  T. F. Gesell and W. M. Lowder (eds).  Proceedings of a Symposium held at Houston, Texas, April 23-28, 1978.  CONF-780422.

Bertolett, A. D. and R. J. Fox.  1974.  Accident-rate sample favors nuclear.  *Electr. World* 182:40-41 (July 15).

Blumer, M. and W. W. Youngblood.  1975.  Polycyclic aromatic hydrocarbons in soils and recent sediments.  *Science* 188:53-55.

Bonnell, J. A., C. J. Schilling and P. M. O. Massey.  1980.  Clinical and experimental studies of the effects of pulverized fuel ash — a review.  *Ann. Occup. Hyg.* 23:159-164.

Bureau of Labor Statistics. 1979. *Occupational Injuries and Illnesses in the United States by Industry, 1976.* U.S. Department of Labor, Washington, D.C.

Campbell, J. A., J. C. Laul, K. K. Neilson and R. D. Smith. 1978. Separation and chemical characterization of finely-sized fly ash particles. *Anal. Chem.* 50: 1032-1040.

Campbell, T. C. 1980. Chemical carcinogens and human risk assessment. *Fed. Proc.* 39:2467-2484.

Chiu, S. Y., L. Fradkin, S. Barisas, T. Surles, S. Morris, A. Crowther and V. DeCarlo. 1980. *Problems Associated with Solid Wastes from Energy Systems.* ANL/EES-TM-118. Argonne National Laboratory, Argonne, Illinois.

Chrisp, C. E., G. L. Fisher and J. E. Lamment. 1978. Mutagenicity of filtrates from respirable coal fly ash. *Science* 199:73-75.

Cochrane, A. L. 1962. The attach rate of progressive massive fibrosis. *Brit. J. Ind. Med.* 19:52-64.

Coleman, J. and G. R. Stewart. 1976. Investigation of accident data for railroad-highway grade crossings. In *Railroad-Highway Crossings, Visibility, and Human Factors*, Transportation Research Record 611, pp. 60-67. Transportation Research Board, National Academy of Sciences, Washington, D.C.

Committee on the Biological Effects of Ionizing Radiation. 1972. *The Effects on Populations of Low Levels of Exposure to Ionizing Radiation.* National Academy of Sciences, Washington, D.C.

Committee on Science and Technology. 1976. *Community Health and Environmental Surveillance System (CHESS): An Investigative Report.* U.S. House of Representatives, 94th Congress, Washington, D.C.

Congressional Research Service. 1977. *National Energy Transportation.* Pub. No. 95-15. Printed by U. S. Senate Committees on Energy and Natural Resources and Commerce, Science and Transportation, Washington. D.C.

Council on Environmental Quality. 1973. *Energy and the Environment: Electric Power.* pp. 42-43. Washington, D.C.

Crouch, E. and R. Wilson. 1979. Interspecies comparison of carcinogenic potency. *J. Toxicol. Environ. Health* 5:1095-1118.

Davis, J.M.G., J. Ohery, and A. LeRoux. 1977. The effect of quartz and other non-coal dusts in coal workers' pneumoconiosis, part II, lung autopsy study. In

*Inhaled Particles IV*, pp. 691-700. W. H. Walton (ed.). Pergamon Press, Oxford.

DeAngelis, D. G. and R. B. Reznic. 1979. *Source Assessment: Residential Combustion of Coal*. EPA 600/2-79-019a. U.S. Environmental Protection Agency, Washington, D.C.

Doll, R., R.E.W. Fisher, E. J. Gammon, W. Gunn, G. O. Hughes, F. H. Tyrer, and W. Wilson. 1965. Mortality of gas workers with special reference to cancers of the lung and bladder, chronic bronchitis, and pneumoconiosis. *Brit. J. Ind. Med.* 22:1-12.

Doll, R. 1972. Mortality of gas workers — final report of a perspective study. *Brit. J. Ind. Med.* 29:394-406.

Dow Chemical Company. 1978. *The Trace Chemistries of Fire — A Source of and Routes for the Entry of Chlorinated Dioxins into the Environment*. Midland, Michigan.

Enterline, P. E. 1964. Mortality rates among coal miners. *Am. J. Public Health* 54:758-768.

Enterline, P. E. 1972. A review of mortality data for American coal miners. *Ann. N. Y. Acad. of Sci.* 200:260-272.

Environmental Protection Agency. 1974. *Health Consequences of Sulfur Oxides: A Report from CHESS, 1970-71*. EPA-650/1-74-004. Research Triangle Park, N.C.

Environmental Protection Agency. 1975. *Scientific and Technical Assessment Report on Particulate Polycyclic Organic Matter*. EPA 600/6-74-001. Washington, D.C.

Environmental Protection Agency. 1977. *Accidents and Unscheduled Events Associated with Non-Nuclear Energy Resources and Technology*. EPA-600/7-77-016. Washington, D.C.

Environmental Protection Agency. 1979. *Radiological Impact Caused by Emissions of Radionuclides into Air in the United States*. EPA 520/7-79-006. Washington, D.C.

Falk, H. L., P. Kotin, and I. Markul. 1958. The disappearance of carcinogens from soot in human lungs. *Cancer* 11:482.

Falk, H. L. and W. Jurgelski, Jr. 1979. Health effects of coal mining and combustion: carcinogens and cofactors. *Environ. Health Perspec.* 33:203-226.

Faoro, R. B. 1975. Trends in concentration of benzene soluble suspended particulate fraction and benzo(a)-pyrene. *J. Air Pollut. Control Assoc.* 25:638-640.

Federal Railroad Administration. 1966-1974. *Accident Bulletins No. 135-143*. U. S. Department of Transportation, Washington, D.C.

Fisher, G. L., C. E. Crisp, and O. G. Raabe. 1979. Physical factors affecting the mutagenicity of fly ash from a coal-fired power plant. *Science* 204:879-881.

Gladney, E. S., J. A. Small, G. E. Gordon, and W. H. Zoller. 1976. Composition and size distribution of in-stack particulate material at a coal fired power plant. *Atmos. Environ.* 10:1071-1077.

Hammond, E. C., I. J. Selikoff, P. L. Lawther, and H. Seidman. 1976. Inhalation of benzpyrene and cancer in man. *Ann. N.Y. Acad. Sci.* 271:116-124.

Hanis, N. M., K. M. Stavraky, and J. L. Fowler. 1979. Cancer mortality in oil refinery workers. *J. Occup. Med.* 21:167-174.

Harris, L. R., J. A. Gideon, S. Berardinelli, L. D. Reed, R. D. Dobbin, J. M. Evans, D. R. Telesca, and R. K. Tanita. 1980. *Coal Liquefaction: Recent Findings in Occupational Safety and Health*. National Institute for Occupational Safety and Health, Rockville, Maryland.

Heise, E. R., P. C. Major, M. S. Mentnech, E. J. Parrish, A. L. Jordon and W. K. C. Morgan. 1977. Predominance of histocompatibility antigens W18 and HL-A1 in miners resistant to complicated coal workers' pneumoconiosis. In *Inhaled Particles IV*, pp 495-505. W. H. Walton (ed.). Pergamon Press, Oxford.

Hoel, D. G., D. W. Gaylor, R. L. Kirschstein, U. Saffiotti and M. A. Schneiderman. 1975. Estimation of risks of irreversible delayed toxicity. *J. Toxicol. Environ. Health* 1:133-151.

Hollingsworth, C. G. 1970. *Mortality Among Disabled Coal Miners*. MS thesis, University of Pittsburgh, Graduate School of Public Health, Pittsburgh, Pennsylvania.

Hubbert, M. K. 1962. *Energy Resources: A Report to the Committee on Natural Resources*. National Academy of Sciences — National Research Council Publ. 1000-D. Washington, D.C.

Kimble, B. J. and M. L. Gross. 1980. Tetrachlorodibenzo-p-dioxin quantitation in stack collected fly ash. *Science* 207:59-61.

Koppenaal, D. W. and S. E. Manahan. 1976. Hazardous chemicals from coal conversion processes? *Environ. Sci. Technol.* 10:1104-1107.

Kubitschek, H. E. and L. Venta. 1979. Mutagenicity of coal fly ash from electric power plant precipitators. *Environ. Mutagen.* 1:79-82.

Laskin, S., M. Kuschner and R. T. Drew. 1970. Studies in pulmonary carcinogenesis. In *Inhalation Carcinogenesis*. M. G. Hanna, Jr., P. Nettesheim, and J. R. Gilbert (eds.). U.S. Atomic Energy Commission, Washington, D.C. CONF-691001.

Lave, L. and E. P. Seskin. 1978. *Air Pollution and Human Health*. Johns Hopkins University Press for Resources for the Future, Baltimore, Maryland.

Lee, M. L., D. W. Later, D. K. Rollins, D. J. Eatough and L. D. Hansen. 1980. Dimethyl and monomethyl sulfate: presence in coal fly ash and airborne particulate matter. *Science* 207:186-188.

Lee, S. D. and J. F. Stara. 1980. *Assessment of Human Health Hazards of Coal Gasification Technology*. Air Pollution Control Association Annual Meeting, June 22-27. Montreal, Canada.

Leikauf, G. and M. Lippmann. 1980. *The Potential Health Significance of Ambient Exposures to Acidic Sulfur Oxide Air Pollutants*. Niagara Falls Regional Meeting, Air Pollution Control Association. October 9-10.

Liddell, F. D. K. 1973. Mortality of British coal miners in 1961. *Brit. J. Ind. Med.* 30:15-24.

Lloyd, J. W. 1971. Long term mortality study of steel-workers V: respiratory cancer in coke plant workers. *J. Occup. Med.* 13:53.

Lloyd, J. W. 1980. Historical perspective of polycyclic aromatic hydrocarbon carcinogenesis: implications for the transition to regenerative energy. In *Health Implications of New Energy Technologies*, pp. 301-306. W. N. Rom and V. E. Archer (eds.). Ann Arbor Science Publishers, Ann Arbor, Michigan.

McBride, J. P., R. E. Moore, J. P. Witherspoon and R. E. Blanco. 1978. Radiological impact of airborne effluents of coal and nuclear plants. *Science* 202: 1045-1050.

Mazumdar, S., C. Redmond, W. Sollecito and N. Sussman. 1975. An epidemiological study of exposure to coal tar pitch volatiles among coke oven workers. *J. Air Pollut. Control Assoc.* 25:382-389.

Meyers, R. E. and R. T. Cederwall. 1975. In *Regional Energy Studies Programs Annual Report*, pp. 46-61. BNL 50478. Brookhaven National Laboratory, Upton, N.Y.

Meyers, R. E., R. T. Cederwall and W. D. Ohmstede. 1979. Modeling regional atmospheric transport and diffusion: some environmental applications. In *Advances in*

*Environmental Science and Engineering*, pp. 118-184. J. R. Pfufflin and Z. N. Ziegler (eds.). Gordon and Breach Science Publishers, New York, N.Y.

Mine Safety and Health Administration, U.S. Department of Labor. 1976-79. *Injury Experience in Coal Mining*. U.S. Government Printing Office, Washington, D.C.

Mining Enforcement and Safety Administration, U.S. Department of Interior. 1971-75. *Injury Experience in Coal Mining*. U.S. Government Printing Office, Washington, D.C.

Morgan, M. G., S. C. Morris, A. K. Meier and D. L. Shenk, 1978. A probabilistic methodology for estimating air pollution health effects from coal-fired power plants. *Energy Systems and Policy* 2:287-310.

Morgan, W. K. C., D. B. Burgess, G. Jacobson, R. J. O'Brien, E. P. Pendergrass, R. B. Reger and E. P. Shoub. 1973. The prevalence of coal workers' pneumoconiosis in U.S. coal miners. *Arch. Environ. Health* 27:221-226.

Morgan, W. K. C. 1980. Pathophysiology of coal workers' respiratory disease. In *Health Implications of New Energy Technologies*, pp. 233-238. W. N. Rom and V. E. Archer (eds.). Ann Arbor Science Publishers, Inc., Ann Arbor, Michigan.

Morris, S. C., P. D. Moskowitz, W. A. Sevian, S. Silberstein and L. D. Hamilton. 1979. Coal conversion technologies: some health and environmental effects. *Science* 206:654-662.

Moskowitz, P. D., S. C. Morris and A. S. Albanese. 1980. The global carbon dioxide problem: impacts of U.S. synthetic fuel- and coal-fired electricity generating plants. *J. Air Pollut. Control Assoc.* 30:353-357.

Naeye, R. L., J. K. Mahon and W. S. Dellinger. 1971. Rank of coal and coal workers' pneumoconiosis. *Am. Rev. Respir. Dis.* 103:350-355.

National Academy of Sciences. 1972. *Particulate Polycyclic Organic Matter*. Washington, D.C.

National Coal Association. 1976. *Coal Traffic Annual*. Washington, D.C.

National Institute of Occupational Safety and Health. 1978. *Recommended Health and Safety Guidelines for Coal Gasification Pilot Plants*. DHEW (NIOSH) No. 78-120, Cincinnati, Ohio.

National Research Council, Panel on Trace Element Geochemistry of Coal Resource Development Related to Health. 1980. *Trace-Element Geochemistry of Coal*

    *Resource Development Related to Environmental Quality
and Health.*  National Academy Press, Washington, D.C.

National Safety Council.  1978.  *Fleet Accident Rates.*
Chicago, Illinois.

Natusch, D. F. S., J. R. Wallace and C. A. Evans.  1974.
Toxic Trace elements:  preferential concentration in
respirable particulates.  *Science* 183:202-204.

Ondov, J. M., R. C. Rugaini and A. H. Biermann.  1978.
Elemental particle-size emissions from coal-fired
powered plants:  use of an inertial cascade
inspection.  *Atmos. Environ.* 12:1175-1185.

Ortmeyer, C. E., E. J. Baier and G. M. Crawford.  1973.
Life expectancy of Pennsylvania coal miners compensated
for disability.  *Arch. Environ. Health* 27:227-230.

Ortmeyer, C. E., J. Costello, W. K. C. Morgan, S. Swecker
and M. Peterson.  1974.  The mortality of Appalachian
coal miners 1963 to 1971.  *Arch. Environ. Health*
29:67-72.

Palmer, A.  1979.  Mortality experience of 50 workers with
occupational exposures to the products of coal hydrogenation processes.  *J. Occup. Med.* 21:41-44.

Peterson, M. and M. Attfield.  1980.  Estimates of bias in a
longitudinal coal study.  *J. Occup. Med.* 23:44-48.

President's Commission on Coal.  1980.  *Recommendations and
Summary Findings.*  Washington, D.C.

Rae, S.  1971.  Pneumoconiosis and coal dust exposure.  *Brit.
Med. Bull.* 27:53-58.

Redmond, C. K.  1976.  Cancer experience among coke
by-product workers.  *Ann. N.Y. Acad. Sci.* 271:102-115.

Redmond, C. K., A. Ciocco, J. W. Lloyd and H. W. Rush.
1972.  Long term mortality study of steel workers VI:
mortality from malignant neoplasms among coke oven
workers.  *J. Occupat. Med.* 14:621-629.

Reger, R. and J. Hancock.  1980.  Coal miners exposed to
diesel-exhaust emissions.  In *Health Implications of
New Energy Technologies*, pp. 213-231.  W. N. Rom and
V. E. Archer (eds.).  Ann Arbor Science Publishers,
Inc., Ann Arbor, Michigan.

Rockette, H. E.  1977a.  *Mortality of Coal Miners Covered by
the United Mine Workers Health and Retirement Funds.*
Pub. No. 77-155.  National Institute of Occupational
Safety and Health, Washington, D.C.

Rockette, H. E.  1977b.  Cause specific mortality of coal
miners.  *J. Occup. Med.* 19:795-801.

Rockette, H. E.  1980.  Mortality patterns of coal miners. In *Health Implications of New Energy Technologies*, pp. 269-281.  W. N. Rom and V. E. Archer (eds.).  Ann Arbor Science Publishers, Ann Arbor, Michigan.

Rogozen, M. B., L. W. Margler, M. K. Martz and D. F. Hausknecht.  1977.  *Environmental Impacts of Coal Slurry Pipelines and Unit Trains*.  OTA-E-60-PTZ.  Office of Technology Assessment, Washington, D.C.

Rom, W., H. Barkman, W. Turner, R. Kanner, W. Wright, M. Nichols and A. Renzetti, Jr.  1980.  Coal workers' respiratory disease in Utah:  a preliminary report. In *Health Implications of New Energy Technologies*, pp. 247-256.  W. N. Rom and V. E. Archer (eds.).  Ann Arbor Science Publishers, Inc., Ann Arbor, Michigan.

Rowe, M. D.  1980.  Human exposure to sulfates from coal-fired power plants.  *J. Air Pollut. Control Assoc.* 30:682-684.

Salmon, E.  1980.  *Comparative Assessment of Health and Safety Impacts of Coal Use*.  DOE/EV-0069.  U.S. Department of Energy, Washington, D.C.

Schlesinger, R. B., M. Lippman and R. E. Albert.  1978. Effects of short-term exposures to sulfuric acid and ammonium sulfate aerosols upon bronchial airway function in the donkey.  *J. Am. Ind. Hyg. Assoc.* 39:275-285.

Schneiderman, M. A., P. Decoufle and C. C. Brown.  1979. Threshold for environmental cancer:  biological and statistical considerations.  *Ann. N.Y. Acad. Sci.* 329:92-130.

Schoppert, D. W. and D. W. Hoyt.  1968.  *Factors Influencing Safety at Highway-Rail Grade Crossings*.  National Cooperative Highway Research Program Report 50. Transportation Research Board, National Research Council, Washington, D. C.

Schottenfield, D., J. F. Haas, J. G. Meikle, B. R. Hart and A. G. Zauber.  1980.  Epidemiological surveillance of petroleum refinery workers.  In *Human Health and Environmental Toxicants*, pp. 81-89.  Academic Press and Royal Society of Medicine, London.

Selikoff, I. J., M. M. Key and D. H. K. Lee (eds.).  1972. Coal workers' pneumoconiosis.  *Ann. N.Y. Acad. Sci.* 200.

Sexton, R. J.  1960.  The hazards to health in the hydrogenation of coal.  *Arch. Environ. Health* 1:208-231.

Suess, M. J.  1975.  The environmental load and cycle of polycyclic aromatic hydrocarbons.  Presented at *Inter-*

*national Conference on Sensing and Monitoring Environmental Pollutants*, Las Vegas, Nevada, September 1975.

Swanson, V. E., J. H. Medlin, J. R. Hatch, J. L. Coleman, G. H. Wood, S. D. Woodruff and R. T. Hildebrand. 1976. *Collection, Analysis, and Evaluation of Coal Samples in 1975.* U.S. Department of Interior, Geological Survey Open File Report 76-468, Washington, D.C.

Sweet, D. V., W. E. Crouse, J. V. Crable, J. R. Carlberg and W. S. Lainhart. 1974. The relationship of total dust, free silica, and trace metal concentrations to the occupational respiratory disease of bituminous coal miners. *J. Am. Ind. Hyg. Assoc.* 35:479-488.

Theodore Barry and Associates. 1971. *Industrial Engineering Study of Hazards Associated with Underground Coal Mine Production, Vol. I.* OFR 4(I)-72(PB207226). Report to U.S. Bureau of Mines, Washington, D.C.

Thomas, T. L., P. Decoufle and R. Moure-Eraso. 1980. Mortality among workers employed in petroleum refining and petrochemical plants. *J. Occup. Med.* 22:97-103.

U.S. Department of Commerce. 1975. *Statistical Abstract of the United States.* Government Printing Office, Washington, D.C.

Vaughn, B. E., K. H. Abel, D. A. Cataldo, J. M. Hales, C. E. Hane, L. A. Rancitelli, R. C. Routson, R. E. Wildung, and E. G. Wolf. 1975. *Review of Potential Impact on Health and Environmental Quality from Metals Entering the Environment as a Result of Coal Utilization.* Pacific Northwest Laboratories, Battelle Memorial Institute, Richland, Washington.

von Hippel, F. 1981. *Global Risks.* Chapter 5, this volume.

Walton, W. H., J. Dodgson, G. G. Hadden and M. Jacobsen. 1977. Effect of quartz and other non-coal dusts in coal workers' pneumoconiosis, part I epidemiological studies. In *Inhaled Particles IV*, pp. 669-690. W. H. Walton (ed.). Pergamon Press, Oxford.

White, O. (ed.). 1979. *Proceedings of the Symposium on Assessing the Industrial Hygiene Needs for the Coal Conversion and Oil Shale Industries.* BNL-51002, Brookhaven National Laboratory, Upton, N.Y.

Wiser, W. H. 1980. Health implications of coal liquefaction and coal gasification technologies. In *Health Implications of New Energy Technologies*, pp. 307-319. W. N. Rom and V. E. Archer (eds.). Ann Arbor Science Publishers, Ann Arbor, Michigan.

Wolff, R. K., S. A. Silbaugh, D. G. Brownstein, R. L. Carpenter and J. L. Mauderly. 1979. Toxicity of 0.4 and 0.8 µg sulfuric acid aerosols in the guinea pig. *J. Toxicol. Environ. Health* 5:1037-1047.

Wool, H. and J. B. Ostbo. 1980. *The Labor Outlook for the Bituminous Coal Mining Industry.* EA-1477, Electric Power Research Institute, Palo Alto, California.

*John P. Holdren, Kent B. Anderson,*
*Peter M. Deibler, Peter H. Gleick,*
*Irving M. Mintzer, Gregory P. Morris*

# 4. Health and Safety Impacts of Renewable, Geothermal, and Fusion Energy

## Introduction

The increased interest of the last decade in environmental consequences of energy sources is not a temporary aberration. Rather, it reflects a growing awareness that rational choices among alternative approaches to obtain energy benefits require consideration of the full cost − environmental and social as well as monetary − that each approach entails. If maximization of human well-being is the goal, as it should be, then it may be as reasonable to reject an energy technology for excessive environmental or social costs as to do so for the more traditional reason − excessive monetary costs. Much of the interest of professionals and the public in energy sources other than fossil fuels and nuclear fission is, in fact, due to the perception that these "conventional" energy sources, although affordable in monetary terms, suffer from serious environmental and social liabilities (Holdren and Herrera, 1971; Freeman et al., 1974; Budnitz and Holdren, 1976; Brooks et al., 1979). The impression is widespread that alternative sources such as renewables, geothermal energy and fusion will have smaller liabilities in these respects.

In reality, of course, no energy source is completely free of environmental liabilities, and systematic and careful assessment is required to determine how the liabilities of other energy sources compare to those of fossil fuels and fission. Such an assessment ideally would include all of the following classes of environmental effects (Budnitz and Holdren, 1976; Holdren, 1978a):

(1) injuries (fatal and nonfatal, occupational and public) from accidents or sabotage;

(2) illnesses (fatal and nonfatal, occupational and public, somatic and genetic) from routine emissions and exposures;

(3) damage to property;

(4) diminution of well-being through disruption of ecosystems or climate;

(5) aesthetic loss and nuisance; and

(6) undesirable change in sociopolitical conditions and processes.

This chapter treats only the first two categories — the "direct" effects of energy technology on public and occupational health and safety — for a variety of nonfossil, nonfission energy sources:  renewables (solar heating and cooling, solar thermal electricity conversion, photovoltaics, wind, hydropower, ocean energy, and biomass), geothermal energy, and fusion. A recent, broader review of environmental aspects of renewables that touches on all but the sixth category of effects is Holdren, Morris, and Mintzer (1980). A useful compendium of analyses of sociopolitical effects of a wide variety of energy options is Unseld et al. (1979).

Direct impacts on public and occupational health and safety have been the most intensively studied of the environmental effects of fossil fuels and fission, and they are certainly the categories of environmental effects most susceptible to quantitative comparisons among different energy sources. It must be emphasized, however, that these "direct" impacts may not always represent the most important of an energy technology's threats to human well-being. In the case of fossil fuels, for example, it is entirely possible that climate change caused by carbon dioxide accumulation in the atmosphere will undermine human well-being on a larger scale than anything attributable to toxic emissions (U. S. Council on Environmental Quality, 1981); and the biggest risk of heavy use of oil is surely the chance that a world war will be fought over access to Middle East supplies (Deese and Nye, 1981). Similarly, the most important environmental/social liabilities of nuclear fission are its contribution to the spread of nuclear weapons among nations and the possibilities of nuclear terrorism it poses (Nuclear Energy Policy Study Group, 1977). These and other global risks of energy supply are treated in detail by von Hippel elsewhere in this volume; we mention them here to remind the reader that environmental comparisons based only on the kinds of effects emphasized in our own chapter are likely to be woefully incomplete.

The next several sections describe briefly the characteristics of renewable, geothermal, and fusion energy sources that give rise to direct impacts on human health and safety. The final section contains quantitative estimates of health and safety impacts of these technologies in a common format, together with a discussion of the methods by which these estimates were obtained.

## Flat-Plate Solar Collectors

Flat-plate solar collectors for water heating or space heating offer the potential for substantial savings of energy with no emissions of air pollutants during the collectors' operation. The materials requirements for such systems, however, may be relatively large, and may entail emission of significant quantities of air pollutants.

Flat-plate collectors can supply low-temperature heat for several tasks, including domestic and commercial water heating, swimming pool heating, and space heating. This discussion focuses on the use of flat-plate collectors for domestic water heating and space heating.

Domestic water heating is the most economical application of flat-plate collectors (with the possible exception of swimming pool heating) and the largest potential application of such devices. A domestic water heating system can reduce the fuel requirement for water heating by about half, using 5-10 $m^2$ of collector. Large collectors will produce less useful energy per unit of collector area and thus will be somewhat less economical (although, up to a point, they still may produce useful energy more cheaply than the backup fuel). Domestic water heating systems also have the advantages of facing a fairly constant year-round load and requiring little additional equipment besides the collectors themselves and a slightly larger hot-water tank.

All of this is in marked contrast to the use of solar collectors for space heating. In most climates in the United States, a well-insulated house has a highly variable demand for heat, ranging from zero for at least a third of the year to 200-300 MJ per day during extreme cold spells. Simply because of the pattern of space-heating demand, meeting a significant portion of it with a solar collector system requires larger collector areas and larger and more expensive storage systems than supplying the same amount of solar energy for water heating, and hence is less economical (Besant, Dumant, and Schoenau, 1979).

In Tables 1–7, the lower end of the range for flat-
plate collectors is based on the materials requirements for
flat-plate collectors operating under sunny U. S. conditions, while the upper end of the range is based on the
requirements for collectors and all auxiliary equipment for
space-heating applications in unfavorable climates (Albers,
Barviec, and Rooney, 1976).  The upper end thus represents a
highly uneconomic application.  The lower figures, on the
other hand, approximate the materials requirements for a
solar water-heating system but do not include the materials
requirements for plumbing to connect the collectors to the
hot-water system, pumps, valves, controls, heat exchangers,
and a large hot-water tank (Holdren, Morris, and Mintzer,
1980).

The materials requirements for flat-plate collectors
vary greatly from one design to another.  Most manufacturers
produce collectors with either aluminum or copper absorber
panels and glass covers.  This is the type of collector on
which the figures in Tables 1-7 are based, but some designs
use steel absorber panels, some use plastic or fiberglass
covers, and still others make the entire collector of a
lightweight plastic extrusion.  Another design uses an
evacuated glass tube containing a smaller tube that functions as both absorber and heat-transfer tube.  Different
designs could produce very different materials requirements
from those assumed here.

Installation and maintenance of flat-plate collector
systems requires significant amounts of labor, but no
special occupational hazards are evident.  No emissions of
air pollutants attend either installation or operation,
although tiny amounts of materials may outgas from the collectors during stagnation periods (when, either by design or
because of mechanical failure, no heat is being removed from
the collectors).  In systems that use antifreeze compounds
(as opposed to draindown) to prevent freezing of the heat
transfer fluid, a small risk of contamination of the potable
water supply exists, but building codes are designed to
minimize this risk (by requiring the use of double-walled
heat exchangers, for example), and it is not counted here.
Also not counted here is any possible water pollution caused
by spills or improper disposal of such antifreeze compounds.

## Passive Solar Heating and Cooling of Buildings

Passive solar building designs can save energy that
would otherwise be needed for heating and cooling of buildings.  The term "passive solar" encompasses a variety of
building techniques with a corresponding variety of materials requirements, potentials for saving energy, and risks.

Virtually all of the hazards associated with passive solar
technologies arise from the acquisition of building materials.   The construction, operation, and maintenance of
passive solar buildings probably present no hazards beyond
those associated with ordinary buildings.

There is no standard definition of a passive solar
building.   Instead there are several competing definitions
and a catalog of design principles.   The design principles
are all aimed at making the building function as a solar
collector during the heating season while minimizing solar
gains during the cooling season.   Among the generally
agreed-upon principles are:   orient the building with its
long axis running east-west, minimize the window area on the
building's north side, provide adequate window area on the
south side, install properly designed overhangs or external
shading devices to keep direct sunlight off the south-facing
windows during the cooling season, and provide sufficient
"thermal mass" to store excess energy for release at night
(or to store the coolness of night air to reduce cooling
loads during the day).   These principles imply several
others:   the building should be sited with consideration of
solar access; it should be oriented toward the south, with
frequently used rooms on the south side and less frequently
used rooms on the north; and heating and cooling needs
should be minimized by using abundant insulation, multiple-
pane glass, and careful caulking and weatherstripping
(Anderson, 1976; Mazria, 1979).

Passive solar technologies are intimately linked with
energy conservation technologies, to the extent that some
definitions of "passive solar" include ordinary conservation
measures.   Yet there is a major practical distinction
between conservation technologies – such as insulation,
weatherstripping, caulking, and insulating glass, all of
which can be added to any new building with essentially no
thought or redesign of the building – and passive solar
designs, which at a minimum require consideration of orientation and solar access, and which commonly entail modification of the building structure (Anderson, 1981).

For the purposes of this chapter, we consider just two
typical passive solar modifications of an ordinary new residential building:   1) additional south-facing glass replacing a well-insulated wall, and 2) additional thermal mass in
the building's interior.   In many respects this represents a
worst-case analysis of passive solar designs, because alternative formulations – using for example, a poorly insulated
house to begin with, or simply rearranging of windows –
could produce larger energy savings and smaller (or zero)
materials requirements.   But the analysis chosen is a more

realistic characterization of the opportunities for passive solar designs in new residences, where the choice is whether to build a well-insulated building that pays no attention to the sun or one modified to take advantage of seasonal variations.

Passive solar technologies can be compared to technologies that produce energy because the passive solar designs can save energy that otherwise would have to be used for space heating and cooling. The passive solar technologies are therefore "worth" the energy they displace. The form, timing, and amount of the energy savings are determined by the energy use before the energy-saving technology is applied (the "base case"). Different assumptions about the base case will produce different results for the value of energy-saving technologies. The results presented here are based on an analysis of a variety of ordinary conservation and passive solar technologies for space conditioning of new single-family houses (Anderson, 1981). They assume a base case of a house with R-30 insulation in the ceiling[1], R-19 insulation in the walls, and double pane windows. They also assume that a 10°F nighttime thermostat setback is used during the heating season. It is important to note that our base case house already has 44 ft$^2$ of south-facing windows; these windows, which represent just one-quarter of the building's total window area, collect much useful solar energy. Our figures for "additional south-facing windows" assume that 100 ft$^2$ of double pane windows are added to this building, that the windows are shaded by a fixed overhang, and that no insulation is applied to the windows at night.

The health and safety risks associated with the passive solar technologies considered here are concentrated almost entirely in the materials-acquisition phase. The use of additional south-facing windows entails additional glass manufacture (in fact, a very large amount of glass manufacture per unit of energy, relative to other technologies). It also requires additional wood (above what would be needed for a stud wall) for the structural framing around the window opening, and wood or aluminum for the window frame itself. Manufacture of these materials entails emissions and occupational hazards, as does the manufacture of any material. But beyond this stage, there is little if any additional health or safety hazard. In terms of risk, installation of windows is not much different than constructing a wall. During the building's lifetime, the windows emit no pollutants and pose little hazard. Perhaps maintaining windows (washing them) is slightly more hazardous than "maintaining" the wall section they replace, but no data on this point are available.

For the thermal mass, the concentration of the risks in the materials acquisition stage is even clearer. Maintenance (painting) of concrete walls is essentially identical to that of wooden ones.

## Solar Thermal Electricity

Several different approaches currently are under development for the conversion of solar thermal energy into electricity. In this section we discuss four of these approaches: solar ponds, power towers, paraboloidal dishes, and parabolic troughs.

The solar pond approach involves the construction of saline ponds approximately one to two meters deep for the collection of low-temperature heat (Office of Technology Assessment, 1978). The heat collected and stored in these ponds may be used to drive low-temperature heat engines for the generation of electricity (Office of Technology Assessment, 1978; California Energy Commission, 1980b).

In the power-tower, paraboloidal-dish and parabolic-trough approaches, heat is collected at higher temperatures than in the solar ponds by using tracking concentrators. Higher conversion efficiencies are achieved at the cost of greater collector complexity. In the power-tower design, a field of steerable mirrors (called heliostats) focuses sunlight onto a receiver-boiler mounted atop a central tower. Health hazards particular to this approach arise from the tower itself (e.g., worker falls, aircraft collisions) and from the possibility of people encountering the concentrated beam (U. S. Energy Research Development Administration, 1977a; U. S. Department of Energy, 1979c; Holdren, Morris, and Mintzer, 1980). The latter could result in the temporary blinding of aircraft pilots or of automobile drivers.

In the parabolic-trough approach, the collectors focus sunlight on a selectively coated pipe mounted along the trough axis. Through this pipe flows a high-temperature working fluid such as liquid sodium, which is pumped to a centrally located heat exchanger and boiler. Working fluid leaks and fires are potential hazards during routine operations. Additional hazards may arise from the large amount of thermal storage medium needed in both the power-tower and the parabolic-trough approaches to achieve high-plant capacity factors.

In the paraboloidal dish concept, a small high-temperature heat engine is located at the focus of a two-axis tracking concentrator. The electricity generated by these distributed dishes is then transferred to a central

switchyard and dispatched from the plant into the surrounding
grid. The primary hazard is one of leakage of the working
fluid from the individual heat engines.

Because all of the high-temperature solar thermal systems are very capital intensive and use only direct beam
radiation, there is a strong economic incentive to locate
them in the sunniest regions. They are likely to be
deployed in large, central station power plants remote from
the load centers which they serve. Construction of these
plants will require large amounts of common construction
materials, especially steel, concrete, aluminum, copper, and
glass. Routine emissions generated in the manufacture of
these materials will be mainly carbon monoxide, hydrocarbons, particulates, oxides of nitrogen, and fluorides.
These emissions will cause measurable public risk to populations downwind of smelting and refining facilities (Davidson
and Grether, 1977; Davidson, Grether, and Wilcox, 1977;
Office of Technology Assessment, 1978; Holdren, Morris, and
Mintzer, 1980).

Decommissioning of these facilities may require special
handling of working fluids and coolants. Most other materials can be disposed of without special precautions. If
the "best available technology" is applied throughout the
solar-electric-energy supply cycle, the total health risks
from construction and operation of these facilities are
expected to be appreciably smaller than the risks anticipated from delivering an equivalent amount of electricity
from coal.

## Terrestrial Photovoltaics

Photovoltaic cells use semiconductor materials to convert sunlight to low-voltage, direct current electricity.
Photovoltaic power systems may be deployed in large, central-
station power plants, sited in remote areas that experience
high levels of insolation. These systems are also amenable
to dispersed applications in which the photovoltaics are
integrated into the walls and roofs of conventional buildings.

Each of the most promising semiconductor materials
poses significant hazards of human exposure to toxic materials (Mintzer, 1980). The three semiconductor materials
closest to large-scale commercial deployment are silicon,
cadmium sulfide and gallium arsenide. Workers in the materials-acquisition and device-fabrication stages of the
photovoltaic energy cycle may be exposed to dusts, fumes,
and aerosols with large fractions of respirable particles
averaging less than one micron in diameter (Gandel and Dil-

lard, 1976; Mintzer, 1980; U. S. Energy Research Development Administration, 1977b; Habegger, Gasper, and Brown, 1980).

Chronic inhalation of small particles of silicon is known to cause silicosis, a progressive scarring of human lung tissue (U. S. Energy Research Development Administration, 1977b; U. S. Department of Energy, 1977). Large quantities of these small particles are generated in the submerged-electrode arc furnace which is commonly used to refine silica or quartzite ($SiO_2$) into metallurgical-grade silicon, a precursor of the polycrystalline silicon used to fabricate silicon photovoltaic cells. Fumes containing these particles diffuse into the work environment and escape up the stack. The introduction of the closed-top arc furnace may significantly reduce both the occupational and public exposure to this risk (Hunt et al., 1978).

Cadmium is a long-term cumulative poison which is known to concentrate in the human kidney. Chronic exposure to airborne particles of cadmium has been associated epidemiologically with increased incidence of proteinuria, emphysema, and hypertension. Chronic ingestion of foodstuffs contaminated with cadmium is believed to be the cause of the disease known in Japan as Itai-Itai (U. S. Environmental Protection Agency, 1974).

Workers in the zinc-smelting and cadmium-refining industries may be exposed to dusts containing significant amounts of cadmium oxide. Individuals working in facilities where cadmium sulfide cells are fabricated by vapor- or spray-deposition processes may be exposed to fumes and aerosols containing cadmium sulfide (CdS) (Gandel and Dillard, 1976). The loss fraction for cadmium in the Jordan process of spray deposition may be as high as 1% by weight. In addition to occupational exposure inside the plants, there is also a residual risk of public exposure to airborne cadmium downwind from smelting, refining, and fabrication facilities (Neff, 1978). Fabrication of front-wall CdS cells by the modified Clevite process of vapor deposition generates significantly less risk of both occupational and public exposure.

Arsenic, a poison of historic as well as literary fame, is toxic if either ingested or inhaled. It was recently designated by the Environmental Protection Agency as a suspected carcinogen. It is most commonly present as the oxide, $As_2O_3$, called white arsenic. Gallium is nontoxic and so will not be discussed in this review.

Worker exposure to $As_2O_3$ occurs in conjunction with arsenic separation during copper and lead smelting as well as during gallium arsenide cell fabrication (Hovel, 1975; Neff, 1978; Mintzer, 1980). Considerable risk exists for slow leakage of fumes containing arsenic from the high-pressure crystallization furnace in which single crystals of gallium arsenide (GaAs) are grown. Standards for occupational exposure to arsenic recently have been reduced from 500 µg/l to a time-averaged exposure of 5 µg/l.

In addition to the risks associated with materials acquisition and refining of the primary semiconductor materials, workers also will be exposed to other toxic chemicals during the fabrication of the devices. Toxic substances encountered during device fabrication include strong acids, dopants, solvents, degreasers, and the fumes from soldering and welding. Processes that involve slicing ingots of single-crystal material into wafers with diamond-blade or multi-wire slurry saws may expose workers to aerosols containing cutting oils and silicon-carbide grit (Gandel and Dillard, 1976; Mintzer, 1980).

Both CdS and GaAs cells pose additional health risks from accidents occurring during operation. Cadmium sulfide cells may volatilize if exposed to high temperatures, allowing cadmium sulfide or cadmium oxide to be released. In dispersed applications, in which these cells are mounted on the walls or roofs of conventional buildings, these cells are vulnerable to the extreme heat generated by building fires. Dangerous levels of acute exposure would occur only if several adjacent buildings equipped with these devices burned simultaneously. Since cadmium exposure is known to have a cumulative long-term effect, there could be a problem caused by chronic exposure among firefighters. If cadmium sulfide cells were deployed on a large scale in residential communities, modifications in the firefighting techniques used in these communities might be necessary (Neff, 1978; Mintzer, 1980).

Because of their high conversion efficiency, gallium arsenide cells are likely candidates for use in photovoltaic collectors with a high optical concentration ratio (Kelly, 1978; Office of Technology Assessment, 1978; Ehrenreich, 1979). In many such designs, active cooling of the arrays is required. In the event of a loss-of-coolant accident, the cells of a single collector or of a series of linked collectors might be permanently damaged and the arsenic might be released in the form of $As_2O_3$. In those designs in which optical concentration is achieved by using acrylic Fresnel lenses, a fire that occurs in one area could spread across an entire array field. In such a fire, an entire central station facility could be disabled and a large amount of arsenic released. Such a release could result in a significant exposure to off-site populations and may result in contamination of valuable land downwind from the facility. Since both cadmium and arsenic are known to pass through food chains and to concentrate in higher organisms, off-site contamination of land or water supplies by either of these elements must be avoided.

The power-conditioning equipment used to boost voltage and to convert the direct-current output of photovoltaic cells to alternating current contains toxic substances. These substances are liable to leakage or release in fires (Holdren, Morris, and Mintzer, 1980). Electricity storage by means of lead-acid or other batteries poses chemical, fire, and explosion hazards.

In addition to the occupational and public risks posed by the manufacture and use of photovoltaic cells, there are also hazards generated by the production of the more common materials used to encapsulate, frame and support photovoltaic modules. Significant amounts of atmospheric emissions occur in the production of the aluminum, steel, glass, and concrete used in the construction of these systems. Workers in the manufacturing facilities are exposed to the occupational risks typical of each of these industries.

The normal operating lifetime of photovoltaic power systems is expected to be measured in decades. Eventually, however, they will degrade. Depending on the semiconductors contained in the cells, some special precautions may be necessary for safe decommissioning of these devices (Holdren, Morris, and Mintzer, 1980). Silicon, because it is biologically inert, will not require special handling. Cells containing cadmium and arsenic, however, must be disposed of in such a way as to guarantee their isolation from the biosphere for an indefinite period. If allowed to leach into soils or water supplies, these elements may migrate into the food web with damaging consequences.

The health hazards posed by large-scale deployment of photovoltaics are significant but manageable with existing technology. The risks posed by the production and use of silicon cells are the least severe. Large-scale use of cadmium or arsenic in these devices will yield both occupational and public-health risks if these materials are allowed to enter the biosphere. Despite the high materials requirements involved in the fabrication of photovoltaic power systems, application of the "best available technologies" for pollution abatement is expected to reduce the life-cycle risks of this technology to levels significantly less than those to be expected if the same amount of electricity were generated from coal.

## Orbiting Photovoltaic Power Systems

Orbiting photovoltaic power systems would employ large arrays of silicon or gallium arsenide photovoltaic cells placed in geosynchronous orbit above the earth's surface. Because the receiving surface of the photovoltaic array would be designed to track the sun, electricity could be generated by these systems continuously. The electrical energy produced by the photovoltaics would be beamed in the form of microwaves to large, ground-mounted receivers, called rectennas. Power-conditioning equipment located at the rectenna sites would convert the energy embodied in the microwaves back to electricity and inject the resulting current into utility grids as baseload power. A "reference system" currently under development by the Department of Energy and the National Aeronautics and Space Administration involves deployment of 60 such satellites at a rate of two per year, each with a rated capacity of 5 GW(e) (U. S. Department of Energy, 1978; Moses, 1979; Herendeen, Kary and Rebitzer, 1979).

The most important components of the current "reference system" design for the space power satellite are a tensioned-array structure fabricated from a graphite composite mate-rial, with gallium-aluminum-arsenide solar cells and an amplifier/transmitter mounted on this array structure. The amplifier/transmitter would utilize a large klystron tube for power amplification and conversion of the direct current output of the photovoltaics to microwave frequencies (Habegger, Gasper, and Brown, 1980). Other major components include a graphite-epoxy transmitting antenna and a directional controller which would "lock on" to a pilot beam generated at the rectenna site. The large tensioned array would be fabricated in geosynchronous orbit, the individual elements extruded by automated manufacturing equipment. The photovoltaic cells would be carried into orbit and "rolled out" like a carpet. Worker/astronauts would attach the photovoltaic cells to the skeleton formed by the tensioned array.

The collector area of the space power satellite may be as large as 30 $km^2$. The rectenna sites are estimated to have approximately 80 $km^2$ of active receiver area. The exclusion zone surrounding each rectenna will increase land area requirements from approximately 55 $km^2$ for the rectennas alone to approximately 100 $km^2$ for the facility as a whole. The design for the rectennas calls for a collection of rectifying diodes mounted on steel mesh plates which are attached to a steel and concrete structure. The energy generated by the photovoltaic arrays will be beamed to the rectenna site at a frequency of 2.45 gigahertz. The beam

density at the center of the transmitting antenna is estimated to be 22 kW/cm$^2$. At the center of the rectenna field
the power density of the beam would be approximately 23 mW/
cm$^2$, while at the edge of the rectenna field the figure
would be about 1 mW/cm$^2$ (U. S. Department of Energy, 1978).

The construction and deployment of orbiting photovoltaic power systems could generate significant health hazards
at each stage of the energy-supply cycle. Because final
agreement has not been reached on a specific design for the
space power satellite and because of the lack of experience
in construction of large-scale projects in space, considerable uncertainty exists as to the magnitudes of the risks
involved in such an enterprise.

Construction of launch facilities, transport rockets
and the ground-mounted rectennas all will require large
volumes of such conventional construction materials as
steel, concrete, aluminum, and copper. Production of these
materials will entail health and safety risks to workers and
will produce air pollutants and water pollutants to which
the general public will be exposed (Teeter and Jamieson,
1980). In addition, manufacture of the GaAs solar cells and
some of the exotic components of the rockets will expose
workers and the public to airborne arsenic and fine particulates of metallic compounds. Since none of these materials
has ever been produced in the quantities required by the
space-power-satellite program, methods for control of toxic
residuals at the requisite scale have not been developed.

Transportation of the necessary materials into space
will generate both occupational and public health risks.
Accidents on launch could result in significant health
effects. Explosion of a heavy-lift launch vehicle with a
full load of liquid hydrogen has the potential to cause
first degree burns 300 meters from the launch site. A worst-
case analysis of potential accidents of this type suggests
that as many as 1000 immediate deaths could result (Habegger,
Gasper, and Brown, 1980).

Placing into high orbit as much as 50 million kg per
satellite, the current "reference system" concepts will
require as many as 100 flights by the heavy lift launch
vehicle, 30 flights of the personnel launch vehicle, 30
flights of the cargo orbiter transfer vehicle, and 25
flights of the personnel orbiter transfer vehicle per 5 GW
satellite (Habegger, Gasper, and Brown, 1980). The exhaust
from this launch series would pollute both troposphere and
stratosphere. The consequences of a large program could
include changes of patterns of cloudiness and precipitation
in the troposphere causing possible negative effects on

agricultural productivity. The consequences could also include changes in the vertical structure of the stratosphere with unknown but possibly nonnegligible effects on climate (Moses, 1979).

Occupational health and safety problems in space will include exposure to cosmic rays, effects of long periods of weightlessness, and hazards associated with failures of the life-support systems. Failure of any of the essential life support systems while personnel are in orbit could cause immediate catastrophic consequences to workers. Both the workers and their equipment will be exposed to high-energy beams of heavy ions, electron-bremsstrahlung, ultraviolet radiation and meteors. The lack of social and recreational opportunities combined with long periods of weightlessness may place additional physiological and psychological stress on the worker-astronauts (Habegger, Gasper, and Brown, 1980).

Early attention to possible health effects of the space power satellite has focused mainly on the 2.45-GHz microwave beam. This beam may be hazardous to workers in the orbiting units, to workers at or near the 100 km$^2$ receivers on the ground, to members of the public in the vicinity of the receivers, and to aircraft passengers flying through the beam. Unscheduled excursions of the microwave beam may expose individuals to power densities approaching the Occupational Safety and Health Administration limits for occupational exposure of 25 mW/cm$^2$. The impacts on human health of long-term low-level exposure to microwave radiation are not well understood. Early studies suggest that chronic exposure to this type of radiation may induce mutagenic, teratogenic, immunologic and neurologic effects in humans (Habegger, Gasper, and Brown, 1980). No threshold level (beneath which exposure is without consequence) has yet been determined.

Workers at the rectenna site may be chronically exposed to microwaves at low power density. Members of the public living outside the exclusion zone at the rectenna site may also be exposed to low-intensity microwaves due to reflections and anomalies in the rectenna field. The health effects of chronic exposure to this type of radiation are not currently understood.

Development of the space power satellite poses an additional series of indirect risks to human health. Many of the components developed for this program have potentially destructive uses as part of advanced weapon systems. The launch and transport vehicles built for the space power satellite program could also be used to deliver military hardware into orbit. The immense generating capacity of the orbiting array could provide the motive power for the advanced particle beam weapons currently under development in both the United States and the U.S.S.R.  In addition, if the current reference design using a pilot beam to guide transmission of the power beam is modified, it may be possible to direct all or part of the energy output of the space power satellite onto military or civilian targets. Because the beam is odorless, colorless, weightless, and smokeless, and the effects of chronic exposure to low-intensity microwaves are difficult to distinguish, it would be very difficult to verify that it was not being used intermittently or consistently as an anti-personnel weapon.

Estimates of the risks from deployment of orbiting photovoltaic power systems are burdened by ranges of uncertainty spanning several orders of magnitude.  All stages of this energy supply cycle will involve very high capital costs and will have the potential for causing significant numbers of premature deaths.  The magnitude of the risks can not be closely specified at this time.  The technology for controlling the risks or mitigating the hazards of this scheme is not now available.  Such control technology is unlikely to be developed on the same time scale as the one proposed by advocates of this technology.

## Wind Systems

Many different designs and sizes of wind energy conversion systems are available for both centralized and dispersed applications.  Wind turbines with power outputs exceeding 1 MW are already being integrated into electric utility grids, and smaller units, in the kilowatt range, are available for individual residential and commercial applications.

The health and safety effects of these systems are unlikely to be serious.  Materials requirements for large wind systems (see Table 1) are not particularly great, and neither, therefore, are the occupational effects and emissions associated with materials acquisition.  Wind energy systems use and produce no unusual materials with potentially toxic characteristics, as do some of the other energy systems.  In addition, labor requirements for construction and operation and maintenance appear to be of the same order of magnitude as those for conventional energy systems.  The jobs themselves may be riskier if considerable work is done while on the towers that support the blades and power equipment.  Trained personnel will do these tasks, however, and the occupational risks to such workers are unlikely to be significantly higher than the risks to workers in other industries (U. S. Department of Labor, 1978b).

Small wind machines for dispersed residential operation may pose greater risks to workers and the public than do large units. Small machines are considerably more materials intensive (Lawrence and Strojan, 1980; U. S. Department of Energy, 1980a) and their installation and maintenance is more likely to be done by less-skilled homeowners than by trained workers. Detailed data on smaller wind generators are insufficient to estimate the occupational and public risks.

Both large and small wind turbines share the liability of possible blade failure, causing the blade or blade fragment to become a projectile. Such incidents are unlikely to be common or particularly hazardous when they occur. Blade failures in dispersed urban operation will be more hazardous than in large arrays sited in windy, unpopulated areas. For any wind turbine, the angular velocity, angle of throw, and size of the blade fragment determine the distance such a fragment will travel. For remote applications, such a distance might be used to site a cluster of machines away from highways or communities.

Electricity produced by wind turbines will be used to displace more expensive fossil fuels. Since the wind is an intermittent source of energy, wind turbines will, at least initially, be operated in a fuel-saving mode similar to run-of-river (non-peaking) operation of hydroelectric systems. Capacity factors are expected to range from 20-50% for low- and high-wind locations (U. S. Department of Energy, 1979d, 1980a). Wind systems are likely to be located in high-wind regions initially, but the risk estimates presented in Tables 3-4 include low-wind regimes.

Operating wind machines as fuel savers means that early wind systems are unlikely to include any significant energy storage schemes such as compressed air, batteries, flywheels, or coupled arrays of wind machines and hydroelectric pumped-storage units. Such schemes pose hazards of their own that will have to be evaluated as they are proposed and their design characteristics become known. If wind energy systems are ever used for intermediate or baseload electricity production, it is possible that sufficient reliability can be achieved by combining large-scale systems that are geographically dispersed, eliminating the need for extensive storage.

## Hydroelectric Systems

Hydropower is the most extensively exploited of all the renewable resources, supplying more than 10% of total U. S. electricity consumption. Although considerable new potential

exists at both developed and undeveloped sites, large amounts
of new hydroelectricity are unlikely to be produced, for two
main reasons. First, new large sites have become scarce.
Second, the construction of new dams for hydroelectric power
is arguably the worst electricity option in terms of damage
to environmental goods and services per unit of electrical
energy produced (Harte and Jassby, 1978; Brooks et al.,
1979). For this latter reason, and because hydroelectric
reservoirs often flood valuable land, new dams are increasingly difficult to site.

Several complications arise when one attempts to calculate generic occupational and public health and safety risks
of hydroelectric systems. First, hydroelectric dams vary
tremendously in size, design, mode of operation, and location, and no single generalized design can be identified.
The installed capacity of hydroelectric dams ranges between
tens of kilowatts and thousands of megawatts, and dam designs
range from massive earth-filled structures to thin-walled
concrete arches. Second, energy production at dams may be
restricted by seasonal irrigation needs upstream and down-
stream, by the need for empty flood control storage in the
reservoir behind the dam, or by industrial or municipal water
supply requirements. Finally, the marginal risks of developing new capacity at existing dams may differ significantly
from the risks present during the construction of new facilities. All of these variables affect the nature, magnitude,
and distribution of the health and safety effects associated
with hydroelectric facilities.

New Dams

In the past, hydroelectric potential was exploited by
building new dams in a river system. For new dams, the
health and safety risks resemble the risks experienced during the design, construction, and operation and maintenance
of most conventional energy systems. Occupational risks
arise from acquiring and transporting the materials for the
dam and power-generating equipment; from constructing the
dam, powerhouse, and associated facilities; and from operating and maintaining the unit. Few of the noxious environmental residuals associated with operating fossil-fuel and
other conventional electricity-generating facilities are
present, although changes in water quality in the reservoir
and in the downstream stretches of the river may affect
alternative uses for the water (such as recreation, water
supply, or irrigation).

Even though the occupational risks of additional capacity from new dams are not unusually large, as already
mentioned, many more new dams are unlikely to be built.

## Existing Dams

The occupational risks associated with adding electric-ity-generating capacity at existing hydroelectric and non-hydroelectric dams are significantly less than the risks of building new dams. The risks of materials acquisition and facility construction are almost entirely eliminated, with the exception of acquiring, fabricating, and installing the power equipment, and of reinforcing and renovating the dam itself. Many old dams, abandoned years ago for economic reasons, are in need of structural inspection and rehabili-tation before they can be used to produce electricity. A program to inspect and renovate these dams may significantly reduce the risk of dam failure — the most serious component of risk to the public.

## Catastrophic Risks

All dams pose the risk of catastrophic failure, threat-ening the lives and property of individuals living in down-stream floodplains. Although such occurrences are rare, they are not unknown and the consequences can be severe. A study of the worst consequences of the sudden failure of a number of major California dams estimated fatalities rang-ing from 11,000 up to as high as 240,000 (Ayyaswamy et al., 1974). Public deaths resulting from catastrophic dam fail-ures differ from public deaths from emissions in terms of lost life-expectancy. Such deaths are likely to result in decades of lost life-expectancy, compared to days to months for public deaths due to aggravation of pre-existing respi-ratory diseases associated with sulfates and particulates.[2] Additional public risks may arise from increased recrea-tional hazards (such as boating and swimming accidents) that occur on the reservoir created behind hydroelectric dams. Calculating these risks accurately is extremely difficult and subjective because of the poor quality of the data and the stage of development of the methodology.

## Calculating the Risks

Surprisingly, materials requirements for hydroelectric systems are poorly documented. The best data come from actual statistics on a series of 25 Tennessee Valley Author-ity dams (Tennessee Valley Authority, 1954), from the Bech-tel materials model (Carasso et al., 1975), and from a study on materials demands in the United States for future energy development by the U. S. Geological Survey (Albers, Barveic, and Rooney, 1976). Historical data on the risks to workers, although theoretically more suited to calculating these risks, are not available in satisfactory quantity or form (Holdren et al., 1979). Estimates of labor requirements for construction and operation and maintenance times are available from the Department of Energy and from the Bechtel model (Carasso et al., 1975; U. S. Department of Energy, 1980b). These estimates were used to calculate the construction risks and operation and maintenance risks in the same manner as for the other technologies, assuming that construction risks fall into the category of general construction (SIC, 15-17) and operation and maintenance risks fall into the category of electric services (SIC, 491) (U. S. Department of Labor, 1978).

Since the occupational risks include the risk of transporting the materials required to build the dam, typically earth and rock, hydroelectric systems have a large component of transportation risk. Even though the majority of dam materials are not transported long distances (usually tens of miles) the sheer mass of materials adds significantly to the overall risk.

Building new large and small hydroelectric dams will have greater occupational health and safety impacts than will retrofitting existing dams with generating equipment. Because new dams also will have considerably greater ecological impacts (Gleick, 1980), attention should focus on the capacity that is available at existing sites. Programs to renovate existing non-hydroelectric dams could also reduce significantly the probability of dam failures — a worthy goal regardless of the magnitude of the energy available at these sites.

### Ocean Energy Systems

Schemes to produce electricity from the ocean were first proposed well over 100 years ago. The two principal concepts currently under extensive development are: (1) running a low-temperature heat engine on the temperature difference between warm water near the ocean surface and the colder waters far below; and (2) tapping the energy available in waves through various devices that convert the vertical motion of waves into mechanical motion useful for driving some type of engine. Of all of the concepts proposed to date, the first, called ocean thermal energy conversion (OTEC), is the closest to commercial operation.[3]

Because the energy available in the ocean is diffuse, and because devices placed in the ocean will experience harsh conditions, large quantities of materials will be required to produce significant amounts of energy. The energy collectors will have to be located offshore, and transmission of the energy to points of demand will require additional materials and facilities.

Ocean Thermal Energy Conversion

There has been considerable research on the utilization of temperature differences between the warm upper layers and cold lower layers of the ocean. The technology for producing electricity involves operating a low-temperature heat engine using tremendous flows of ocean water and enormous heat exchangers. A working fluid such as ammonia, suitable for operation in a low temperature thermal cycle, is required. The materials requirements in Table 1 span a range of theoretical designs. Although no particularly esoteric materials are likely to be used, considerable fabrication will be required for the heat exchangers and the water-delivery pipes. This extra handling of the materials will increase the overall occupational risks. The use of ammonia as a working fluid will pose additional risks should routine or accidental releases occur.

For the purposes of this analysis, we have assumed that the construction of OTEC plants involves equal components of ship-building and routine power-plant construction. Any construction that must be done on site in the open ocean will add to the risks faced by workers. Similarly, operation and maintenance is assumed to be a combination of electric services and water transportation services but will be considerably riskier since it will occur in the open ocean and may involve extensive diving and underwater repair. Labor requirements for construction, operation, and maintenance have been estimated by contractors developing and studying OTEC system designs (Lockheed Missiles and Space Company Inc., 1975; Perry, Marland, and Zelby, 1978).

The public risks from OTEC systems are not expected to be large, although there are several possible areas in which risks could be incurred. Major collisions at sea involving passenger ships, although unlikely, could result in significant loss of life. Accidents involving biocides used to clean piping and the heat exchangers could affect members of the public, although the direct effects of such accidents are likely to be on local ecosystems. Similarly, routine or accidental spills of ammonia could affect the public if such spills occur on or close to land.

The greatest uncertainty in the public risks associated with ocean thermal energy systems arises from the climatic effects that may occur if they are deployed in large numbers. These effects could arise for two reasons: (1) changes in the surface temperature of large areas of ocean could affect precipitation and temperatures on nearby land masses; and (2) large quantities of cold water from the deep layers of the ocean may, when brought up to the surface, release carbon dioxide to the atmosphere. The complexities of ocean-atmosphere $CO_2$ exchange make this phenomenon as yet poorly understood, and neither it nor the possible resultant effect on climate can be quantified.

## Wave Energy Systems

A number of schemes have been proposed for tapping the energy available in the waves. Four major designs are being investigated and some of these have been produced as experimental models (Ross, 1979). The economic cost of producing and maintaining large numbers of these devices may be a significant barrier to their deployment, assuming a mature technology can be developed. Construction of these devices could be done on land, and the units deployed like buoys or offshore tanker-loading points. Maintenance of the devices is likely to be both difficult and dangerous.

Because wave-energy systems are still in the design stage, no materials numbers or estimates of labor requirements for construction, operation, and maintenance are available. As a result, no risk estimates are possible. The nature of these devices, however, suggests that occupational risks are likely to be quite significant.

### Fuels from Biomass

The term "biomass" covers a diverse array of photosynthetically derived materials. Biomass has always been used as a source of food and materials; now it is playing an increasingly important role as an energy source. Some forms of biomass are suitable for use as solid fuels; all forms can be converted into liquid or gaseous fuels (synfuels). Biomass resources include concentrated wastes that routinely require management and disposal (municipal solid wastes, sewage, manure at large feedlots, wastes from the food processing and wood products industries); wastes that are generated in a dispersed pattern and are not routinely collected for purposes of waste management (crop residues, logging residues, manure from small feedlots and grazing animals); and biomass that is specially grown or collected for man's use (harvesting of standing forests, intensive cultivation of biomass crops).

The conversion of concentrated wastes to energy will have beneficial effects for public health by helping to solve current waste-disposal problems. The collection of dispersed residues and the production of new-growth biomass for energy, in contrast, will have mainly adverse health effects. Agricultural and forestry operations provide suitable analogs for most of the occupational categories that will be employed in these endeavors (Morris, 1980). Agricultural operations achieve a level of occupational health and safety that is well above the average level for all workers in the United States. Forestry operations, by contrast, suffer from a rather high level of occupational risk. In data compiled by the Federal Department of Labor, forestry is one of the highest risk occupations in terms of total work-days lost due to accidents (U. S. Department of Labor, 1978a). Whether the very high level of risk reported by the Department of Labor for conventional forestry operations is directly applicable to silvicultural operations geared to biomass-energy production, however, must be questioned. Forestry operations for producing biomass energy will probably be highly mechanized, and little tree climbing work will be required. Mechanized pulpwood-harvesting operations achieve significantly lower accident levels than is characteristic of the forestry industry as a whole. The National Safety Council (NSC) accident-rate data for the forestry industry show a value for work-days lost that is only one-third as big as that reported by the Department of Labor (NSC, 1978). The NSC's sample group is made up of member companies, and is largely skewed to the largest operations in the industry as a whole, which is the sample group for the Department of Labor statistics. These large companies are the biggest users of the most modern mechanized equipment, so the NSC data probably better reflect the level of occupational risk that can be expected from silvicultural-energy operations. This risk level is still worse than the average for all jobs in the United States, but it is well within the range of other risky jobs.

While the occupational hazards of growing and collecting biomass residues are well known, it is difficult to determine the seriousness of the public health hazards of these activities. The most serious source of concern associated with most of these activities derives from the increased use of agricultural chemicals, such as pesticides, herbicides, and fertilizers, necessary to protect cultivated crops and to replace nutrients embodied in the biomass (Larson, 1979). Another potentially serious public health effect from biomass-residue production is associated with the non-commercial harvesting of trees for use as firewood in residential applications. Wood-cutting accidents can cause serious injuries and deaths. It is worth noting that this particular public-health risk accrues directly to the people who benefit from the use of the energy produced, a circumstance that is not typical of most of the public-health risks considered here.

Most dry forms of biomass can be burned directly to produce heat, steam, or electricity. The wood products industry currently uses more than a quad per year ($10^{18}$ J/yr) of its wastes (bark, shavings, sawdust, pulping liquor) for process heat and the cogeneration of heat and electricity, and firewood use in residential applications is rapidly approaching the quad per year level (Tillman, 1978; High, 1980).  Direct combustion of biomass has the most serious implications for public health of any biomass energy technology, especially if combustion is carried out in the urban environment.  While biomass combustion produces low levels of sulfur-oxide emissions compared to oil or coal combustion, it produces high levels of particulates and comparable levels of other combustion emissions (oxides of nitrogen, carbon monoxide, hydrocarbons) (Morris, 1980).  A significant fraction of the particulates derived from biomass combustion are in the respirable size range (<1 micron diameter) (Cooper, J., 1980), and these particles, which are mostly particulate carbon, may have traces of polycyclic aromatic hydrocarbons (PAHs) bound to them.  The health impacts of fine particulate carbon are only beginning to be studied (Budiansky, 1980), while many PAHs are well known carcinogens.  The occupational risks associated with industrial wood combustion are likely to be comparable to those associated with coal combustion.

Wood stoves and fireplaces also present a greater fire hazard to homes than other heating modes (Shelton, 1979), possibly as much as doubling the risk of a fire where wood burning is the primary heating source.  The most important causes of this increased fire hazard are believed to be improper installation and maintenance of wood-burning equipment, so this hazard may be amenable to straightforward technical solutions.

Two basic approaches are available for the production of synfuels from biomass:  biological conversion and thermochemical conversion.  Biological conversion technologies produce virtually no air pollutants, although fuel combustion to provide process heat may be a source of air emissions (Morris, 1980).  The thermochemical conversion technologies will produce some airborne emissions, but at a substantially lower level than is the case with direct biomass combustion.  The combustion of biomass-derived synfuels, too, should lead to substantially lower levels of emissions, especially of particulates, than solid biomass combustion.  In almost every case, the total fuel-cycle emissions from biomass-synfuels schemes should be less for a given quantity of energy produced than the fuel-cycle emissions from solid biomass combustion (Morris, 1980).

Synfuels production, especially when thermochemical conversion technologies are used, may produce waste water

contaminated with highly toxic chemicals. These wastes
present a hazard that is similar to that faced by workers in
the petrochemicals industry. Synfuels technologies may have
the effect of reducing the public's health risk from biomass
energy production at the expense of increasing the occupational risk.

## Geothermal Energy

Our discussion of geothermal technologies is based on
one vapor-dominated and two liquid-dominated Known Geothermal Resource Areas (KGRAs) in the United States.[4] The
generic health and safety issues discussed, however, will be
present to some degree at any geothermal development. The
Geysers field, one of the world's few vapor-dominated areas,
has operated for two decades and currently generates in
excess of 900 MW(e) (McIlraith, 1980). In the accompanying
calculations, data are used also for two liquid-dominated
KGRA's, Heber in the Imperial Valley of southern California
and the Baca Ranch of New Mexico. Neither plant is yet
operating, but they will constitute the first United States
commercial use of the liquid-dominated resource for electricity generation.

The two greatest concerns for occupational and public
health and safety are hydrogen sulfide ($H_2S$) and noise.
Other noncondensable gases (primarily ammonia), radon, and
water quality are health and safety issues of lesser magnitude.

Hydrogen sulfide is a highly toxic gas considered
dangerous at concentrations in the range of 200 to 1000
parts per million (ppm) by volume (Layton, 1980). At concentrations in excess of 1000 ppm, pulmonary edema (fluid
accumulation in the lungs) is followed by respiratory paral-
ysis that may result in death. At lower concentrations,
$H_2S$ irritates the mucous membranes of the sinuses, and eye
injury may result from concentrations as low as 50 ppm. The
U. S. National Institute of Occupational Safety and Health
(NIOSH) recommended an occupational exposure standard of
10 ppm for a forty-hour week (NIOSH, 1977).

The mean atmospheric residence time of $H_2S$, about
18 hours, is sufficient to permit complete conversion of $H_2S$
to sulfur dioxide ($SO_2$) in the troposphere (Thompson, 1976).
The unfortunate result of this conversion of $H_2S$ to $SO_2$ may
be decreased ambient air quality. This problem has not been
taken into account in most studies of geothermal development. It is common to examine only ambient concentrations
of $H_2S$. Conversion of $H_2S$ to $SO_2$ will require greater

attention if geothermal development expands rapidly in areas such as the Imperial Valley.

Limited occupational health data available for The Geysers KGRA indicate that more than half of all reported incidents involve the handling of either the chemicals used in abatement processes (such as sodium metavanadate, anthra quinone disulfonic acid, and copper and ferric sulfates), or chemical residues and byproducts resulting from abatement (Hahn, 1979). The data are too limited to support detailed quantitative analysis.

The human health effects of high noise levels, other than loss of hearing, are not well understood. One health official hypothesizes that stress-related coronaries at the Geysers may be partially due to occupational noise exposure (Hahn, 1980).

At the vapor-dominated geothermal systems, steam venting is the noisiest activity. Noise levels are 65 to 75 dBA during well maintenance and up to 125 dBA at 15 m (95 dBA if muffled) during well testing (Case et al., 1977). At the liquid-dominated KGRA's, the loudest noise will be associated with plant operation and the occasional well drilling necessary to continued field development. These noise levels will be about 75 to 85 dBA at 15 m and 40 to 55 dBA at 0.8 km (Morris and Hill, 1980).

Barring the occurrence of human settlement at the Heber or Baca Ranch plant boundaries, noise is not anticipated to be of public concern at either KGRA (Morris and Hill, 1980; U. S. Department of Energy, 1980d).

Ammonia ($NH_3$) and radon are the only noncondensable gas constituents other than $H_2S$ that may pose a health problem. $NH_3$ removal is not currently planned for future plants, although exposure to the gas has produced acute effects in workers during drilling operations at The Geysers (Hahn, 1979).

Radon ($^{222}Rn$) is present in geothermal fluid in concentrations of roughly 10 to 100 microcuries/MWh(e) (Layton, 1980). Radon emission rates at The Geysers exceed those of tested Imperial Valley wells by a factor of three. One recent study of the radon emissions at The Geysers found no cause for occupational or public health concern (Anspaugh, 1978). The Environmental Impact Statement for the Baca development makes no mention of radon (Morris and Hill, 1980; U. S. Department of Energy, 1980d).

Water quality downstream of geothermal plants may be adversely affected either by reduced flow resulting from removal of water for cooling purposes or by accidental spills of geothermal fluid with high concentrations of dissolved solids and a variety of trace constituents. While the latter cause of decreased water quality can not be entirely controlled, the former cause is not likely to be a problem at lower levels of electricity generation.

## Fusion

Thermonuclear fusion, the process that powers the sun and the hydrogen bomb, may well be brought to fruition as a controlled terrestrial energy source in the next thirty years (Holdren, 1978b). Early fusion reactors almost certainly will use the deuterium-tritium reaction, for which the deuterium (the stable heavy hydrogen isotope) is readily obtainable from seawater and the tritium (unstable, super-heavy hydrogen, almost nonexistent in nature) can be produced from lithium in the fusion reactor itself. Lithium is available both from terrestrial deposits and from seawater. Health and safety impacts of acquiring fusion fuels should be modest, owing to the extraordinarily small quantities of fuel required per unit of energy delivered. For example, a fusion reactor rated at 1000 MW(e) and operating at a capacity factor of 80% would use about 1000 kg of lithium and 100 kg of deuterium per year, compared to about 3 billion kg of coal or 200,000 kg of uranium oxide to generate the same amount of electricity in present day power plants.

The technological difficulty of harnessing fusion in a controlled fashion arises mainly from the very high temperature (around 100 million °C) needed to make the fusion reaction proceed at a satisfactory rate. Two classes of approaches are being pursued for providing this temperature and confining the reacting fuels under such conditions — magnetic confinement and inertial confinement — and both almost certainly will require large quantities of construction materials (larger even than for fission reactors, Holdren, 1978b). Materials posing special occupational hazards, such as beryllium, may be needed in large quantities for some reactor designs.

Popular accounts sometimes portray fusion as completely free of the radiological hazards that generate so much concern in the case of fission, but it is not. Radioactive tritium is not only a primary fuel for deuterium-tritium reactors but also would be produced in appreciable quantities even in more advanced systems relying mainly on the deuterium-deuterium reaction. The tritium inventory will pose hazards to workers at the reactors, will be subject to

routine leakage, and could be released in larger quantities
in the event of an accident. Secondly, energetic neutrons
produced in both deuterium-tritium and deuterium-deuterium
reactions can produce a wide variety of radioactive isotopes
by neutron activation of the materials surrounding the
reaction chamber. These activation products will deliver
radiation doses to workers operating and maintaining fusion
reactors, they might be susceptible to release in severe
accidents, and the long-lived isotopes in any case will have
to be treated as radioactive waste when the activated components reach the end of their useful lives.

These potential hazards, then, bear some qualitative
resemblance to those of fission; but there are important
quantitative differences in fusion's favor, and these probably can be made even larger by intelligent design. In a
first-generation fusion reactor, in the design of which no
effort has been devoted to minimizing the tritium inventory,
for example, the quantitative hazard potential of the tritium is 50 to 100 times smaller than that of the comparably
volatile fission products in a fission reactor of the same
generating capacity (Holdren, 1978b). Minimizing tritium
inventory by design probably can shrink its hazard 5 to 10
times more, and it would be perhaps 50 times lower in a
deuterium-deuterium fuel cycle.

Activation products in a fusion reactor made of stainless steel would represent a *theoretical* hazard about 100
times greater than that of the tritium, but it is unclear
whether even a very severe accident could release a substantial fraction of these materials (radioactive iron, cobalt,
manganese, molybdenum, and so on, embedded in the steel
structure itself) into the environment. If a large release
does turn out to be possible, the hazard could approach that
calculated in the "Rasmussen Report" (U. S. Nuclear Regulatory Commission, 1975) for severe accidents at fission
light-water reactors (Holdren, 1981a). On the other hand,
consideration of the similarly hard-to-release quantities of
plutonium (and its relatives) in fission reactors – particularly the breeder reactors that most resemble fusion in
longevity of fuel supply – restores a 10- to 30-fold advantage to fusion. More importantly, if materials less susceptible to neutron activation than stainless steel prove suitable in other respects for fusion reactor application (as
seems likely to be the case), then fusion would have a very
large safety advantage over fission irrespective of whether
plutonium is considered on the fission side and irrespective
of what fraction of fusion activation products could be
released in an accident. Vanadium and titanium seem to
be promising candidate fusion-reactor materials in this
respect.

Comparison of the hazard of fusion activation products as long-lived radioactive waste with that of fission wastes reveals a margin of 10- to 100-fold in fusion's favor for the *worst* choices of fusion-reactor materials and an advantage of 1,000 to 10,000 for fusion if the better materials can be used (Haefele et al., 1977; Holdren, 1978b). An essential difference between fusion and fission, which underlies these numbers, is that the radioactive products of fission are direct and unavoidable consequences of the energy- and fuel-producing reactions themselves, whereas in fusion the main radioactive materials occur in side reactions susceptible to manipulation through (for example) choice of structural materials.

Finally, mention must be made of fusion-fission "hybrid" energy systems, in which a fusion core is surrounded by a blanket where fusion neutrons induce fission reactions and/or breed fissile fuel (Lidsky, 1975). Since a fission breeder can at best produce fuel at a rate sufficient to feed itself and a *few* "client" convertor reactors, perhaps a quarter to a third of the total number of reactors in use would have to be the expensive breeders. A fusion-fission hybrid reactor, on the other hand, apparently could produce enough fissile fuel to support 10 to 20 "client" fission convertor reactors, so that the great majority of reactors in use could be these cheaper convertors. The impacts of such a system on health and safety seem unlikely to be very different than those of a pure fission system, since nearly all of the energy would be coming from the fission part. (Only if fission breeders were much more dangerous than the fission convertors that would replace them in a system fueled by hybrids would a significant health and safety advantage be attributable to the use of hybrids. See Holdren, 1981b.)

## Quantitative Comparisons

This section presents some quantitative information relevant to the direct impacts of the above described energy sources on human health and safety, in a format that facilitates comparisons among these sources. Estimates of analogous effects produced by the use of fossil fuels and nuclear fission are provided as benchmarks, but of course other papers in this volume treat these energy sources in much more detail.

We pointed out in the introduction that the "direct" effects of energy sources on human health and safety, with which we are here concerned, may in the case of some energy sources pose smaller hazards to human well-being than do the "indirect" effects caused by energy's disruptions of ecological, geophysical, and sociopolitical conditions and pro-

cesses. We must now add that the subset of the direct
effects for which decent quantitative estimates are available or readily derived, and which are therefore the focus
of this section, are for many energy sources almost certainly not even the most important of these direct effects.
Specifically, most of the data and estimates we present here
are for occupational deaths and injuries in the construction
and operation of energy systems (including, under the head-
ing of construction, the acquisition of materials and the
fabrication of components), and for occupational and public
deaths and injuries caused by transport of energy-related
materials (construction materials, components, and fuels).
By contrast:

- the data on occupational illnesses are much
  scantier and less reliable than those on accidents;

- the data base on which to build estimates of
  accident risks to the public other than from
  transport is inadequate even for hydropower
  (see above) and more so for the other technologies we are considering;

- concerning public illness caused or aggravated
  by emissions of air pollutants, dose-response
  relations of any plausibility are available in
  the literature only for ionizing radiation and
  for sulfur oxides in the presence of particulates, but not for oxides of nitrogen, hydrocarbons, or trace metals; and

- dose-response relations for public disease from
  water pollutants other than radionuclides are
  not available at all.

It is therefore only with the strongest reservations that we
provide in this section yet another tabulation of health and
safety impacts that, for some of the energy sources considered, doubtless leaves out more than it includes. We do
so because even the incomplete quantification of impacts
that the present state of the art permits is enough to provide some useful insights, indicating what are *not* critical
problems as well as calling attention to issues in need of
more work.

## Basic Approach

The quantitative estimates of health and safety impacts
presented here are normalized in all cases to correspond to
one exajoule (1 EJ = $10^{18}$ J = 0.948 quadrillion Btu) of
energy delivered in one of three stated end-use forms —
heat, fuel, or electricity. This format encourages direct

comparison of alternative ways of obtaining a given energy benefit. We do not consider comparisons between the impacts of getting different end-use forms (or tabulations of impact per unit of energy with no specification at all of end-use form) to be very meaningful, because the main end-use forms are in general not interchangeable without additional processing that entails both economic costs and further impacts.[5] Presenting the information in this way, we hope, will discourage such prevalent but essentially meaningless comparisons as between the risks of getting an exajoule of liquid fuel and the risks of getting an exajoule of electricity.

Underlying most of our estimates are data culled from the literature [see the earlier review, Holdren, Morris, and Mintzer (1980), as well as the notes in the tables that follow] concerning materials requirements for construction of the facilities needed to harness the various energy sources considered. Since employment figures for the various primary materials industries are available in national statistics, as are incidence rates of fatal and nonfatal occupational accidents and injuries in these industries, the materials figures can be translated into estimates of the occupational damages attributable to materials acquisition for the energy facilities in question. Additional occupational damages arise in the transport of these materials, in their fabricaton (in some cases) into components, and in the actual construction of the facilities.

Part of the risk to public health and safety from energy technologies also is proportional in various ways to the quantities of materials used. Materials acquisition, for example, produces emissions to air and water, and quantitative data at least for the air emissions (per million metric tons of various materials, on a nationally aggregated basis) are available. In principle, these data could be combined with models relating emissions to ambient concentrations and with dose-response relations to estimate public health consequences. (In present practice, the errors and uncertainties in carrying out such a procedure are so great — see the additional discussion below — that we refrain from doing so here and simply list emissions per exajoule.) Additionally, the transport of materials for energy facilities poses risks to public as well as to occupational safety, and these public risks can be estimated by combining ton-miles of transport by different modes with the corresponding accident statistics, as discussed further below.

Further occupational and public risks, not generally proportional to materials use, occur in connection with the routine operation and maintenance of energy facilities.

Estimating these on the occupational side requires knowing the worker-years devoted to operation and maintenance (which are necessarily little more than educated guesses for many of the technologies considered here) and the accident statistics for the relevant occupations. Where fuels are involved (true only of biomass and fusion among the energy sources considered here, with the quantities being negligibly small in the fusion case), transport becomes a source of occupational and public risk in routine operation as well as in construction. (Operation of energy facilities can pose accident risks to the public other than in fuel transport; these possibilities were discussed above for the various energy sources we have considered, but we have too little information to attempt any systematic quantitative comparisons.)

Emissions in routine operation also are a source of public risk, with biomass and geothermal the only sources among those we are considering for which routine emissions of air pollutants per exajoule are both potentially significant and estimable. (Emissions from fusion in routine operation may be significant but cannot now be meaningfully estimated; as with routine emissions from fission reactors, they presumably can be held, at a cost, to virtually any level demanded.)

Finally, the decommissioning of energy facilities at the end of their useful lifetimes will pose occupational risks and, in some cases, will produce emissions with potential effects on public health. These risks may be roughly proportional to materials use in the facilities to be decommissioned, but we have too little data to venture quantitative estimates here.

Comparative Data

Table 1 shows materials use, in thousands of metric tons per exajoule of delivered energy, for renewable, geothermal, and fusion energy sources. Data for delivery of liquid fuels based on petroleum and for delivery of electricity from fossil fuels and light-water fission reactors are given for comparison. Shown in Table 2 for the same energy sources are labor requirements, subdivided into (a) materials acquisition, fabrication, and transport, (b) construction, and (c) operation and maintenance (including acquisition and transport of fuel, where applicable). The units are thousands of worker-years per exajoule of delivered energy.

Table 3 shows occupational deaths and working-days-lost to injuries and illnesses in the acquisition of materials

Table 1. Materials use ($10^3$ MT/$10^{18}$ J)[a]

| | Steel | Nonferrous metals[b] | Concrete[c] | Glass | Plastics |
|---|---|---|---|---|---|
| **Heat** | | | | | |
| Flat-plate collectors[d] | 43-520 | 43-280 | | 65-370 | 9.3-93 |
| Solar ponds[e] | | | 0-600 | | |
| South windows[f] | | | | | |
| Thermal mass[g] | | 640-1300 | 80,000-200,000 | 1100-2300 | |
| **Fuels** | | | | | |
| Biomass synfuels[h] | 4.1-25 | 0-3.3 | 25-570 | 0.07-0.52 | 0.08-6.5 |
| Refined oil products[i] | 2-6 | 0-10 | 1-5 | | |
| **Electricity** | | | | | |
| Solar-thermal electric[j] | 430-2000 | 6.3-140 | 970-43,000 | 8.3-370 | 4.7-110 |
| Photovoltaic[k] | 0-1200 | 0-1800 | 140-16,000 | 80-470 | 0-8.7 |
| Space photovoltaic[l] | 350 | 36-37 | 310 | 0-4.5 | 1.5-1.8 |
| Wind[m] | 160-530 | 7.6-15 | 200-1700 | | 18-70 |
| Hydroelectric[n] | 30-62 | 0.68-2.3 | 400-2250 | | |
| Ocean thermal[o] | 33-570 | 16-100 | 1300-3100 | | 17-21 |
| Coal/biomass[p] | 37-67 | 1.0 | 150-220 | | |
| Geothermal, vapor dominated[q] | 66-190 | 0.76-2.5 | 160-360 | | |
| Geothermal, liquid dominated[r] | 230-690 | 2.5-8.9 | 520-1300 | | |
| Fusion[s] | 140-210 | 5-12 | 300-750 | | |
| LWR[t] | 40-60 | 1.3 | 250-400 | | |

Table 1. (continued)

ᵃAll systems are assumed to have a 30-year lifetime, except as noted. MT = metric ton.

ᵇNon-ferrous metals are primarily aluminum and copper. All of this material is treated as aluminum in subsequent calculations, except as noted.

ᶜConcrete is a mixture of cement (typically 20% by weight), sand, gravel, and water.

ᵈValues at the lower end of the range refer to collectors only, operated in sunny climates, assuming an annual output of 860 kWh (thermal)/m², and an operating lifetime of 30 years (OTA, 1978). Values at the upper end of the range represent total system requirements (Albers, Barviec, and Rooney, 1976).

ᵉCalculated values assume 18 MJ/m² per day incidence and a collector achieving 33% efficient conversion to delivered heat (OTA, 1978).

ᶠCalculated values assume 100 ft² of additional triple-pane windows save 2 to 4 GJ/year of resource energy; panes are 3/32 of an inch thick; building life is 30 years; heating system efficiency is 75%; cooling system coefficient of performance is 3.5. Savings in building loads are based on Place et al. (1980), extended to triple-pane glass. Aluminum requirements are from Fentron Industries, Inc. (1980) and Ramsey and Sleeper (1970), assuming windows are 2 feet by 4 feet. Wood could be substituted for this aluminum, with a requirement of $1.8-3.6 \times 10^6$ MT/1018 J (Ramsey and Sleeper, 1970; Pella Inc., 1980). In either case, structural differences between plain walls and walls with windows would require an additional $1.5-3.0 \times 10^6$ MT/1018 J of wood (Ramsey and Sleeper, 1970; Ching, 1975). These windows have no night-time insulation, which would increase energy savings greatly.

ᵍCalculated values are based on Place et al. (1980), using the same assumptions as in note (e) above. Volume of partition walls is estimated at 3.75 m³ resulting in an annual resource-energy savings of 1 to 2.5 GJ.

ʰValues are based on Bailie (1976); USERDA (1977c); and Waste Management Inc. (1976), and cover the range for the following types of conversion technologies; biogasification, ethanol fermentation, thermal gasificiation, and hydrocarbon synthesis.

Table 1. (continued)

[i]Values are based on large-scale refineries geared to gasoline production (Carasso et al., 1975; Albers, Barviec, and Rooney, 1976; Smith, Weyant and Holdren, 1975).

[j]Values are based on USFEA (1974); Albers, Barviec, and Rooney (1976); Hildebrandt and Vant-Hull (1977); Caputo (1977); OTA (1978); and Lawrence (1979), and cover the range for power-tower, trough, and parabolic disk collectors with load factors of 0.41-0.54.

[k]Values are based on USFEA (1974); Albers, Barviec, and Rooney (1976); Caputo (1977); OTA (1978); and Ehrenreich (1979), and cover the range for flat-plate and concentrating collector systems with load factors of 0.41-0.54. The high end of the range for non-ferrous metals reflects designs using aluminum for framing and structural supports; while the high end of the range for steel reflects designs using steel frames and supports.

[l]Values are based on Teeter and Jamieson (1980); USDOE (1978); and Moses (1979), and cover the two alternative "reference system" concepts being developed by the National Aeronautical and Space Administration (NASA). One system uses silicon solar cells, the other uses gallium arsenide cells. The high end of the ranges for non-ferrous metals and glass are for the silicon cell design. Significant quantities of additional materials, some of which are exotic, will also be required by current concepts for the space power satellites.

[m]Values are based on large-scale [>1 MW(e)] devices (USERDA, 1977d; Sathaye et al., 1977; USDOE, 1980c). The high end of the range for concrete reflects the use of a concrete tower and foundation; the high end of the range for steel reflects the use of a steel tower.

[n]Values are calculated based on USDOE (1980a); Tennessee Valley Authority (1954); Carasso et al. (1975); and Albers, Barviec, and Rooney (1976), assuming a system lifetime of 60 years and annual load factors of 0.5. In addition to the concrete, 33,000-40,000 MT/$10^{18}$ J of earth and rock are required for the dam construction.

[o]Values are based on USDOE (1980a); MITRE/METREK (1977); Lockheed (1975); Albers, Barviec, and Rooney (1976); and USFEA (1974).

**Table 1.** (continued)

[p]Values are based on coal- and wood-fired power plants (Albers, Barviec, and Rooney, 1976; Smith, Weyant, and Holdren, 1975; USERDA, 1977c).

[q]Values for materials requirements include materials used in well drilling and in plant construction. Materials requirements for well drilling are derived from USDOE (1980d), based on the Bechtel model (Carasso et al., 1975). The original data refer to onshore drilling for natural gas. An error bound of -20% to +75% has been added to account for the greater diameter and depth of geothermal wells. Materials requirements for plant construction are based on McIlraith (1980) for a 110 MW(e) unit. An error bound of ±20% has been added, and non-ferrous metals, not mentioned in the reference, are assumed to be 1-5% of the total steel used in the plant.

[r]The number of wells required for an annual production of $10^{18}$ J(e) is based on DeHoven (1980); Cooper, A. (1980); and USDOE (1980d), with an error bound of ±20%. Materials used in well construction are calculated as per note (p) above (USDOE, 1980d), as are materials used in plant construction, using data from DeHoven (1980).

[s]Values are based on a variety of conceptual fusion-reactor designs (Hartley et al., 1976; Cameron et al., 1979), and assume a 30-year lifetime and 70% capacity factor, plus an allowance for periodic replacement of radiation-damaged structures.

[t]Values are based on large-scale power plants [1000 MW(e)] with annual load factors of 0.7 (Albers, Barviec, and Rooney, 1976; Smith, Weyant, and Holdren, 1975).

Table 2. Employment ($10^3$ WYr/$10^{18}$ J)[a]

| | Materials acquisition, fabrication, and transportation | Construction | Operation and Maintenance | Total |
|---|---|---|---|---|
| **Heat** | | | | |
| Flat-plate collectors[b] | 3.2-39 | 53-67 | 25-50 | 81-156 |
| South windows[c] | 41-110 | | | 41-110 |
| Thermal mass[d] | 160-420 | | | 160-420 |
| **Chemical Fuel** | | | | |
| Biomass, waste conversion[e] | 0.12-2.2 | 3.3 | 3.2-78 | 6.7-84 |
| Biomass, forestry[f] | 0.12-2.2 | 3.3 | 63-140 | 67-140 |
| Biomass, cultivation[g] | 0.12-2.2 | 3.3 | 31-210 | 47-210 |
| Oil refining[h] | 0.32-0.76 | 0.91 | 2.55 | 3.5-4.3 |
| **Electricity** | | | | |
| Solar-thermal electric[i] | 14-160 | 30 | 30 | 74-220 |
| Photovoltaic[i] | 20-130 | 13 | 30 | 63-180 |
| Space photovoltaic[j] | 7.3-14 | 110 | 0.21 | 110-120 |
| Wind[k] | 6.2-20 | 3.4-23 | 3.7-16 | 13-49 |
| Hydroelectric[l] | 1.4-6.5 | 5.6-9.5 | 0.05-4.8 | 6.9-21 |
| Ocean thermal[m] | 3.7-31 | 4.3-45 | 0.4-7.8 | 8.4-83 |
| Biomass wastes[n] | 0.92-2.7 | 6.8 | 8.7-45 | 16-55 |
| Biomass, forestry[o] | 0.92-2.7 | 6.8 | 99-140 | 110-140 |
| Biomass, cultivation[p] | 0.92-2.7 | 6.8 | 51-240 | 58-250 |
| Geothermal, vapor dominated[q] | 1.4-7.0 | 2.7-4.1 | 11-16 | 18-32 |
| Geothermal, liquid dominated[q] | 4.7-27 | 14-31 | 28-48 | 47-96 |
| Fusion[r] | 3.0-9.2 | 24-48 | 15-29 | 42-87 |
| Coal[h] | 0.92-2.7 | 6.8 | 34 | 42-44 |
| LWR[h] | 1.2-2.9 | 9.6 | 7.7 | 18-20 |

Table 2. (continued)

[a]Values in the first column (i.e., materials acquisition, fabrication, and transportation) are calculated by multiplying the material requirements for each technology from Table 1 by the employment requirements in Table 3. Values in the other columns are based on information in the technical literature, as referenced in the following notes. WYr = worker years.

[b]Values for construction, and operation and maintenance (O&M), are based on figures for domestic water heating systems. Interviews with solar water heating contractors suggest that installation of a typical system for a new single-family home requires about 40 worker-hours and O&M may take 0.5-1 worker-hours/year for a system that delivers 10 GJ/year.

[c]No labor requirement is shown for construction or O&M because it is assumed that there is no significant difference in labor requirements to install a window than to build a wall of equal area, and no O&M is required for windows.

[d]No labor requirement is shown for construction or O&M because it is assumed that there is no significant difference in labor requirements between building and maintaining a wall of concrete and building and maintaining a stud wall of equal area. (For construction this may not be true.)

[e]Values for construction labor are calculated assuming that the total construction-labor requirement for a biomass conversion plant per unit of steel requirement is the same as the construction labor-to-steel ratio for an oil refinery [see footnote (h) below]. O&M labor requirements for biomass conversion plants are based on Ashare, Wise, and Wentworth (1977); Raphael Katzen Assoc. (1978); OTA (1979); Bliss and Blake (1977); Kohan et al. (1979); and Desrosiers (1979).

[f]Values for construction labor and conversion-plant labor are as per note (e) above. O&M labor requirements for logging are from Intergroup Consulting Economists (1976).

[g]Values for construction labor and conversion-plant labor are as per note (e) above. O&M labor requirements for farming are from USDOC (1979), Peart, Ladisch, and Zink (1979), and Salo et al. (1977).

[h]Values for construction and O&M labor are from Smith, Weyant, and Holdren (1975).

Table 2. (continued)

[i]Values for construction and O&M labor are from Caputo (1977) and OTA (1978).

[j]Values for construction and O&M labor are from Caputo (1977) and Habeggar, Gasper, and Brown (1980).

[k]Values for construction and O&M labor are from USERDA (1977d), Sathaye et al. (1977), USDOE (1980c), and USFEA (1974).

[l]Values for construction and O&M labor are from USDOE (1980a) and Carasso et al. (1975).

[m]Values for construction and O&M labor are from USDOE (1980a), MITRE/METREK (1977), Lockheed (1975), and USFEA (1974).

[n]Values for construction-labor requirements are assumed to be the same as those for a coal-fired plant (Smith, Weyant, and Holdren, 1975). Values for O&M labor in the power plant are from Smith, Weyant, and Holdren (1975), and Kohan et al. (1979).

[o]Values for construction and power-plant labor requirements are as per note (n) above. Values for logging-labor requirements are as per note (f) above.

[p]Values for construction and power-plant labor requirements are as per note (n) above. Values for silvicultural-labor requirements are from Salo et al. (1977).

[q]Values for construction and O&M labor requirements are based on USDOE (1980d), and extrapolated to other sites on a per-unit-of-energy-produced basis.

[r]Fusion requires 3.5 times more steel and 1.6 times more concrete than fission (see Table 1). To be conservative, values for construction and O&M labor requirements are assumed to be from 2.5 times (the average of 1.6 and 3.5) to 5.0 times (twice the average) as great as the corresponding values for fission.

Table 3. Occupational deaths, injuries, and illnesses from materials acquisition[a]

| Occupational category | SIC code | 10³ worker-yr per 10⁶ MT | Deaths per 10³ worker-yr | WDL per 10³ worker-yr | Deaths per 10⁶ MT | WDL per 10⁶ MT |
|---|---|---|---|---|---|---|
| **Steel** | | | | | | |
| Iron mining[b] | 101 | 0.30 | 0.40 | 630 | 0.12 | 189 |
| Coal for steel[c] | 12[d] | 0.29 | 0.75 | 964 | 0.22 | 280 |
| Primary steel manufacturing[b] | 33[d] | 7.6 | 0.13 | 1220 | 0.99 | 9270 |
| | | 8.2 | | | 1.3 | 9700 |
| **Aluminum** | | | | | | |
| Bauxite mining[e] | 105[d] | 0.24 | 0.40 | 500 | 0.0096 | 120 |
| Aluminum manufacturing[b] | 33[d] | 27.8 | 0.18 | 913 | 5.00 | 25400 |
| | | 28 | | | 5.0 | 26000 |
| **Concrete** | | | | | | |
| Sand and gravel mining[f] | 144 | 0.038 | 0.28 | 1280 | 0.011 | 49 |
| Cement manufacturing[g] | 324 | 0.41 | 0.23 | 840 | 0.094 | 344 |
| Ready-Mix concrete[h] | 3273 | 0.20 | 0.07 | 1270 | 0.014 | 254 |
| | | 0.65 | | | 0.12 | 650 |
| **Glass** | | | | | | |
| Flat glass[i] | 321 | 15 | 0.07 | 910 | 1.1 | 13,700 |
| Plastics[j] | 2821 | 4.9 | 0.05 | 390 | 0.24 | 1,910 |
| Fabricated metals[k] | 34 | 28 | 0.05 | 600 | 1.5 | 16,800 |

Table 3. (continued)

[a]Occupational effects data are from National Safety Council (1978). Data on nonfatal worker-days lost (WDL) are averages for 1975-1977. Fatality rates are for 1977 only, and should be considered as only rough indicators. Where data are not available for the three- and four- digit SIC industries, more highly aggregated parent categories are used.

[b]Production data (U. S. Department of Commerce, 1978b) and employment data (U. S. Department of Labor, 1978b) are for 1974.

[c]Productivity data are for 1974 (U. S. Department of Commerce, 1978c, Table 1281). Fatality data (U. S. Department of Commerce, 1978c, Table 1276) and illness and injury data (U. S. Department of Labor, 1978a) are for 1974.

[d]Where data for three- and four-digit industries within the SIC group 33 were available, these values were used in the calculations.

[e]Production data are for 1974 (Hayes, 1976, Table 1308). Employment data are for 1970 (U. S. Department of the Interior, 1970), and are scaled to 1974 values by multiplying by 1.07, the increase in production during this period.

[f]Production and employment data are for 1974 (U. S. Department of Commerce, 1978c, Tables 1271, 1276).

[g]Production and employment data are for 1974 (U. S. Department of Commerce, 1978c, Tables 1292, 1376).

[h]Production and employment data are for 1977 (U. S. Department of Commerce, 1978a).

[i]Production data (U. S. Department of Commerce, 1976) and employment data (U. S. Department of Labor, 1978a) are for 1975.

[j]Production and employment data are for 1975 (U. S. Department of Commerce, 1978a).

[k]Production and employment data are for 1972 (U. S. Department of Commerce, 1978e, Table 7a).

and in materials fabrication, broken down by Standard Industrial Classification (SIC) codes (U. S. Department of Labor,
1978) and presented as products of labor intensity (thousand
worker-years per million metric tons) times incidence rates
(deaths and working-days-lost per thousand worker-years).
These data have been combined with labor requirements
(Table 2) and incidence rates for transport, construction,
and operation and maintenance to produce the estimates shown
in Table 4 of total occupational effects for all the energy
sources considered, expressed as deaths and working-days-
lost per delivered exajoule and per thousand worker-years.

   The treatment of component fabrication in this connection needs some elaboration. Data generally are not available for the amount of labor that goes into component fabrication (to be distinguished from on-site construction labor)
for the various energy technologies. We obtained a range of
estimates by assuming that a low value of 20% and a high
value of 80% of all the metals required for each technology
passed through the fabricated metals industry, for which
labor required and occupational damages per million tons of
metal are known.

   The treatment of transport risks also needs elaboration. The great bulk of the types of materials considered
here move within the United States by rail or truck, and we
considered only these two modes. For each material, data on
the transport industry were used to determine, on a national
average basis, the fractions of the total tonnage moving by
truck and by train.[6] Hazard data on occupational deaths and
working-days-lost per million tons of freight moved by truck
and train were then used to determine the effects attributable to transport of the various materials and, hence, to
the energy technologies in which the materials are used.
This procedure assumes implicitly that occupational deaths
and injuries in transport occur roughly in proportion to
tonnage handled rather than in proportion to ton-miles,
which is equivalent to assuming that most of the risk occurs
in freight handling (loading and unloading, coupling and
decoupling of freight cars, and so forth) rather than "on
the road." If all the materials moved a similar average
distance, of course, tons and ton-miles would be in the same
proportion for each material and the distribution of risk
between loading/unloading and actual transport would be
irrelevant. In reality, all the materials except sand and
gravel for concrete probably do move roughly equal distances.

   Most of the public risks from transport of materials
and fuels for energy occur in transit rather than in freight
handling. For the calculations reported here, we assumed

Table 4. Occupational effects[a]

| | Fatalities | | Lost work days | |
|---|---|---|---|---|
| | $D/10^{18}$ J | $D/10^3$ WYr | $10^3$ WDL/$10^{18}$ J | WDL/$10^3$ WYr |
| **Heat** | | | | |
| Flat-plate collectors[b] | 18-28 | 0.18-0.22 | 55-109 | 0.68-0.7 |
| South windows[c] | 5.3-12 | 0.11-0.13 | 39-94 | 0.89-0.94 |
| Thermal mass[c] | 36-88 | 0.21-0.23 | 220-560 | 1.4 |
| **Chemical Fuel** | | | | |
| Biomass, waste conversion[d] | 1.6-15 | 0.18-0.24 | 3.9-40 | 0.48-0.58 |
| Biomass, forestry[e] | 22-35 | 0.25-0.33 | 87-120 | 0.86-1.3 |
| Biomass, cultivation[f] | 10-53 | 0.21-0.25 | 24-140 | 0.51-0.67 |
| Oil refining[g] | 1.1 | 0.28-0.31 | 1.8-2.0 | 0.47-0.51 |
| **Electricity** | | | | |
| Solar-thermal electric[h] | 16-41 | 0.19-0.22 | 53-220 | 0.72-1.0 |
| Photovoltaic[h] | 12-31 | 0.17-0.19 | 47-160 | 0.75-0.89 |
| Space photovoltaic[i] | 32 | 0.27-0.29 | 86-91 | 0.76-0.78 |
| Wind[h,j] | 2.9-12 | 0.22-0.24 | 13-43 | 0.88-1.0 |
| Hydroelectric[h,k] | 5.0-8.1 | 0.39-0.72 | 48-64 | 3.1-7.0 |
| Ocean thermal[l] | 3.7-36 | 0.43-0.44 | 9.2-79 | 0.95-1.1 |
| Biomass wastes[h] | 3.8-11 | 0.21-0.24 | 11-34 | 0.62-0.69 |
| Biomass, forestry[m] | 34-41 | 0.29-0.31 | 140-160 | 1.1-1.3 |
| Biomass, cultivation[n] | 16-67 | 0.27-0.28 | 45-190 | 0.76-0.78 |
| Geothermal, vapor dominated[o] | 10>16 | 0.50-0.55 | 39-63 | 2.0-2.2 |
| Geothermal, liquid dominated[o] | 26-46 | 0.48-0.55 | 110-200 | 2.1-2.3 |
| Fusion[h] | 10-20 | 0.23-0.24 | 30-60 | 0.69-0.71 |
| Coal[p] | 35 | 0.80-0.83 | 58-60 | 1.4 |
| LWR[q] | 4.8-5.0 | 0.25-0.27 | 14-16 | 0.77-0.80 |

**Table 4.** (continued)

[a] Calculated data for occupational effects include contributions from materials acquisition, metals fabrication, transportation of materials, construction of facilities, and routine operation and maintenance (O&M). Risks of materials acquisition are calculated by multiplying the materials requirements from Table 1 by the occupational effects of materials production from Table 3. Risks of fabricating metals are calculated by the same procedure, assuming that 20-80% of the total metals go through the fabrication stage. Risks of transporting materials are calculated as explained in the text. Risks of construction and O&M are calculated by multiplying labor requirements from Table 2 by data on occupational risks of labor given by SIC categories in USDOL (1978a) and National Safety Council (1978). Construction labor is assumed to be general construction, SIC categories 15-17, except as noted. SIC categories for O&M labor and other assumptions used in the calculations are given in the following footnotes.

[b] O&M labor is assumed to be in Services, SIC group 70-89.

[c] No incremental construction or O&M labor is assumed to be required for south windows and thermal mass (see Table 2).

[d] O&M labor is assumed to be in Petroleum Refining, SIC group 291.

[e] O&M labor for tree harvesting is assumed to be in Saw Mills and Planing Mills, SIC industry 2421. This industry includes "establishments primarily engaged in...producing...wood chips" (USOMB, 1972), and was chosen over SIC 2411 (Logging Camps and Logging Contractors) because logging for energy production will probably use highly mechanized techniques including possibly whole-tree harvesting and in-forest chipping. O&M labor in the synfuels plants is as per note (d), above.

[f] O&M labor for agriculture and short-rotation silviculture is assumed to be in Agricultural Production, SIC Group 01. O&M labor in the synfuels plants is as per note (d) above.

[g] O&M labor is divided between Oil and Gas Field Services, SIC group 13, and Petroleum Refining, SIC group 291.

[h] O&M labor is assumed to be in Electrical Services, SIC group 491.

Table 4. (continued)

[i]Construction labor and O&M labor are divided between Contract Construction, SIC groups 15-17, and Water Transportation Services, SIC group 44.

[j]The high end of the risks from materials acquisition, fabrication, and transportation assumes a steel tower. The low end of the risks from these categories assumes a concrete tower.

[k]In addition to the risks of transporting the materials shown in Table 1, significant transportation risks arise from acquiring and moving earth and rock. This risk is approximately one-sixth as great as the risks of acquiring and transporting the required concrete.

[l]Construction labor is assumed to be divided between Contract Construction, SIC groups 15-17, and Ship and Boat Building, SIC group 373. O&M labor is assumed to be divided between Electrical Services, SIC group 491, and Water Transportation Services, SIC group 44.

[m]O&M labor for tree harvesting is as per note (e) above. Power plant labor is in Electrical Services, SIC Group 491.

[n]O&M labor for agriculture and short-rotation silviculture is as per note (f) above. Power plant O&M labor is in Electrical Services, SIC group 491.

[o]Construction labor is divided between Contract Construction, SIC groups 15-17, and Wellfield Development, SIC industry 1381. O&M labor is divided among Chemicals and Allied Products, SIC group 28, Well Services, SIC group 138, and Electrical Services, SIC group 491.

[p]O&M labor is divided between Coal Mining, SIC group 12, and Electrical Services, SIC group 491.

[q]O&M labor is divided between Mining, SIC group 1099, and Electrical Services, SIC group 419.

that all the public risk occurs *en route*, hence is proportional to ton-miles.  Sand and gravel for concrete were
assumed to move an average distance of 30 miles, and fuels
and all other materials were assumed to move an average distance of 300 miles.  The resulting estimates of public
deaths attributable to transportion of materials associated
with the various energy sources are shown in Table 5.

Table 6 shows the emissions of particulates, $SO_x$, $NO_x$,
CO, and hydrogen fluoride associated with materials production.  These data have been combined with materials requirements and with data about emissions during routine operation
of the energy technologies to generate the total emissions
estimates shown in Table 7.

These emissions estimates cannot be readily converted
into estimates of deaths and illnesses attributable to air
pollution, and we have not tried to do so here.  The first
step in carrying out such a conversion is to relate emissions to ambient concentrations to which human populations
are exposed.  Doing so requires *either* a detailed model
accounting for atmospheric transport and atmospheric chemistry *or* a statistical analysis correlating historical emissions with observed concentrations of the pollutants of
interest.  Both approaches are difficult and very imperfect
at the present state-of-the-art, and the results in either
case depend intimately on the topographical and meteorological characteristics of the particular region in which the
emissions take place.  Thus emissions totals of the sort
presented in Table 7 are not a useful starting point for
such work; one must disaggregate the emissions by region on
a rather fine geographic scale.  Once such a procedure has
been carried out and the results have been combined with
information about population density to determine actual
human exposures, one still needs a dose-response relation
to determine the number of illnesses and fatalities expected
to result.  But dose-response relations valid for prolonged
exposure to low concentrations of air pollutants are very
difficult to obtain (see, e.g., Ehrlich, Ehrlich, and Holdren, 1977, Ch. 10, or Lave and Seskin, 1977, for brief discussions of the reasons) and are available presently in
usable form only for oxides of sulfur in the presence of
particulate matter.

Even in that case, the uncertainties are very large, as
can be illustrated by contrasting the conclusions of different major reviews of the subject.  The Biomedical and Environmental Assessment Division of the Brookhaven National
Laboratory gives a median estimate of 3.25 excess deaths/year
per 100,000 people exposed to an average concentration of
sulfate of 1 $\mu g/m^3$, with an uncertainty range that extends

Table 5.  Public deaths from transportation of materials[a]

|  | Deaths/$10^{18}$ J |
|---|---|
| Flat-plate collectors | 0.5 - 6 |
| Solar-thermal electric | 5 - 100 |
| Photovoltaic | 0 - 60 |
| Wind | 1 - 8 |
| Hydroelectric | 1 - 7 |
| Ocean thermal | 4 - 10 |
| Biomass | b |
| Geothermal |  |
|    Vapor dominated | 1 - 2 |
|    Liquid dominated | 2 - 8 |
| Fusion | 1 - 4 |
| LWR | 1 - 2 |
| Space photovoltaic | b |
| Solar ponds | 0 - 2 |
| Coal (transport of fuel itself) | 17 - 100 |

[a]Due to uncertainties in the data, these values are calculated to one significant figure only.  See text for details of calculations.  Data sources are U. S. Department of Commerce (1978d, 1979) and U. S. Department of Transportation (1980a, b).

[b]Transportation risks could not be calculated from available data, but are potentially large.

Table 6. Emissions from materials acquisition (kg/MT of commodity produced)[a]

| Commodity | Particulates | Sulfur oxides | Nitrogen oxides | Carbon monoxide | Hydrogen fluoride |
|---|---|---|---|---|---|
| **Steel** | | | | | |
| Iron and steel mills[b] | 0.3-150 | ND[c] | ND | 800-1200 | 0.01-0.3 |
| Coke for steel-making[d] | 2 | 2 | 0.02 | 0.95 | 2 |
| Totals | 2.3-150 | 2 | 0.02 | 800-1200 | 2 |
| **Aluminum** | | | | | |
| Primary Al production[e] | 6-300 | ND | ND | ND | 0.3-10 |
| Secondary Al production[f] | 5-70 | ND | ND | ND | ND |
| Totals[g] | 6-260 | | | | 0.3-10 |
| **Concrete** | | | | | |
| Sand and gravel mining[h] | 0.05 | negl. | negl. | negl. | negl. |
| Cement production[i] | 130-170 | 0-30 | 1.3 | ND | ND |
| Concrete batching[h] | 0.005-0.05 | ND | ND | ND | ND |
| Totals[k] | 26-34 | 0-6 | 0-1 | | |
| **Flat glass** | | | | | |
| Sand and gravel mining[h] | 0.05 | negl. | negl. | negl. | negl. |
| Flat glass manufacturing[l,m] | 0-1 | 0.1-2.4 | 4 | <0.1 | <0.1 |
| Totals | 0.1-1 | 0.1-2 | 4 | <0.1 | <0.1 |
| Plastics[n] | 2.5-5.0 | ND | ND | ND | ND |

Table 6. (continued)

[a] Data on emission factors are from U. S. Environmental Protection Agency (1979). Sulfur oxides ($SO_x$) and nitrogen oxides ($NO_x$) figured as $SO_2$ and $NO_2$.

[b] Range covers uncontrolled to controlled emissions and includes weighted averages of emissions from open hearth (24%), basic $O_2$ (56%), and electric furnaces (20%). Distribution of particulates centered on small particles: 45-75% are 0-5 μ.

[c] ND = No data.

[d] Data are for uncontrolled emissions from byproduct coke furnaces. Sulfur is present as $H_2S$ in coke ovens, assumed fully converted to $SO_2$.

[e] Data for particulates include fluoride particulates present primarily as $CaF_2$. Distribution of particles centered on small diameters: 60-70% are 0-5 μ.

[f] Data are for secondary aluminum production using reverberatory furnace.

[g] Totals reflect weighted average of emissions: 83% from primary Al production, 17% from secondary Al production.

[h] Data are for uncontrolled emissions. Particulates are primarily large-diameter particles: 97% > 1 μ, 93% > 60 μ.

[i] Data are for uncontrolled emissions. Range covers cement from both wet and dry processes.

[j] Range covers controlled and uncontrolled emissions.

[k] Concrete is assumed to contain 20% cement by weight.

[l] Range covers both controlled and uncontrolled operations.

[m] Calculations assume 1 MT of sand processed per MT of glass produced.

[n] Data are for emissions from general plastics production.

Table 7. Energy system emissions ($10^3$ MT/$10^{18}$ J)[a]

| | Particulates | Sulfur oxides | Nitrogen oxides | Carbon monoxide | Hydrogen fluoride |
|---|---|---|---|---|---|
| **Heat** | | | | | |
| Flat-plate collectors[b] | 0.37-150 | 0.093-1.9 | 0.26-1.5 | 34-620 | 0.093-1.0 |
| South windows[b] | 4.0-340 | 0.11-5.4 | 4.5-8.8 | 0.22 | 0.4-13 |
| Thermal mass[c] | 2100-6800 | 0-1200 | 0-200 | 0 | 0 |
| Wood stoves | 1000 | 26 | 64 | 19,000-26,000 | |
| **Chemical Fuels** | | | | | |
| Biomass fuels, non-transport[d] | 6.6-190 | 30-130 | 78-550 | 12-49 | 0.0082-0.083 |
| Biomass fuels, transportation[e] | 47-260 | 53-140 | 130-790 | 440-4200 | 0.0082-0.083 |
| Oil fuels, non-transport[f] | 11-42 | 58-540 | 160-250 | 29-160 | 0.004-0.11 |
| Oil fuels, transportation[g] | 47-110 | 53-550 | 190-760 | 450-4300 | 0.004-0.11 |
| **Electricity** | | | | | |
| Solar-thermal, electric[b,h] | 27-1800 | 0.12-260 | 0.042-45 | 360-2500 | 0.93-4.2 |
| Photovoltaic[b,h] | 190-1000 | 2.5-97 | 0.36-18 | 0.0083-1500 | 2.5-19 |
| Space photovoltaic[b] | 9.1-73 | 0.7-2.6 | 0.007-0.336 | 280-420 | 0.71-1.1 |
| Wind[b] | 5.8-140 | 0.3-11 | 0.0032-1.7 | 130-640 | 0.32-1.2 |
| Hydroelectric[b] | 11-86 | 0.06-14 | 0.0006-2.3 | 24-74 | 0.06-0.12 |
| Ocean thermal[b] | 34-220 | 0.07-20 | 0.0007-3.1 | 26-680 | 0.07-2.3 |
| Biomass[i] | 69-8300 | 150-430 | 300-2200 | 220-3300 | 0.074-0.14 |
| Geothermal, vapor dominated[j] | 4.5-41 | 19-130 | 0.001-0.38 | 53-220 | 0.13-0.62 |
| Geothermal, liquid dominated[j] | 14-150 | 0.88-250 | 0.005-1.3 | 180-830 | 0.46-1.5 |
| Fusion[b] | 8.2-60 | 0.28-200 | 0.003-0.75 | 110-250 | 0.28-0.54 |
| Coal[k] | 140-1300 | 350-1200 | 410-820 | 48-150 | 0.074-0.14 |
| LWR[l] | 7.0-23 | 2.7-6.2 | 1.0-2.2 | 33-73 | 0.08-1.3 |

Table 7. (continued)

[a]All values are calculated by summing emissions from materials acquisition and routine operations for systems producing $10^{18}$ joules in the stated energy form. Emissions from materials acquisition are calculated by multiplying the materials requirements in Table 1 by the emissions factors in Table 6. O&M emissions are drawn from the literature, as documented in the following footnotes. $SO_2$ emissions are figured as $SO_2$, $NO_x$ emissions as $NO_x$, and $H_2S$ emissions (from steel production) are assumed fully converted to $SO_2$.

[b]Values are for emissions during materials acquistion only. Emissions of the tabulated pollutants during routine operations are negligible.

[c]Values are calculated for operation only, assuming a wood stove efficiency of 50% (i.e., half of the energy content of the wood is delivered to the house as useful heat), which corresponds to an efficient heating unit (Leonard, 1979; Cooper, J., 1980).

[d]Values for emissions during conversion to fuels are based on Jones et al. (1978), Kohan et al. (1979), and USEPA (1979). Values for combustion emissions are from USEPA (1979) and Sittig (1975).

[e]Values for emissions during conversion to fuels are as per note (d) above. Values for combustion emissions are from Pefley, Aldeman, and Suga, (1980) and OTA (1980), assuming a vehicle mileage of 15-30 miles per gallon.

[f]Values for emissions during oil refining are calculated from Smith, Weyant and Holdren (1975). Values for combustion emissions are as per note (d) above.

[g]Values for emissions during refining are as per note (f) above. Vehicle combustion emissions are as per note (e) above.

[h]Ranges are calculated by assuming: (1) materials based on the use of aluminum frames and structures; (2) materials based on the use of steel frames and structures.

**Table 7.** (continued)

[i] Values for combustion emissions are from Kohan et al. (1979), USEPA (1979), Gorman et al. (1977), and Ritschard et al. (1978).

[j] Values for emissions from barite and bentonite procurement are assumed to be the same as those for concrete. Emissions during operations for vapor-dominated resources are from Reed and Campbell (1975) and Griffen and McClure (1974). Operating emissions for liquid-dominated resources are from USDOE (1980d), Ermak, Nyholm and Gudikson (1979), Westec Service, Inc. (1979), Bechtel Corporation (1976), Morris and Hill (1980), and Anspaugh (1978).

[k] Values for combustion emissions are from Smith, Weyant, and Holdren (1975), assuming high-sulfur coal (2.5-3%), and stack-gas cleaning to remove 80-90% of the $SO_x$ and 99-99.5% of the particulates.

[l] Values for operating emissions are from Smith, Weyant, and Holdren (1975).

from zero to 13 (Hamilton, 1979). The National Academy of Sciences gives a figure of 0.2 excess deaths/year per 100,000 people per $\mu g/m^3$, with an uncertainty range from 10 times smaller to 2 times larger (National Academy of Sciences, 1975). When the Brookhaven group combines its median estimate with an analysis of emissions, ambient concentrations, and associated population exposures for the whole United States, it estimates that each thousand metric tons of sulfur dioxide emitted in the U. S. produces an average of 2.5 excess deaths. The corresponding figure using the National Academy of Sciences dose-response relation would be 0.15 excess deaths per thousand metric tons of $SO_2$. The difference in these estimates is even larger than the numbers just provided suggest, however, because Brookhaven assumes that each death represents the loss of 5 to 15 years of life expectancy while the National Academy assumes that each death represents the loss of only weeks to months of life expectancy. (Brookhaven is assuming that sulfate *causes* a non-negligible part of cardiovascular and respiratory disease; the Academy finds the data in support of this view unpersuasive and assumes that sulfate only *aggravates* pre-existing disease, killing in air-pollution episodes people who already were near death.)

This difference in the available "best estimates" of the public-health consequences of sulfur emissions — a factor of 15 in number of "excess deaths" and a factor of about 100 in mean loss of life expectancy per death (10 years versus 1 month) — is enormous. If one combines the Brookhaven estimate with, say, an intermediate emissions figure of 200,000 MT of $SO_2$ per exajoule (typical, according to Table 7, of chemical fuels from oil or electricity from biomass), one gets, on a national average basis, 500 excess deaths per exajoule with a loss of life expectancy of 10 years per death. If one uses the Academy dose-response relation instead, one gets 30 excess deaths with a loss of life expectancy of 1 month per death. The former figure represents an impact much bigger than the occupational fatalities tabulated for the same energy sources in Table 4; the latter figure is comparable to the corresponding occupational fatalities in number, but much smaller in impact because of the small loss of life expectancy per death on the public side.

## Some Summary Observations

No energy source presently known or imagined — not excepting conservation, renewables, or fusion — is entirely free of impacts on human health and safety. These impacts may be occupational or public, fatal or nonfatal, direct (injuries and illnesses caused by effluents and accidents) or indirect (impacts caused through the disruption of bio-geophysical and sociopolitical conditions and processes).

In general, occupational impacts are more easily quantified than public, injuries more easily quantified than illnesses, fatalities more easily quantified than nonfatal damages, and direct impacts more easily quantified than indirect. Analysts tend to become preoccupied with those components of harm that can be convincingly quantified, but often the largest potential damages are in the categories resistant to quantification.

The importance of a threat to health or safety depends not only on the most probable level of damage associated with the threat but also (among other factors) on the maximum conceivable damage, on the size of the uncertainties associated with the most probable and maximum values, on the real or perceived controllability of the threat, and on whether or not the people threatened are the same ones who choose and use the energy source in question.

No single index can capture these diverse attributes of threats to health and safety, which makes comparing such threats from one energy source to the next (or even different threats from a single energy source) like comparing apples and oranges — it is unavoidably a matter of taste as well as of judgement. This observation does not mean there is no role for analysis but simply that, once analysts have described the threats (in all their dimensions) as best they can, the decisions about which threats to accept in exchange for benefits, which to abate, and which to avoid are as inevitably and properly a *political* matter as any other social choice where individual values and preferences conflict.

With all the caveats implied by the foregoing observations, we can venture some conclusions about the health and safety impacts of the renewable, geothermal, and fusion energy sources we have mainly been considering here.

First, the most easily estimated impacts — occupational accidents — fall within a range for all the energy sources that is similar to the range for these effects in the cases of fossil fuels and nuclear fission. By conventional economic measures, these damages are modest compared to other costs of energy supply; as numbers of deaths per exajoule, they are modest compared to the numbers of fatalities society tolerates in connection with the use of the energy involved; they are susceptible to reduction by identifiable technical and managerial measures; and the people at risk are direct beneficiaries of the activity producing the threat (being employed by it) and are in a good position to be compensated by the users of the energy for any unusual health and safety burdens. This class of impacts, then, provides little basis for altering energy choices made on other grounds.

Second, special occupational hazards that cannot now be estimated quantitatively would be associated with orbiting solar power stations, with photovoltaic-cell manufacture where particularly toxic substances are involved, and perhaps with some processes employed to produce synfuels from biomass. These possibilities warrant continued attention.

Third, accident hazards to the public from the transport of fuels and materials for energy facilities are neither entirely insignificant nor staggeringly large for most of the energy sources considered. Only in the case of certain biomass schemes is it plausible that public risks from transport would approach those of coal, but no detailed estimates for these biomass cases seem to be available. (Conceivably there could be a significant risk to the public associated with the transport into orbit of materials for satellite power stations, but this cannot be estimated at present.) Other public accident risks that are plausibly significant but not presently quantified are dwelling fires due to heating with wood, falls from roofs during owner installation and maintenance of solar collectors, windmill accidents, and accidents at fusion reactors. All of these seem likely to be relatively susceptible to managerial and technical "fixes."

Fourth, threats to public health from routine emissions to air and water are highly uncertain but possibly significant for some of the sources considered. Among air pollutants, only sulfur oxides in the presence of particles can be associated at present with a quantitative dose-response relation, and even in this case the uncertainty is enormous. If the pessimists are correct about the dose-response relation, sulfur emissions pose the largest of the quantifiable direct threats to public health and safety for all the energy sources considered. Clearly, it is critically important to determine who is correct about sulfur. (Of course, the sulfur threat for all of the energy sources will be less than that for coal, irrespective of dose-response relation, assuming all sources of emissions are subject to the same fractional degree of control. Achieving such controls on small biomass combustors may be more difficult than doing so on large coal boilers, however.) Public-health threats from emissions of oxides of nitrogen and particles to the atmosphere and from emissions of organics and other compounds to water are not presently quantifiable but deserve the closest continuing investigation.  If these threats turn out to be important, they will be most so, among the energy sources considered here, for biomass and geothermal.

In summary, notwithstanding the truism that no energy source is completely free of environmental liabilities, and notwithstanding the large uncertainties that surround some classes of these liabilities, it seems that many of the energy sources considered here will pose direct threats to health and safety modest compared to those of coal and oil and compared to those associated with the end-uses of the energy supplied.  Probably more important, however, is that few if any of the energy sources considered here pose *indirect* threats to health and safety remotely approaching those of oil, coal, and nuclear fission.  These indirect threats, as discussed in detail by von Hippel elsewhere in this volume, almost certainly far outweigh the direct ones we have been considering here.

## Acknowledgement

This article is based in part on work supported as follows:  a series of contracts from the Office of Environmental Assessments, U. S. Department of Energy, to the Energy and Environment Division, Lawrence Berkeley Laboratory; a series of contracts from the Development Division, California Energy Commission, to the Energy and Resources Group, University of California, Berkeley; and a consulting arrangement between the senior author and the Magnetic Fusion Energy Division of the Lawrence Livermore National Laboratory.

## Notes

[1]"R-values" are measures of resistance to heat flow. They have units of $(Btu/hr/°F/ft^2)^{-1}$.  The inverse of the sum of the R-values of the components of a cross-section of part of a building's envelope gives the overall heat transfer coefficient for that part of the envelope.  This inverse is called a "U-value", and has units of $Btu/hr/°F/ft^2$. A ceiling with R-30 insulation (corresponding to about nine inches of fiberglass) will allow heat to flow through it at the rate of 1/30 = 0.03 $Btu/hr/ft^2$ of ceiling per degree of difference between the inside and outside temperatures.

[2]Analysts who believe that sulfates and particulates *cause* rather than merely aggravate respiratory disease estimate greater loss of life expectancy — see discussion on Comparative Data.

[3]Tidal power stations, of which an example is in commercial operation at La Rance, France, are estuarine rather than true "ocean" energy systems.  Such tidal power plants

are similar to hydroelectric plants in the nature of their occupational and public health and safety risks. The number of potential sites for such stations is in any case extremely limited, because of the high tidal range needed to make them economically interesting.

[4]The term "Known Geothermal Resource Area" refers to geothermal fields in which exploratory drilling has confirmed the presence of an economically producible resource.

[5]For example, jet fuel will not run a radio transmitter and electricity will not run a jet plane. The convention that three units of fuel are "equivalent" to one unit of electricity, based on the efficiency of typical fuel-burning power plants, has no general usefulness for either economic or environmental assessment; converting the three units of fuel into the one unit of electricity requires incurring additional economic and environmental costs (hence the two quantities are not equivalent for purposes of economic or environmental comparison); and, if one were starting with electricity and wanted liquid fuel, even the energy "equivalency" would be different than the conventional 1:3 (getting the fuel from electrolysis of water would give perhaps two units of fuel for three of electricity).

[6]The materials are assumed to be transported by either railroads or trucks. This assumption introduces a small error for those materials that are transported partly by one mode and then transferred to another.

## References

Albers, J. P., W. J. Barviec, and L. F. Rooney. 1976. *Demand for Nonfuel Minerals and Materials by the United States Energy Industry, 1975-90.* U. S. Geological Survey Professional Paper 1006A. U. S. Government Printing Office.

Anderson, B. 1976. *Solar Home Book.* Cheshire Books, Harrisville, N. H.

Anderson, K. 1980. *A Comparison of Economic Costs, Materials and Labor Requirements, Occupational Risks, and Emissions of Several Air Pollutants Associated with Various Energy Conservation, Energy Supply, and Passive Solar Design Alternatives for Space Conditioning in New Residences.* Energy and Resources Group, University of California, Berkeley, California (In press).

Anspaugh, L. R. 1978. *Final Report on the Investigation of the Impact of the Release of Rn, its Daughters, and Precursors at the Geysers Geothermal Field and Surrounding Area.* Lawrence Livermore Laboratory.

Ashare, E. D. L. Wise, and R. L. Wentworth. 1977. *Fuel Gas Production from Animal Residue.* Dynatech R/D Company, Report COO/2991-10. National Technical Information Service, Springfield, Virginia.

Ayyaswamy, P., B. Hauss, T. Hseih, A. Mocati, T. E. Hicks, and D. Okrent. 1974. *Estimates of the Risks Associated with Dam Failure.* UCLA-ENG-7423, March 1974. UCLA Engineering.

Bailie, R. C. 1976. *Technical and Economic Assessment of Methods for Direct Conversion of Agricultural Residue to Usable Energy.* West Virginia University, Morgantown. TID-28552.

Bechtel Corporation. 1976. *Conceptual Design of Commercial 50 MWe (Net) Geothermal Power Plants at Heber and Niland, California - Final Report.* Report SAN-1R4-1. San Francisco, California.

Besant, R. W., R. S. Dumant, and G. J. Schoenau. 1979. The passive performance of the Saskatchewan Conservation House. In *Proceedings of the 3rd National Passive Solar Conference.* Report CONF-790118. U. S. Department of Energy, National Technical Information Service, Springfield, Virginia, pp. 713-719.

Bliss, C. and D. O. Blake. 1977. *Silvicultural Biomass Farms. Volume V. Conversion Processes and Costs.* MITRE/METREK Division. Report MTR-7347 (V.5). National Technical Information Service, Springfield, Virginia.

Brooks, H., E. Ginzton, K. Boulding, R. Cannon, E. Gornowski, J. Holdren, H. Houthakker, H. Kohn, S. Lewand, L. Lischer, J. Neess, D. Rose, D. Sive, and B. Spinrad. 1979. *Energy in Transition 1985-2010.* Final Report of the Committee on Nuclear and Alternative Energy Systems. Washington, D. C. National Academy of Sciences. Also published in 1980 by W. H. Freeman and Co., San Francisco.

Budiansky, S. 1980. New attention for atmospheric carbon. *Environ. Sci. and Technol.* 14:1430-1432.

Budnitz, R. J. and J. P. Holdren. 1976. Social and environmental costs of energy systems. *Ann. Rev. Energy* 1:553-580.

California Energy Commission. 1980. *Proposed 1980 Residential Building Standards.* Report P400-80-037. Sacramento, California.

California Energy Commission. 1981. *Electricity Tomorrow: Challenges and Opportunities for California, 1981.*

Biannual Report to the Governor and the Legislature. Sacramento, California (January 1981).

Cameron, E., R. W. Conn, G. L. Kulcinski, and I. Sviatoslav-sky. 1979. *Minerals Resource Implications of a Tokamak Fusion Reactor Economy*. Report UWFDM-313. Nuclear Engineering Department, University of Wisconsin, Madison, Wisconsin.

Caputo, R. 1977. *An Initial Comparative Assessment of Orbital and Terrestrial Central Power Systems*. Jet Propulsion Lab Report 900-780. Pasadena, California, California Institute of Technology.

Carasso, M., J. Gallagher, K. Sharma, J. Gayle, and R. Barany. 1975. *The Energy Supply Planning Model*. Bechtel Corporation Report 10900-900 75-31, 2 volumes. San Francisco, California.

Case, G. D., T. A. Bertolli, J. C. Bodington, T. A. Choy, and A. V. Nero. 1977. *Health Effects and Related Standards for Fossil-Fuel and Geothermal Power Plants*. Vol. 6. Lawrence Berkeley Laboratory Report LBL-5287. National Technical Information Service, Springfield, Virginia.

Ching, F.D.K. 1975. *Building Construction Illustrated*. Van Nostrand Reinhold Company, New York.

Cooper, A. 1981. Geothermal Engineer, Chevron Oil Company. Conversation with author. January 15, 1981.

Cooper, J. A. 1980. *Environmental Impact of Residential Wood Combustion Emissions and Its Implications*. Presented at the Wood Energy Institute Wood Heating Seminar VI, February 25-28, Atlanta, Georgia.

Curtis, B., B. Andersson, R. Kammerud, W. Place, and K. Whitley. 1979. *Thermal Mass: Its Role in Residential Construction*. Report LBL-9290. Lawrence Berkeley Laboratory, Berkeley, California.

Curtis, B. 1981. Personal Communication. Lawrence Berkeley Laboratory, Berkeley, California (January).

Davidson, M. and D. Grether. 1977. *The Central Receiver Power Plant: An Environmental, Ecological and Socio-economic Analysis*. Report LBL-6329. Lawrence Berkeley Laboratory, Berkeley, California.

Davidson, M., D. Grether, and K. Wilcox. 1977. *Ecological Considerations of the Solar Alternative*. Report LBL-5927. Lawrence Berkeley Laboratory, Berkeley, California.

Deese, D. A. and J. S. Nye (eds.). 1981. *Energy and Security*. Ballinger, Cambridge, Massachusetts.

DeHoven, N. 1980. Heber project manager for Southern California Edison. Personal Communication (January 13).

Desrosiers, R. E. 1979. *Process Designs and Costs Estimates for a Medium BN Gasification Plant Using a Wood Feedstock.* Solar Energy Research Institute. Report SERI/TR-33-151. National Technical Information Service, Springfield, Virginia.

Ehrenreich, H. 1979. *Principal Conclusions of the American Physical Society Study on Solar Photovoltaic Energy Conversion.* American Physical Society, New York, N. Y.

Ehrlich, P. R., A. H. Ehrlich, and J. P. Holdren. 1977. *Ecoscience: Population, Resources, Environment.* W. H. Freeman and Company, San Francisco, California.

Ermak, D. L., R. A. Nyholm, and P. H. Gudiksen. 1979. *Imperial Valley Environmental Project: Air Quality Assessment.* Lawrence Livermore Laboratory. Report UCRL-52699.

Fentron Industries, Inc. 1980. *Series 2000 and 2000TB Hinged and Pivoted Windows; Series 3000 Sliding Windows — High Performance Window Systems for Hospital, Institutional, Monumental, and Commercial Applications.* Brochure.

Freeman, S. D., P. Baldwin, M. Canfield, S. Carhart, J. Davidson, J. Bunkerley, C. Eddy, K. Gillman, A. Makhijani, K. Saulter, D. Sheridan, and R. Williams. 1974. *A Time to Choose: America's Energy Future.* Final Report of the Energy Policy Project of the Ford Foundation. Ballinger, Cambridge, Massachusetts.

Gandel, M. G. and P. A. Dillard. 1976. *Assessment of Large-Scale Photovoltaic Materials Production.* Report No. LMSC HREC-D496940. Lockheed Missiles and Space Company, Sunnyvale, California.

Gleick, P. H. 1980. *The Environmental Consequences of Hydroelectric Development: The Issue of Size.* ERG-80-7. Energy and Resources Group, University of California, Berkeley.

Gorman, P. G., L. J. Shannon, M. P. Schrag, and D. E. Fiscus. 1977. *St. Louis Demonstration Project Final Report: Power Plant Equipment, Facilities and Environmental Evaluations.* Midwest Research Institute Project No. 4033-L, Kansas City, Missouri.

Griffin, D. P. and H. K. McClure. 1974. *Emissions of Non-condensable Gases and Solid Materials from the Power Generating Units at the Geysers Power Plant.* Report 7485. Pacific Gas & Electric Company, San Ramon, California.

Habegger, L. J., J. R. Gasper, and C. D. Brown. 1980. *Health and Safety: Preliminary Comparative Assessment of the Satellite Power System and Other Energy Alternatives.* Report DOE/ER-0053. Argonne National Laboratory, Argonne, Illinois.

Haefele, W., J. P. Holdren, G. Kessler, and G. L. Kulcinski. 1977. *Fusion and Fast Breeder Reactors.* Report RR-77-8. International Institute for Applied Systems Analysis, Laxenburg, Austria.

Hahn, J. L. 1979. Occupational hazards associated with geothermal energy. *Geother. Resources Council Trans.* 3:283-286.

Hahn, J. 1980. California Department of Health Services, Berkeley, California. Meeting with author (January 8).

Hamilton, L. D. 1979. Health effects of electricity generation. In *Proceedings of Conference on Health Effects of Energy Production,* September 12-14, 1979. Chalk River Nuclear Laboratories, Ontario, Canada.

Harte, J. and A. Jassby. 1978. Energy technologies and natural environments: The search for compatibility. *Ann. Rev. Energy* 3:101-146.

Hartley, J. N., L. E. Erickson, R. L. Engel, and T. J. Foley. 1976. *Materials Availability for Fusion Power Plant Contruction.* Report BNL-2016, Battelle Pacific Northwest Laboratories. National Technical Information Service, Springfield, Virginia.

Hayes, E. T. 1976. Energy implications of materials processing. *Science* 191:661-65.

Herendeen, R. A., T. Kary, and J. Rebitzer. 1979. Energy analysis of the solar power satellite. *Science* 205(4405):451-54.

High, C. 1980. New England returns to wood. *Natur. Hist.* 89:14-32 (February).

Hildebrandt, A. and L. Vant-Hull. 1977. Power with heliostats. *Science* 197:1139-46.

Holdren, J. P. 1978a. Environmental impacts of energy production and use: a framework for information and analysis. In *Energy Information* (W. Hogan, ed.). Institute for Energy Studies, Stanford, California.

Holdren, J. P. 1978b. Fusion energy in context: Its fitness for the long term. *Science* 200:168-180.

Holdren, J. P. 1978c. Fusion power and nuclear weapons: A significant link? *Bull. Atomic Scien.* 34:4-5 (March).

Holdren, J. P.  1980.  *Cross-Cutting Issues in Integrated Environmental Assessment of Energy Alternatives: Distribution of Costs and Benefits.*  Working Paper ERG-WP-80-13.  Energy and Resources Group, University of California, Berkeley, California.

Holdren, J. P.  1981a.  Contribution of activation products to fusion accident risk:  Part 1.  A Preliminary investigation.  *Nucl. Technol./Fusion* 1:79-89.

Holdren, J. P.  1981b.  Fusion-fission hybrids:  Environmental aspects and their role in hybrid rationale.  *J. Fusion Energy* 1:197-209.

Holdren, J. P. and P. Herrera.  1971.  *Energy.*  Sierra Club Books, New York.

Holdren, J. P., K. Anderson, P. H. Gleick, I. Mintzer, G. Morris, and K. R. Smith.  1979.  *Risk of Renewable Energy Sources:  A Critique of the Inhaber Report.*  ERG-79-3.  Energy and Resources Group, University of California, Berkeley, California.

Holdren, J. P., G. Morris, and I. Mintzer.  1980.  Environmental aspects of renewable energy sources.  In *Annual Review of Energy* (J. Hollander, ed.).  Vol. 5, pp. 241-291.  Annual Reviews, Inc., Palo Alto, California.

Hovel, H.  1975.  Solar cells.  In *Semiconductors and Semimetals.*  Vol. 11.  Academic Press, London.

Hunt, L. P., V. D. Dosaj, J. R. McCormick, and A. W. Rauchholz.  1978.  Advances in the Dow-Corning process for silicon.  In *Conference Record of the Thirteenth I.E.E.E. Photovoltaic Specialists Conference,* June 5-8, 1978, Washington, D. C.  Institute of Electrical and Electronic Engineers, New York, N. Y.

Intergroup Consulting Economists.  1976.  *Economic Pre-Feasibility Study:  Large Scale Methanol Fuel Production from Surplus Canadian Forest Biomass.  Vol. 2.*  Fisheries and Environment, Ottawa, Ontario.

Jones, J. L., W. S. Fong, F. A. Schooley, and R. L. Dickenson.  1978.  *Mission Analysis for the Federal Fuels from Biomass Program.  Volume V, Biochemical Conversion of Biomass to Fuels and Chemicals.*  SRI International Report TID-29093.  National Technical Information Service, Springfield, Virginia.

Kelly, H.  1978.  Photovoltaic power systems:  A tour through the alternatives.  *Science* 199:634-640.

Kestin, J., R. DePippo, H. Ezzut Khalifa, and D. J. Ryley (eds.).  1980.  *Sourcebook on the Production of Electricity from Geothermal Energy.*  U. S. Department of

Energy Report DOE/RA/28320-2.   Government Printing Office, Washington, D. C.

Kohan, S. M., P. M. Barkhordar, F. A. Schooley, and R. L. Dickenson. 1979. *Mission Analysis for the Fuels from Biomass Program. Volume IV. Thermochemical Conversion of Biomass to Fuels and Chemicals.* (SRI International) Report SAN-0115-T3. National Technical Information Service, Springfield, Virginia.

Larson, W. E. 1979. Crop residues: energy production of erosion control? *J. Soil and Water Conserv.* 34:74-76.

Lave, L. B. and E. P. Seskin. 1977. *Air Pollution and Public Health.* Johns Hopkins Press for Resources for the Future, Baltimore, Maryland.

Lawrence, K. A. 1979. *A Review of the Environmental Effects and Benefits of Selected Solar Technologies.* Solar Energy Research Institute Report SERI/TP-53-114R. National Technical Information Service, Springfield, Virginia.

Lawrence, K. A. and C. L. Strojan. 1980. Environmental effects of small wind energy conversion systems. In *Proceedings of the Second U. S. Department of Energy Environmental Control Symposium,* CONF-800334/2, pp. 228-241.

Layton, D. (ed.). 1980. *An Assessment of Geothermal Development in the Imperial Valley of California. Volume 1 - Environment, Health and Socioeconomics.* Lawrence Livermore Laboratory Report DOE/EV-0092. National Technical Information Service, Springfield, Virginia.

Leitner, P. 1978. *An Environmental Overview of Geothermal Development: The Geysers-Calistoga KGRA - Volume 3, Noise.* Lawrence Livermore Laboratory Report UCRL-52496. National Technical Information Service, Springfield, Virginia.

Leonard, E. M. (ed.). 1979. *Wood Burning for Power Production.* Report LA-7924-MS. Los Alamos Scientific Laboratory, Los Alamos, New Mexico.

Lidsky, L. M. 1975. Fission-fusion systems: Hybrid, symbiotic, and Augean. *Nucl. Fusion* 15:151-173.

Lockheed Missiles and Space Company, Inc. 1975. *Ocean Thermal Energy Conversion (OTEC) Power Plant Technical and Economic Feasibility.* LMSC-D056566, Vols. I and II.

Mazria, E. 1979. *The Passive Solar Energy Book.* Rodale Press, Emmaus, Pennsylvania.

McIlraith, T. E.  1980.  Geothermal power and problems. *Proceedings of the Ninth Turbomachinery Symposium* 105-118.

Mintzer, I.  1980.  *Integrated Assessment Issues Raised by the Environmental Effects of Photovoltaic Energy Systems*.  Report ERG 80-5.  Energy and Resources Group, University of California, Berkeley, California.

MITRE/METREK Division.  1977.  Annual Environmental Analysis Report.  *A Preliminary Environmental Analysis of Energy Technology Using the Assumptions of the National Energy Plan, Vol. IV.  Simulation Data Base (Draft)*.  McLean, Virginia.

Morris, G.  1980.  *Issues Raised by the Environmental Impacts of Biomass Energy Systems*.  Report ERG 80-6.  Energy and Resources Group, University of California, Berkeley, California.

Morris, W. and J. Hill (eds.).  1980.  *An Assessment of Geothermal Development in the Imperial Valley of California.  Volume 2 — Environmental Control Technology*.  Lawrence Livermore Laboratory Report DOE/EV-0092.  National Technical Information Service, Springfield, Virginia.

Moses, H.  1979.  Impacts of satellite power system technology.  *Energy* 4:799-809.

National Academy of Sciences, Commission on Natural Resources.  1975.  *Air Quality and Stationary Source Air Pollution Control*.  Prepared for the Committee on Public Works of the United States Senate.  U. S. Government Printing Office, Washington, D. C.

National Fire Data Center.  1978.  *Fire in the United States*.  U. S. Department of Commerce.  Government Printing Office, Washington, D. C.

National Institute for Occupational Safety and Health, U. S. Department of Health Education and Welfare.  1977.  *Criteria for a Recommended Standard: Occupational Exposure to Hydrogen Sulfide*.  NIOSH-77-158.

National Safety Council.  1978.  *Work Injury and Illness Rates*.  Report 125.58.  1978 edition.  National Safety Council, Chicago, Illinois.

Neff, T. L.  1978.  Comparative social costs and photovoltaic prospects.  In *Conference Record of the Thirteenth I.E.E.E. Photovoltaic Specialists Conference, June 5-8, 1978, Washington, D. C.*  Institute of Electrical and Electronic Engineers, New York, N. Y. pp. 1001-03.

Nuclear Energy Policy Study Group. 1977. *Nuclear Power Issues and Choices*. Ballinger, Cambridge, Massachusetts.

Office of Technology Assessment. Congress of the United States. 1978. *Application of Solar Technology to Today's Energy Needs*. Washington, D. C.

Office of Technology Assessment, Congress of the United States. 1979. *Gasohol-A Technical Memorandum*. Report OTA-TM-E-1. U. S. Government Printing Office, Washington, D. C.

Office of Technology Assessment, Congress of the United States. 1980. *Energy from Biological Processes Vol. II - Technical and Environmental Analyses*. Report OTA-E-128. U. S. Government Printing Office, Washington, D. C.

Peart, R. M., M. R. Ladisch, and H. R. Zink. 1979. Gasification of corncobs in a producer gas generator. Presented at *Technology for Energy Conservation Conference*, Tuscon, Arizona, January 23-25, 1979. Purdue University, Agricultural Engineering Department.

Pefley, R., H. Adelman, and T. Suga. 1980. *Methanol/Ethanol/Gasoline Blend Fuels Demonstration with Stratified Charge Engine Vehicles (Final Report)*. University of Santa Clara Report. Prepared for the California Energy Commission.

Pella, Inc. 1980. *Pella Residential/Light Construction Catalog-Windows and Sliding Glass Doors*.

Perry, A. M., G. Marland, and L. W. Zelby. 1978. Net energy analysis of an OTEC system. In *Proceedings of the 5th Ocean Thermal Energy Conversion Conference*. Volume I (February 20-27).

Place, W., R. Kammerud, B. Andersson, B. Curtis, W. Carroll, C. Christensen, and M. Hannifan. 1980. *Human Comfort and Auxiliary Control Considerations in Passive Solar Structures*. Report LBL-10034. Lawrence Berkeley Laboratory, Berkeley, California.

Ramsey, C. G. and H. R. Sleeper. 1970. *Architectural Graphic Standards*. John Wiley and Sons, Inc., New York, N. Y. (6th ed.).

Raphael Katzen Associates. 1978. *Grain Motor Fuel Alcohol Technical and Economic Assessment Study*. Cincinnati, Ohio. Report HCP/J6639-01. U. S. Government Printing Office, Washington, D. C.

Reed, M. J. and G. E. Campbell. 1975. Environmental impact of development in the Geysers Geothermal Field, U.S.A.

In *Proceedings of the 2nd U. N. Symposium on Develop-ment and Use of Geothermal Resources - Vol. II.* U. S. Government Printing Office, Washington, D. C.

Reno, V. 1980. Shakedown for the envelope house: A physi-cal exam. *Solar Age* 5:14-21 (November).

Ritschard, R. L., K. F. Haven, M. Henriquez, J. Kay, and W. Walzer. 1978. *Characterization of Solid Waste Conversion and Cogeneration Systems.* Report LBL-7883. Lawrence Berkeley Laboratory, Berkeley, California. National Technical Information Service, Springfield, Virginia.

Ross, D. 1979. *Energy from the Waves.* Pergamon Press, Ltd., Oxford, England.

Salo, D. J., R. E. Inman, B. J. McGurk, and J. Verhoeff. 1977. *Silvicultural Biomass Farms. Vol. III, Land Suitability and Availability.* MITRE/METREK Division Report MTR-7347 (Vol. III). National Technical Infor-mation Service, Springfield, Virginia.

Sathaye, J. A., H. Ruderman, R. Sextro, P. Benenson, L. Kunin, P. Chan, J. Kooser, Y. Ben Dov, B. Green, and R. Clear. 1977. *Analysis of the California Energy Indus-try.* Report LBL-5928. Lawrence Berkeley Laboratory. Berkeley, California.

Shelton, J. W. 1979. *Wood Heat Safety.* Garden Way Publish-ing, Charlotte, Vermont.

Sittig, M. 1975. *Environmental Sources and Emissions Hand-book.* Noyes Data Corporation, Park Ridge, N. J.

Smith, K., J. Weyant, and J. Holdren. 1975. *Evaluation of Conventional Power Systems.* Report ERG 75-5. Energy and Resources Group, University of California, Berkeley, California.

Teeter, R. R. and W. M. Jamieson. 1980. *Preliminary Mate-rials Assessment for the Satellite Power System.* Report DOE/ER-0038. Battelle Columbus Laboratories, Columbus, Ohio.

Tennessee Valley Authority. 1954. *Engineering Data, TVA Water Control Projects and Other Major Hydro Develop-ments in the Tennessee and Cumberland Valleys,* Vol. I. Technical Monograph 55.

Thompson, R. 1976. Behavior of hydrogen sulfide in the atmosphere and its effects on vegetation (Tucker, Fayne, and Anderson, eds.). In *Geothermal Environmental Seminar - 1976: Lake County, California.* Shearer Graphic Arts, Lakeport, California.

Tillman, D. A. 1978. *Wood as an Energy Resource*. Academic Press, New York, N. Y.

U. S. Council on Environmental Quality. 1981. *Global Energy Futures and the Carbon Dioxide Problem*. U. S. Government Printing Office, Washington, D. C.

U. S. Department of Commerce. 1976. *Flat Glass Quarterly*. Office of Industrial and Trade Administration. American Statistical Index 1976 Report No. 2506-9.6. U. S. Government Printing Office, Washington, D. C.

U. S. Department of Commerce, Office of Industrial and Trade Administration. 1978a. *U. S. Industrial Outlook 1978*. U. S. Government Printing Office, Washington, D. C.

U. S. Department of Commerce, Bureau of Economic Analysis. 1978b. *Business Statistics, 1977*. U. S. Government Printing Office, Washington, D. C.

U. S. Department of Commerce. 1978c. *Statistical Abstract of the United States, 1978*. U. S. Government Printing Office, Washington, D. C.

U. S. Department of Commerce. 1978d. *Analysis of Accident Data and Hours of Service of Interstate Commercial Motor Vehicle Drivers*. U. S. Bureau of Motor Carrier Safety, Washington, D. C.

U. S. Department of Commerce. 1978e. *Census of Manufacturers, 1972*. U. S. Government Printing Office, Washington, D. C.

U. S. Department of Commerce. 1979. *Statistical Abstract of the United States*. 100th edition. Bureau of the Census.

U. S. Department of Energy. 1977. *Environmental Developmental Plan: Photovoltaics*. DOE/EDP-0003. National Technical Information Service, Springfield, Virginia.

U. S. Department of Energy. 1978. *Preliminary Environmental Assessment for the Satellite Power System*. Office of Energy Research-Satellite Power Systems Project Office. DOE/ER-0021. Vols. 1 and 2. National Technical Information Service, Springfield, Virginia.

U. S. Department of Energy. 1979a. *Energy Budget Levels Selection, Technical Support Document for Notice of Proposed Rulemaking on Energy Performance Standards for New Buildings*. DOE/CS-0119. Office of Conservation and Solar Energy. Office of Buildings and Community Systems.

U. S. Department of Energy. 1979b. Energy performance standards for new buildings; proposed rule. 10 CFR 435. *Federal Register 44*, No. 230, pp. 681-68181.

U. S. Department of Energy. 1979c. *Environmental Readiness Document: Solar Thermal Power Systems.* DOE/ERD-0019. National Technical Information Service, Springfield, Virginia.

U. S. Department of Energy. 1979d. *Technology Assessment of Wind Energy Conversion Systems.* LA-8044-TASE. Los Alamos National Laboratory.

U. S. Department of Energy, Assistant Secretary for Environment. 1980a. *Technology Characterizations: Environmental Information Handbook.* DOE/EV-0072. U. S. Government Printing Office, Washington, D. C.

U. S. Department of Energy. 1980b. *Summary of Solar Energy Technology Characterizations.* DOE/EV-0099.

U. S. Department of Energy. 1980c. *Technology Assessment of Wind Energy Conversion Systems.* DOE/EV-0103.

U. S. Department of Energy. 1980d. *Geothermal Demonstration Program-50MW Power Plant, Boca Ranch, New Mexico — Final Environmental Impact Statement.* DOE/EIS-0049. National Technical Information Service, Springfield, Virginia.

U. S. Department of the Interior. 1970. *Mineral Facts and Problems.* Bureau of Mines Bulletin 650. U. S. Government Printing Office, Washington, D. C.

U. S. Department of Labor. 1978a. *Occupational Injuries and Illnesses in the United States by Industry, 1975.* Bureau of Labor Statistics Bulletin 1981. U. S. Government Printing Office, Washington, D. C.

U. S. Department of Labor. 1978b. *Employment and Earnings, 1909-1975.* Bureau of Labor Statistics. U. S. Government Printing Office, Washington, D. C.

U. S. Department of Transportation. 1980a. *Analysis of Motor Carriers of Property, 1978.* Federal Highway Administration, Washington, D. C.

U. S. Department of Transportation. 1980b. *1979 Accident/ Incident Bulletin 148.* Federal Railroad Administration, Washington, D. C.

U. S. Energy Research Development Administration. 1977a. *Solar Program Assessment: Environmental Factors, Solar Thermal Electric Systems.* ERDA-77-47/4. U. S. Government Printing Office, Washington, D. C.

U. S. Energy Research Development Administration. 1977b. *Solar Program Assessment: Environmental Factors, Photovoltaics.* ERDA-77-47/3. U. S. Government Printing Office, Washington, D. C.

U. S. Energy Research Development Administration.  1977c.
*Solar Program Assessment: Environmental Factors, Fuels
for Biomass.* ERDA-77-47/7.  U. S. Government Printing
Office, Washington, D. C.

U. S. Energy Research Development Administration.  1977d.
*Solar Program Assessment: Environmental Factors for
Wind Energy Conversion.* ERDA-77-47/6.  U. S. Govern-
ment Printing Office, Washington, D. C.

U. S. Environmental Protection Agency.  1974.  *Scientific
and Technical Assessment Report on Cadmium.* Report
60016-75-003.  U. S. Government Printing Office, Washington, D. C.

U. S. Environmental Protection Agency.  1979.  *Compilation of
Air Pollutant Emissions Factors* (3rd edition, including
supplements 1-9).  Report AP-42.  U. S. Government
Printing Office, Washington, D. C.

U. S. Federal Energy Administration.  1974.  *Project Independence Blueprint, Final Task Force Report: Solar
Energy.* OTA, Congress of the U. S., Washington, D. C.

U. S. Nuclear Regulatory Commission.  1975.  *Reactor Safety
Study.* WASH-1400, NUREG-75/014.  National Technical
Information Service, Springfield, Virginia.

U. S. Office of Management and Budgets.  1972.  Statistical
Policy Division.  *Standard Industrial Classification
Manual: 1972 Edition.* U. S. Government Printing
Office, Washington, D. C.

U. S. Public Health Service.  1978.  *Facts of Life and Death.*
U. S. Government Printing Office, Washington, D. C.

Unseld, C. T., D. E. Morrision, D. L. Sills, and C. P. Wolf
(Eds.).  1979.  *Sociopolitical Effects of Energy Use
and Policy.* Supporting Paper 5.  Study of Nuclear
and Alternative Energy Systems.  National Academy of
Sciences, Washington, D. C.

Waste Management, Inc.  1976.  *A.S.E.F. Solid Waste to
Methane Gas Title I: Preliminary Engineering.* Report
CONS/2770-1.  National Technical Information Service,
Springfield, Virginia.

Westec Service, Inc.  1979.  *Final Environmental Impact
Report: North Brawley Ten Megawatt Geothermal Demonstration Facility.* San Diego, California.

# 5. Global Risks from Energy Consumption

## Introduction

Global risks are among the most uncertain risks associated with energy technologies but are also, perhaps, the most important since they affect relationships between nations and hence, in a relatively direct way, affect the probability of war.

In this paper some of the global risks associated with current and frequently proposed future levels of consumption of energy from oil, coal, fission, fusion, and "renewable sources" are discussed. The dangers involved are all quite serious and relatively near term. These include: world war over Persian Gulf oil, climate change due to the buildup of atmospheric $CO_2$, the accelerated proliferation of nuclear weapons, and competition between food and energy for land and water. It will, therefore, be urged that much greater emphasis be placed on examining how we use energy and how to reduce energy waste. At the levels of consumption which economically justified levels of energy efficiency could bring about, enough flexibility could develop in our choice of a future energy supply mix so that the associated global risks could be reduced dramatically.

## Petroleum

There can be little disagreement that the current level of dependence on petroleum for energy in the United States is dangerous and must be transitory. It is only because the per capita use of petroleum in the rest of the world is so much less than it is in the United States that we have the possibility of shifting to other energy sources in an orderly way.

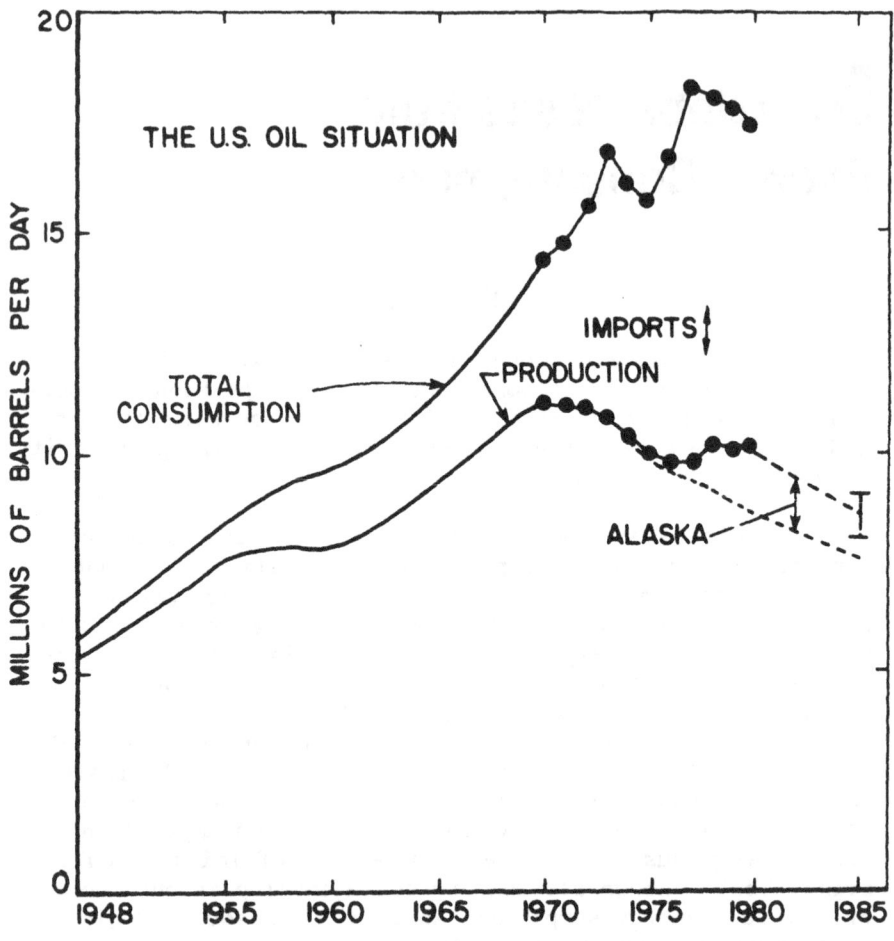

Figure 1.   The U. S. oil situation.

The remaining resource of recoverable conventional oil is about 400 bbl or 50 metric tons (MT) for each of the four billion people in the world.[1]  In the United States we may have up to twice this world average per capita oil resource (USGAO, 1979), but we consume about 4 MT per capita per year (USDOE/EIA, 1980).  At this rate we will consume the equivalent of our entire remaining endowment of oil resources in the next 10-30 years.  We have found that we can only sustain a rate of oil consumption anywhere near our current level by persuading other nations, in one way or another, to give us a share of *their* oil.  Today about 40% of U.S. petroleum consumption is sustained by imports (Fig. 1) and, according to most governmental and industrial projections, domestic production will continue to fall.

The current worldwide distribution of oil production and consumption is not stable — even at an average world per capita consumption rate of about 0.6 MT per year.  Very few regions other than the Persian Gulf will be able physically to maintain their oil production at the current levels for long, and the concentration of approximately one-half of the world's oil resources in a region populated by less than 2% of the world's people (Fig. 2) is a source of increasing world tension.  The non-Communist oil-importing nations, in particular, have found their economies suddenly vulnerable to political developments in this very unstable region, which for good measure, lies directly adjacent to the Soviet Union.

This vulnerability will not be easy to overcome since total fossil fuel consumption of the non-Communist world tripled between 1947 and 1978 with oil replacing coal as the dominant fossil fuel during this post-World War II period.[2]  During this same period, the Persian Gulf became a major locus of world oil production.  In 1947, the United States and the Middle East accounted for 60 and 10%, respectively, of world oil production (API, 1975, Table IV.1).  In 1978, the corresponding percentages were 16 and 34% (BP, 1979, p. 6).

The levels of tension resulting from the dependence of the non-Communist industrialized nations on oil imports from the Persian Gulf are, of course, dangerous for world peace.  It is certainly a principal cause for the new U.S. interest in building up its war-fighting capability, both conventional (the Rapid Deployment Force) and nuclear (the MX missile).

## Other Fossil Fuels

To many people the answer to the petroleum problem is to shift back to the more abundant, albeit less convenient,

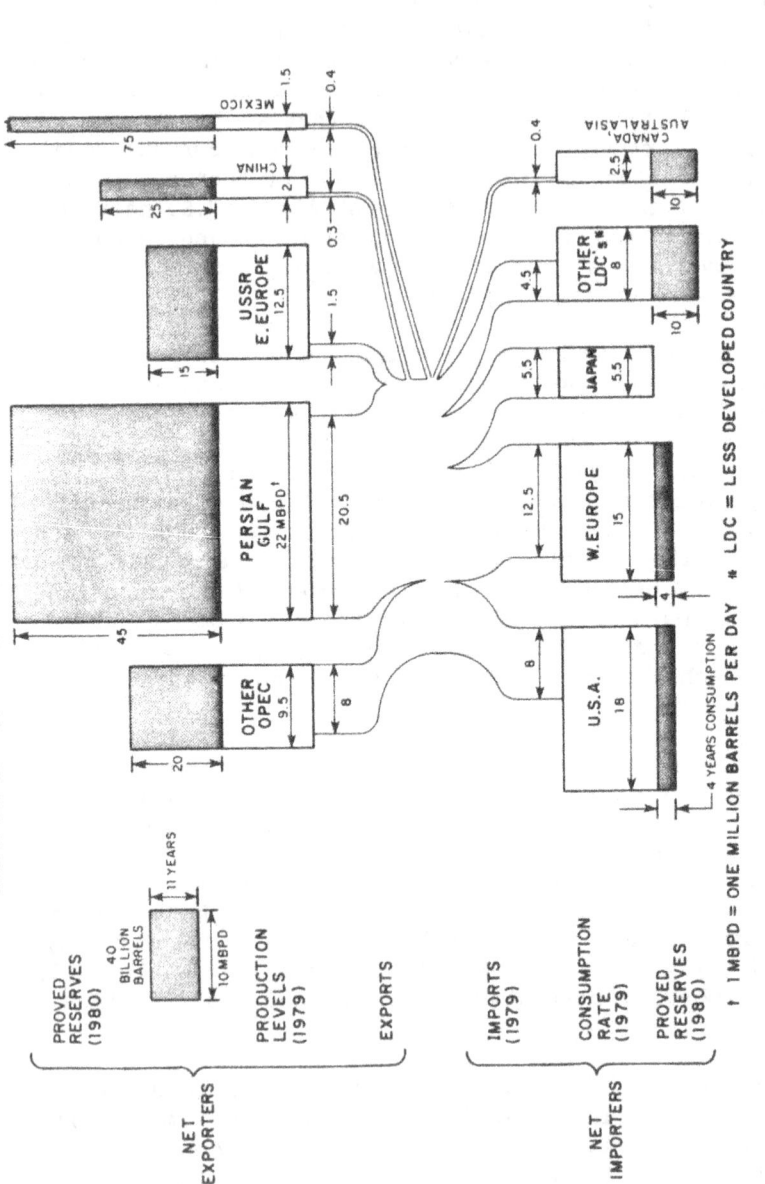

Figure 2. The world oil situation in 1979. The production and consumption data in Figure 2 are obtained principally from BP (1979). The reserve data are taken from Auldridge (1980). Most numbers are rounded to the nearest one-half million barrels per day (MBPD). Oil consumption by the OPEC and "other LDC" nations was estimated from 1978 data (USDOE/EIA, 1978, Table 2). Both numbers were increased by 0.5 MBPD to bring 1979 world production and consumption into balance.

fossil fuels — notably coal. Here we run into another global problem, however: the buildup of carbon dioxide in the atmosphere.

Today there are 170 MT of carbon in the atmosphere for each person in the world. About ten times that much carbon exists underground in mineable fossil fuels (Baes et al., 1976) and at current worldwide fossil fuel consumption rates, we are releasing this carbon into the atmosphere at a rate of 1.4 MT per capita per year.[3]

In the short term (a few decades), carbon is apparently accumulating at approximately equal rates in the surface layers of the ocean and in the atmosphere (Broecker et al., 1979). It appears, therefore, that at the current rate of carbon dioxide buildup, man could double the level of carbon dioxide in the atmosphere in about 250 years. If the world per capita consumption rate of fossil fuels were increased to the U.S. level in 1979 (6 times world average) and mix [50% oil, 30% natural gas, and 20% coal (BP, 1979)] using coal and coal-derived liquid and gaseous fuels, then at the current world population level, this length of time would be reduced to less than 25 years.[4]

In the real world, global fossil fuel consumption will neither stay constant nor increase instantaneously. Figures 3a and 3b show, respectively, two fossil fuel consumption scenarios, and the resultant increases of atmospheric $CO_2$ calculated by Baes et al. (1976). The high scenario is a classical "boom and bust" scenario, which assumes that the release of carbon dioxide due to the consumption of fossil fuels will continue to grow approximately at the 4.3% annual rate that prevailed between 1860 and 1975 (with brief interruptions during the World Wars and the 1929-1933 crash). The growth only stops when the limits on the world's resources of economically mineable fossil fuels are approached around the year 2060; then a period of relatively rapid decline begins. The peak rate of fossil fuel consumption projected for 2060 is extraordinary — corresponding to a rate of carbon dioxide release 15 times higher than the 1975 level. In absolute terms, 80 billion MT of carbon would be released per year or 10 MT per capita for a world population of 8 billion. From another perspective, however, this peak rate of fossil fuel consumption is not extraordinary at all: it corresponds to a world per capita rate of coal consumption equivalent only to current U.S. per capita fossil fuel energy consumption.

In the low scenario of Fig. 3a, the $CO_2$ emission rate peaks in 2025 at about 2.5 times the current level, followed by a symmetrical decline in emissions after 2025 as nonfossil

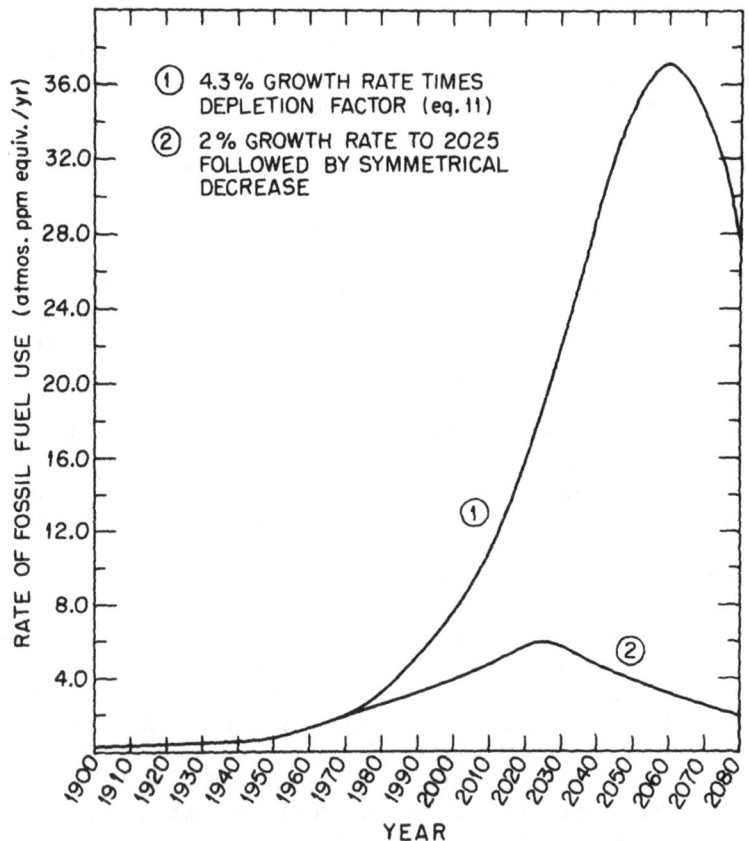

**Figure 3a. Possible limiting scenarios for the use of fossil fuels (Baes et al., 1976, p. 37).**

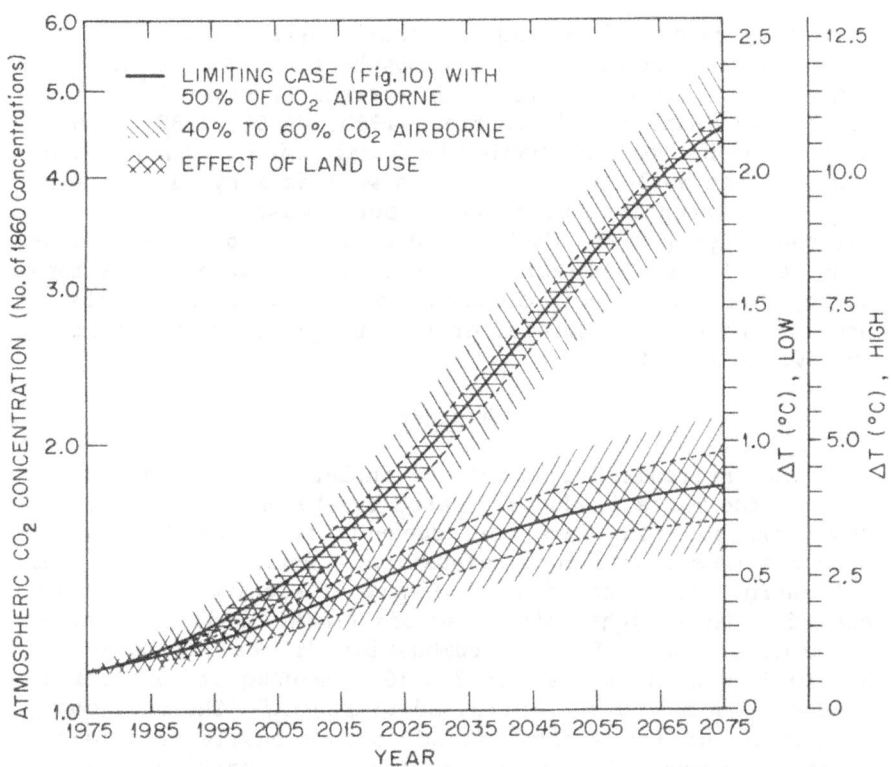

Figure 3b. Projected atmospheric $CO_2$ concentrations and possible changes in the average surface temperature (Baes et al., 1976, p. 40).

energy sources take over.  The pre-2025 low growth scenario
corresponds to an approximately constant global per capita
level of fossil fuel energy consumption, if there is a doubling of the world's population and a shift to coal during
that same period.  (About 1.3 times as much $CO_2$ would be
released per unit energy consumed in 2025 if 100% of the fossil fuel consumed were coal instead of the present 50-20-30%
mix of petroleum, natural gas, and coal.)  The low scenario
predicts somewhat less than a doubling and the high scenario
predicts somewhat more than a quadrupling of preindustrial
$CO_2$ levels.

Most calculations suggest that a quadrupling of the
carbon dioxide content of the atmosphere would cause a warming of the global climate by an average of several degrees
centigrade (Manabe and Stouffer, 1980; USDOE, 1980).  This
would probably be accompanied by local climate changes that
would affect world agriculture, as well as many natural systems, in currently unpredictable but almost certainly significant ways (USDOE, 1980).  A decision to continue to consume fossil fuels subject only to their resource limitations
would, therefore, be a decision to set no weight on the
probable major consequences of the changes in global climate
that would result.

## Fission

The environmental impacts of nuclear energy are reduced
because the waste products created by the energy release are
about one million times more concentrated than the waste
products from fossil fuel combustion.  About 30 MW-d of thermal energy are released per kilogram of uranium loaded into
one of today's light-water reactors (IAEA, 1980).  The corresponding number for the combustion of coal is about
$3 \times 10^{-4}$ MW-d/kg of fuel or $3 \times 10^{-5}$ MW-d/kg of combustion
products including the entrained nitrogen.[5]  The very concentration of the energy stored in fissionable materials
creates, however, its own set of problems — particularly the
problem of nuclear weapons.

Surely, the greatest threat to the future of civiliza-
tion today lies in the enormous stockpile of nuclear weapons
that are continuously being added to and refined by the
United States and the Soviet Union in their mindless nuclear
arms race.  According to estimates by the U. S. Congressional
Office of Technology Assessment (OTA, 1979), by 1985 U. S.
strategic nuclear forces will possess about 14,000 nuclear
warheads with a total explosive power of 3.5 billion tons of
TNT, and Soviet Union strategic nuclear forces will possess
about 9,000 nuclear warheads with a total explosive power of
10 billion tons of TNT.  In addition, each side possesses

10-20 thousand tactical or "theatre" nuclear warheads.  For comparison, the total tonnage of bombs dropped in World War II is estimated at 3 million tons (Garwin, 1980).

The danger posed by this nuclear arms race is being increased by the continuing spread of nuclear weapons and weapons manufacturing capabilities to many other nations. Although the addition to the total destructive potential already in the arsenals of the world's megadeath "super-powers" will be relatively small for many years, it takes only a few nuclear weapons to kill millions of people.

Unfortunately, despite the protestations of the nuclear industry to the contrary (see e.g., Starr, 1978), the spread of nuclear weapons technologies has been closely linked to the spread of civilian nuclear technologies in the past and is likely to continue to be so in the future.  The French nuclear program was so ambiguous in the early years, for example, that many of the scientists involved believed it had only civilian purposes (Scheinman, 1965).  China developed its nuclear weapons on a technological foundation that was established with the assistance of the Soviet Union under an agreement which was made in 1957 and dissolved a few years later – possibly because of Chinese interest in nuclear weapons (OTA, 1977).  Apparently, India produced its 1974 nuclear explosion with plutonium that was created in a research reactor provided by Canada (SIPRI, 1975).  Israel is widely believed to have, at least, the ability to rapidly construct nuclear weapons with plutonium produced from a French-supplied research reactor that is under no international safeguards (SIPRI, 1972).  South Africa is also commonly believed to have, or be close to having, a nuclear weapons capability that uses highly enriched uranium produced using technology developed with assistance from West Germany (Rogers and Cervenka, 1978).  Pakistan is known to be developing nuclear weapons using equipment and knowledge procured clandestinely from the nuclear industry in Europe (Oberdorfer, 1979; BBC-TV Panorama, 1980).  Argentina has an operating nuclear power reactor provided by West Germany. Although this reactor is under international safeguards, Argentina has not yet signed the Nonproliferation Treaty, and the Chairman of its National Atomic Energy Commission has stated publicly that his technologists are capable of constructing nuclear weapons (OTA, 1977).  Iraq recently used her "oil weapon" to force France to keep a commitment to supply Iraq with research reactor fuel containing weapons grade uranium (Wade, 1980).  Iraq insisted on this; despite the fact that France had shown that Iraq's twin research reactor would operate satisfactorily on low enriched uranium (IAEA, 1980).

Of course, banning nuclear power would not put the
nuclear weapons genie back into the bottle, but history suggests that civilian nuclear energy programs provide a convenient cover as well as the training, technology, and
nuclear material necessary for the construction of nuclear
weapons (Feiveson, 1972).  If the international nuclear
energy establishment is successful in commercializing the
plutonium breeder reactor, the potential numbers of nuclear
weapons will increase vastly, and separated nuclear weapons
material will be circulating in such large amounts that it
is likely we will soon be facing the threat of nuclear armed
terrorist groups who won't be susceptible to deterrence by
the threat of nuclear retaliation.

A one million kW(e) breeder reactor operating on the
plutonium fuel cycle would discharge about 1 MT of plutonium
each year (Feiveson, von Hippel, and Williams, 1979).  If
plutonium breeders were used to supply the world with primary energy at the same rate that fossil fuel does today,
5000 MT of plutonium would be discharged each year or enough
[at 10 kg of plutonium apiece (Taylor, 1975)] to make one-
half a million Nagasaki bombs — one for every 8000 people in
the world.  The diversion of even one ten-thousandth of this
plutonium by terrorists would make possible the devastation
of 50 cities a year.  It is sobering to note, therefore,
that the U. S. Government has been able to keep track of the
plutonium in its weapons program to an accuracy of only
about one part in a hundred.[6]

It is easy to demonstrate that a commitment to a plutonium economy can be postponed for decades until the level of
our long-term commitment to nuclear power can be settled.
There is sufficient uranium in the earth's deposits of high
grade uranium ore to sustain our current generation of
nuclear reactors (which do not involve commerce in separated
plutonium) in any numbers that electricity demand growth can
justify well into the next century (Feiveson, von Hippel,
and Williams, 1979).  Unfortunately, however, the world's
energy research and development establishment became committed to the plutonium breeder more than a decade ago.  At
that time it appeared that the breeder would cost little
more than conventional nuclear power reactors; the redou-
bling of the demand for electric energy every 10 years
appeared to be a law of nature [between 1950 and 1970 U. S.
electricity consumption increased by a factor of 4 — two
doublings — and world electricity consumption grew by a
factor of 5 (Doblin, 1975)], which would inevitably lead to
electricity demands that only the breeder could conceivably
satisfy, and the problems of nuclear weapons proliferation
and nuclear terrorism were clouds on the horizon, which
appeared "no bigger than a hand."  Now all these conditions

have changed, and it appears quite possible that the plutonium breeder may never be needed.  Yet, the spokesmen and
public relations departments of much of the U.S. electricity
industry continue to urge a national commitment to deploy
plutonium breeder reactors with rhetoric which becomes ever
more strident.[7]

## Fusion

Fusion is another way of releasing nuclear energy and
is likely to share with fission many of the same problems of
maintaining the separation between military and civilian
technologies.  Indeed, the easiest fusion reaction to
ignite, the deuterium-tritium reaction, releases approximately 5 times as many neutrons per unit of energy released
as nuclear fission and has, therefore, been discussed as a
possible basis for a fissile fuel production facility that
could "breed" more excess plutonium or other chain reacting
material than fission breeder reactors (see e.g., Bethe,
1979).

## Solar Energy

The problems associated with our currently dominant
commercial energy technologies have helped stimulate the
renewed interest in solar energy technologies.  Other
stimuli are the relatively uniform distribution of the solar
resource, the possibility of exploiting it on a relatively
small scale, and the increased costs of "conventional"
energy supplies.

The most abundant form of solar energy is, of course,
direct sunlight.  The average rate at which energy in sunlight falls on U. S. buildings, alone, is equal to one-half
of the current rate of U. S. fossil fuel consumption.[8]
Direct solar energy could be captured and redistributed in
amounts equal to tens of times current human fossil energy
use without serious global effects (Williams, 1978).  Some
indirect forms of solar energy such as wind power could also
be exploited on a considerably smaller but still significant
scale.[9]

The large-scale exploitation of other forms of indirect
solar energy would not necessarily have such benign results,
however.  Consider, for example, the potential implications
of a very large increase in the use of biomass (wood, grass,
etc.) as fuel.  Today biomass provides approximately one-
sixth as much fuel energy worldwide as do fossil fuels.  It
would take the energy content of almost 10% of the earth's
gross annual biomass production – twice as much as is harvested today to provide humans with food and fiber[10] – to

equal the current level of world fossil fuel consumption. Sustaining a population of 8 billion, at the level of today's U. S. per capita fossil fuel energy use, would take approximately the earth's entire annual biomass production. Biomass productivity could be increased greatly in certain areas, but it is obvious that exploitation of biomass energy at even the current level of fossil fuel use would have global implications. "Energy plantations" could, for example, compete for land and water with food or fiber producing activities. Since more carbon is stored in living plants than in the atmosphere, the harvesting of standing biomass could also significantly increase the $CO_2$ in the atmosphere.[11]

## Energy Efficiency

Our examination of the global problems associated with energy supply technologies raises the question: Why do we use so much energy anyway? This question is always fruitful because it seems that whenever one studies in some detail a particular energy end-use, one always finds that at least one-half of the energy is wasted due to inefficiencies that would cost much less to rectify than the value of the wasted energy at current prices.

Ross and Williams (1981) have recently published an energy efficiency analysis of the entire U.S. economy. They consider only cost-effective energy efficiency improvements, including a shift to 45 mpg passenger cars and to buildings that are one-third as energy intensive as today. They conclude that an economy with twice the current U.S. per capita income could be supported at a per capita level of energy consumption lower by one-quarter than today's. A National Academy of Science (NAS, 1978) study has come to a similar conclusion.

Opportunities for energy efficiency improvements are not limited to the United States. One of the reasons why the forests in many areas of the Third World are being depleted (Eckholm, 1975), for example, is because the efficiencies of Third World cooking stoves are so low.[12]

## Conclusions

It would appear that many of the very serious global risks that are associated with current and projected levels of energy consumption are being undertaken to support energy waste rather than energy needs. A direct way to reduce these risks would, therefore, be to increase the efficiency of energy use. U.S. security might be increased, for example, if we trained, re-equipped, and re-deployed the Rapid

Deployment Force into our homes with the mission of reducing U.S. residential energy waste. Similarly, funds that are proposed for the construction of the MX intercontinental missile system might be much more effectively used to improve our security if they were spent to retool our automobile factories for the production of 60 mpg automobiles.

## Notes

[1]One barrel of crude petroleum weighs about 0.136 MT. Most estimates of ultimately recoverable world crude oil resources fall in the range of 1600 to 2300 billion bbl. As of 1975, an estimated 336 billion bbl had been produced (OTA, 1980a). The annual rate of production since then has been about 22 billion bbl per year (USDOE/EIA, 1980) which would bring the total production through 1980 to about 450 billion bbl.

[2]In 1947, total world consumption of coal, oil and natural gas outside of the Communist nations was the energy equivalent of 1.3 billion MT of oil, with coal accounting for 60% (USDOI, 1976). In 1978, the corresponding level of energy consumption was the energy equivalent of 4.2 billion MT of oil, with oil accounting for 60% and coal only 20% (BP, 1979). It has been assumed here that coal has two-thirds the heating value of oil per ton.

[3]In 1978, the world consumed the fossil fuel energy equivalent of $6.1 \times 10^9$ MT of oil [50% oil; 30% coal; 20% natural gas (USDOI, 1976)]. This is about 1.4 MT of oil equivalent per capita per year for a 1978 global population of 4.3 billion (UN, 1979). Oil is about 87% carbon by weight, and natural gas and coal contain respectively 0.8 and 1.4 times as much carbon per unit of stored energy as oil (Albanese and Steinberg, 1980). On average, therefore, the combustion of the energy equivalent of 1 MT of petroleum in 1978 released 0.94 MT of carbon in $CO_2$ to the atmosphere. The flaring of natural gas and the manufacturing of cement in 1976 each released about 2% as much $CO_2$ to the atmosphere as did fossil fuel use (Albanese and Steinberg, 1980).

[4]The factor of 6 between United States and world average per capita energy consumption would result in a factor of 12 in $CO_2$ production because coal contains 1.3 times as much carbon per unit energy as the current world fossil fuel mix and because the conversion of coal to liquid and gaseous synthetics would have an efficiency of about 0.6 (Albanese and Steinberg, 1980).

[5]The ratio of waste stream masses is reduced to a factor of 250 if the wastes associated with uranium mining and enrichment are included. In 1977, the average uranium ore being mined was only about 0.15% uranium. In the

isotopic enrichment process that precedes the manufacture of
fuel for today's commercial light-water power reactors
(enrichment from 0.7 to about 3% $^{235}$U), approximately five-
sixths of the uranium ends up in the depleted (0.2% $^{235}$U)
uranium "tails" stream at the enrichment plant.

[6]In 1977, the U. S. Energy Research and Development
Administration (ERDA) reported that "ERDA plants dating from
the establishment of the Atomic Energy Commission in 1946
showed a cumulative Inventory Difference through September 30, 1976, of 1,490 kilograms of plutonium and 690 kilograms of uranium-235 in uranium enriched to 20 percent or
more." [ERDA Press Release, "ERDA Issues Report on Inventory Differences for Strategic Nuclear Materials," August 4,
1977.] The U. S. inventory of plutonium can be estimated to
be on the order of 100 MT according to the following chain
of argument: As of 1976 the inventory of $^{90}$Sr at the ERDA
Hanford and Savannah River sites — the locations at which
the Department of Energy produces its plutonium — was 285
million Ci (Krugman and von Hippel, 1977). Assuming that
the wastes averaged 15 years old, this would correspond to
an original production of approximately 400 million Ci of
$^{90}$Sr (half-life, 30 years). About 3 Ci of $^{90}$Sr are produced
by the fission of 1 gm of uranium in reactors of the type
(thermal neutron) used for the production of weapons plutonium. The total amount of uranium fissioned would therefore
have been approximately 135 MT. If all of the uranium had
been fissioned in plutonium production reactors with a production of 1 gm of plutonium per gram of uranium fissioned,
U. S. plutonium production during this period would have
been approximately 135 MT. [Lamarsh (1976) estimates 1 gm
$^{239}$Pu per gram of uranium fissioned in a small plutonium
production reactor.] In fact, some of the uranium was used
to provide neutrons for the production of tritium, which is
also used in nuclear weapons, so that actual cumulative
U. S. plutonium production would be somewhat lower — but
still on the order of 100 MT.

[7]See e.g., the flyer titled "A War We Can Win: the
Clinch River Breeder Reactor Project" that was being distributed during 1980 by the Breeder Reactor Corporation. In
this flyer Paul Harvey, "the world's largest one-man news
network," explains to the American public, "the quick way
for us to win this energy war is with 'nuclear weapons.'
The United States now has available breeder reactors...The
National Academy of Sciences, in a study sponsored by our
government, determined that we need *all* our energy options...
But the administration, intimidated by nervous Nellies in
its own Environmental Protection Agency, has suspended
licensing...Nearly every enlightened nation in the world is
building breeders — except ours...we may lose by default —
the nuclear war we could so easily win."

The Breeder Reactor Corporation was originally established to build the Clinch River demonstration breeder reactor and receives most of its funding from the federal government.

[8]U.S. buildings cover an area of ground of about 10 billion $m^2$, and the annual average level of "insolation" in the United States is about 170 $W/m^2$ (Rabl and von Hippel, 1981). The total annual insolation on the U. S. building area is, therefore, about $40 \times 10^{15}$ Btu, which is approximately one-half of U.S. annual energy use (USDOE/EIA, 1980). Of course, only a small fraction of this energy could be collected and used to displace fossil fuels.

[9]Thompson (1981) estimates that an average of 3.5 times the current U. S. electricity production could be produced using wind turbines spaced about 20 rotor diameters apart over that one-sixth of the North American land area which has an average wind power density exceeding 400 $W/m^2$. This is equivalent to the current rate of U. S. fossil fuel consumption (assuming a fuel to electrical energy conversion efficiency of 40%).

[10]In 1978, the world produced an estimated 1.5 billion MT of grain [29% wheat, 24% corn, 24% rice, 13% barley, 5% soybeans, and 3% oats (UN, 1979)]. Associated with this grain production was about 2.4 billion tons (dry weight) of crop residue (Burwell, 1978). The world also supported about 2.8 billion domesticated food-producing grazing animals [45% cattle, 39% sheep, and 16% goats (UN, 1979)] which consumed about 3 billion MT of dry biomass including much of the grain and crop residues. Assuming that one-half of the food for these animals was derived from forage, the total of grain, grain crop residues, and forage would come to about 6 billion MT dry biomass. In 1977, an estimated 2.5 billion $m^3$ (1.3 billion MT) of wood were harvested for fiber [lumber, paper, etc. (UN, 1979)]. An approximately equal amount of logging residue was left in the forest. [OTA (1980b) estimates that U. S. logging residues, not including stumps, currently have a dry weight equal to approximately 55% of the harvest.] The total dry weight of plant materials harvested and left annually as residues in human agriculture and forestry activities, therefore, comes to about 8 billion MT or about 5% of the estimated annual primary production of the earth's land plants. [The global annual primary production of land biomass is estimated to be $1.72 \times 10^{11}$ MT of dry organic matter (Rodin et al., 1975) and to have an energy content equal to about 70 billion MT tons of petroleum.]

[11]There are about 650 billion MT of carbon stored in the atmosphere (Baes et al., 1976). According to Rodin, Bazilevich, and Rozov (1975), "the total phytomass of the

land is estimated to be $2.4 \times 10^{12}$ MT dry weight." About one-half of this phytomass would be carbon, and 56% is located in the tropical zone. Pimental (1980) estimates that the carbon in the world's soil humus is 1.34 billion MT, of which 16% is in the tropic zone. Estimates in USDOE (1980) of total organic carbon stored in tropical plants and soil are respectively three and two times smaller, however.

[12]According to a comprehensive study of energy use in an Indian village (Reddy and Subramanian, 1979), it was found that the energy content of the wood consumed for cooking purposes was $8 \times 10^9$ J per capita per year — twice the annual per capita primary energy consumption for cooking in the United States (Blue et al., 1979).

## References

Albanese, A.S. and M. Steinberg. 1980. *Environmental Control Technology for Atmospheric Carbon Dioxide*. DOE/EV-0079. U.S. Department of Energy. Washington, D.C.

American Petroleum Institute (API). 1975. *Basic Petroleum Data Book*. Washington, D.C.

Auldridge, L. 1980. World oil flow slumps, reserves up. *Oil and Gas J.*, December 29, pp. 78, 79.

Baes, C.F. Jr., H.E. Goeller, J.S. Olson, and R.M. Rotty. 1976. *The Global Carbon Dioxide Problem*. ORNL-5194. Oak Ridge National Laboratory, Oak Ridge, Tenn.

BBC-TV Panorama. *The Birth of the Islamic Bomb*. June 15, 1980.

Bethe, H.A. 1979. The fusion hybrid. *Phys. Today* 32(5): 44-51.

Blue, J.L., K.H. Lowe, B.J. Hurlbut, G.E. Liepins, A.B. Rose, M.A. Smith, and M.G. Strohlein. 1979. *Buildings Energy Use Data Book, Edition 2*, p. xxi. ORNL-5552, Oak Ridge National Laboratory, Oak Ridge, Tenn.

British Petroleum (BP). 1979. *BP Statistical Review of the World Oil Industry*. London.

Broecker, W.S., T. Takahashi, H.J. Simpson, and T.H. Peng. 1979. Fate of fossil fuel carbon dioxide and the global carbon budget. *Science* 206:409-418.

Burwell, C.C. 1978. Solar biomass energy: an overview of U. S. potential. *Science* 199:1041-1048.

Doblin, C.P. 1979. *Historical Data Series, 1950-1976*. WP-79-87. International Institute for Applied Systems Analysis, Laxenburg, Austria.

Eckholm, E.   1979.   *Planting for the Future: Forestry for Human Needs.*   Worldwatch Institute Report No. 26. Washington, D.C.

Feiveson, H.A.   1972.   *Latent proliferation: The international security implications of civilian nuclear power* (Ph.D. Thesis, Woodrow Wilson School of Public and International Affairs, Princeton University, 1972).

Feiveson, H.A., F. von Hippel, and R.H. Williams.   1979. Fission power: an evolutionary strategy.   *Science* 203: 330-337.

Garwin, R.L.   1980.   New weapons/old doctrines: strategic warfare in the 1980's.   *Proc. Amer. Phil. Soc.* 124: 261-265.

International Atomic Energy Agency (IAEA).   1980.   International fuel cycle evaluation.   Report of Working Group 8.   *Advanced Fuel Cycle and Reactor Concepts*, p. 98.   Vienna, Austria.

Krugman, H. and F. von Hippel.   1977.   Radioactive wastes: a comparison of U.S. military and civilian inventories. *Science* 197:883-885.

Lamarsh, J.R.   1976.   On the construction of plutonium – producing reactors by small and/or developing nations, reprinted in *Export Reorganization Act of 1976.*   Hearings before the U.S. Senate Committee on Government Operations, January 19, 20, 29, 30 and March 9, 1976, pp. 1326-1355.

Makhijani, A. and A. Poole.   1975.   *Energy and Agriculture in the Third World.*   Ballinger Press, Cambridge, Massachusetts.

Manabe, S. and R.J. Stouffer.   1980.   Study of climatic impacts of $CO_2$ increase with a mathematical model of the global climate.   In *Report of the Workshop on Environmental and Societal Consequences of a Possible $CO_2$-Induced Climate Change*, p. 127.   CONF-7904143.   U.S. Department of Energy.   National Technical Information Service, Springfield, Virginia 22161.

Oberdorfer, D.   1979.   Pakistan: the quest for atomic bomb. *Washington Post*, August 27, 1979, pp. A-1, A-22.

Office of Technology Assessment (OTA).   1977.   *Nuclear proliferation and safeguards.*   p. 101.   U. S. Government Printing Office, Washington, D.C.

Office of Technology Assessment (OTA).   1979.   *The Effects of Nuclear War.*   U.S. Government Printing Office, Washington, D.C.

Office of Technology Assessment (OTA). 1980a. *World petro-leum availability 1980-2000*. Technical Memorandum. U. S. Government Printing Office, Washington, D.C.

Office of Technology Assessment (OTA). 1980b. *Energy from Biological Processes*. U.S. Government Printing Office, Washington, D.C.

Pimental, D. 1980. Increased $CO_2$ effects on the environment and in turn on agriculture and forestry. In *Report of the Workshop on Environmental and Societal Consequences of a Possible $CO_2$-Induced Climate Change*. CONF-7904143. U.S. Department of Energy. National Technical Information Service, Springfield, Virginia 22161.

Rabl, A. and F. von Hippel. 1981. *The Solar Radiation Resource*. Princeton University, Center for Energy and Environmental Studies Report (to be published, 1981).

Reddy, A.K.N. and D.K. Subramanian. 1979. The design of rural energy centers. *Proc. Indian Acad. Sci.* C2, Part 3.

Rodin, L.E., N.I. Bazilevich, and N.N. Rozov. 1975. Productivity of the world's main ecosystems. In *Productivity of World Ecosystems*. U.S. National Academy of Sciences. Washington, D.C.

Rogers, B. and Z. Cervenka. 1978. *The Nuclear Axis*. Times Books. New York.

Ross, M. and R.H. Williams. 1981. *Our Energy: Regaining Control*. McGraw-Hill, New York.

Scheinman, L. 1965. *Atomic Energy Policy in France Under the Fourth Republic*. Princeton University Press, Princeton, N. J.

Starr, C. 1978. Nuclear power and weapons proliferation – the thin link. *Technol. and Soc.* March, 1978. p. 4.

Stockholm International Peace Research Institute (SIPRI). 1972. *The Near-Nuclear Countries and the NPT*, p. 27. Humanities Press, New York.

Stockholm International Peace Research Institute (SIPRI). 1975. *SIPRI Yearbook 1975*, p. 16. MIT Press, Cambridge, Mass.

Taylor, T.B. 1975. Nuclear safeguards. *Ann. Rev. Nucl. Sci.* 25:407-421.

Thompson, G. 1981. *The Prospects for Wind and Wave Power in North America*. Princeton University, Center for Energy and Environmental Studies Report, No. 117.

United Nations (UN). 1979. *World Statistics in Brief.* New York, N.Y.

U.S. Department of Energy. Energy Information Administration (USDOE/EIA). 1978. *International Petroleum Annual.* DOE/EIA-0042 (78). U.S. Government Printing Office, Washington, D.C. Table 2.

U.S. Department of Energy. Energy Information Administration (USDOE/EIA). 1980. *Monthly Energy Review.* DOE/EIA-0035 (80/12). U.S. Government Printing Office, Washington, D.C.

U.S. Department of Energy (USDOE). 1980. *The Role of Tropical Forests on the World Carbon Cycle.* CONF-800350. National Technical Information Service, Springfield, Virginia 22161.

U.S. Department of Energy (USDOE). 1980a. *Report of the Workshop on Environmental and Societal Consequences of a Possible $CO_2$-Induced Climate Change.* CONF-7904143. National Technical Information Service, Springfield, Virginia 22161.

U.S. Department of the Interior (USDOI). 1976. *Energy Perspectives 2.* U.S. Government Printing Office, Washington, D.C.

U.S. Government Accounting Office (USGAO). 1979. *Analysis of Current Trends in U.S. Petroleum and Natural Gas Production.* EMD-80-24. Washington, D.C.

U.S. National Academy of Science (NAS). 1978. U.S. energy demand: some low energy futures. Report of Demand and Conservation Panel of the Committee on Nuclear and Alternative Energy Systems. *Science* 200:142-152.

Wade, N. 1980. France, Iraq, and the bomb. *Science* 209: 1001.

Williams, J. 1978. Global climatic disturbance due to large-scale energy conversion systems. In *Multidisciplinary Research Related to the Atmospheric Sciences* (Boulder, Colorado, National Center for Atmospheric Research).

_William D. Schulze, David S. Brookshire,_
_Ralph C. d'Arge_

# 6. Economic Valuation of the Risks and Impacts of Energy Development

## Introduction

The traditional approach for evaluating energy technologies, purely on the grounds of financial or economic feasibility, has given way to a set of much broader societal concerns. Since the choices to be made concerning technologies, (e.g., fast breeder reactors vs. greater use of coal vs. solar energy) will determine the future quality of life, this broader perspective seems valid. Economic analysis has a clear role in quantifying two aspects of these concerns — those relating to environmental impacts and those relating to risks. This chapter is an attempt to describe the economic state of the art in quantifying what, in traditional benefit-cost analysis, have often been considered intangibles (environmental quality, wilderness experiences, etc.).

The perceived inability of benefit-cost analysis to include broad social concerns has resulted in a number of attempts to quantify risks and environmental impacts in what, from the perspective of economics, are confused and misleading ways. A prime example of this type of study is the Inhaber report (1978) wherein various risks to life of alternative energy technologies are directly compared. Inhaber argues, for example, that, in terms of deaths per unit of energy, nuclear energy is safer than solar home heating. His calculations include lives lost in such activities as uranium mining and in the manufacture of materials for solar collectors as well as risks of nuclear accidents and risks undertaken in installing rooftop collectors. Is it correct from an economic perspective to add up all of these deaths from whatever source? The answer is no. The uranium miner is paid higher wages to accept the risky job of underground

mining; a cost which is eventually passed through as a higher
price for nuclear power. Similarly, markets internalize many
of the risks of installing solar collectors on roofs. Higher
wages are normally paid for riskier jobs in all such industries (see Thaler and Rosen, 1976) so standard feasibility
tests (a comparison of costs where the cheapest source of
energy is the best) already adjust for these *voluntarily
accepted risks* undertaken by employees. Riskier technologies
will cost more because employees in labor markets will demand
and get higher wages to accept such risks. However, not all
risks are internalized by such markets. In particular, no
market pays citizens living near a nuclear power plant to
accept the risk of a nuclear accident. Such a phenomenon is
termed an externality by economists because no organized markets exist to internalize the burden of such risks in monetary terms. Thus, the cost of nuclear power as calculated
using standard feasibility analysis does not include all
costs to residents. Most economists now argue that this
external social cost should be included for purposes of
benefit-cost analysis.

From the perspective of the formal field of ethics, this
last point, that some risks are involuntary, is of great
importance. Few ethical systems would view compensated-
voluntary risks as "wrong" in the moral sense. However,
uncompensated-involuntary risks may be viewed under some
circumstances as morally wrong. This is especially true for
those ethical systems which focus on protecting individual
rights. Thus, locating a nuclear power plant next to an
objecting and fearful neighborhood (even if such fears are
groundless) can be viewed as doing harm to individual rights.
Alternatively, some ethical systems look to the good of the
whole and might argue that those in the objecting neighborhood should make a sacrifice in the national interest. In
any case, the difference between compensated-voluntary risk
and uncompensated-involuntary risk has clear significance
both from an economic perspective and from an ethical perspective (the latter class of risk constitutes an externality
and raises issues of protection of individual rights).

Thus, from the perspective of both economics and phi-
losophy, Inhaber has made a serious error in simply adding
all risks for purposes of social decision making — he is
mixing apples and oranges. Different classes of risk have
vastly different implications. The following section discusses these issues in depth.

The second possible contribution economic analysis can
make to energy decisions relates to economic evaluation of
environmental effects. Quantifying the aesthetic value of
visibility in the Southwest (which may be impaired by new

coal-fired power plants) or valuing wildlife populations which may be disrupted by strip mining of coal in dollar terms has required the development of new techniques. The most broadly applied methodology dealing with the difficult problem of environmental valuation is the "bidding game" or contingent valuation study. This technique is described in the third section, together with a summary of six separate studies which attempt to determine the economic value of certain environmental attributes. The final two sections discuss certain problems associated with benefit-cost analysis of both local and global energy impacts.

## The Economics and Ethics of Valuing Risk

A number of ethical questions persistently trouble economic policy analysis — which usually takes the form of a benefit-cost study. One of the most vexing is the problem of public safety. Many "costs" take the form of risks to human life. Benefits result from reducing such risks or increasing public or private safety. But, how are such safety benefits to be estimated in dollar value for human life? Economists have approached this issue recently by scrupulously avoiding any notion of valuing a *particular* human life. In fact, if an economic measure is used, the value of particular life can be taken as infinite, since to induce a particular rational individual to accept a risk of *certain death* would require infinite compensation (no value is large enough). However, individuals do, in fact, accept compensation for small risks of death. Examples abound. Driving to work entails a small risk presumably compensated as part of wages or salaries. Jobs which are riskier than others can usually be shown to pay more, all other things equal. Thus, a TV antenna installer voluntarily risks falling from rooftops, but presumably demands a *priori* compensation for the additional risk he undertakes. Studies of wages and risk have shown that differing groups and individuals require between $340 (Thaler and Rosen, 1976) to as much as $1,000 (Smith, 1974) more in annual income to *voluntarily* accept increased annual job related risks of death of about one in one thousand (0.001). On this basis, economists argue that a program which reduces risk to 1,000 people by 0.001 and consequently expects to save one life (0.001 × 1,000), is worth between $340,000 and $1 million.

The problem is more complicated than this, however. In observing actual expenditures for safety, enormous differences are apparent. Many traffic safety programs — more barricades, traffic lights, etc. — could save one life per year at a cost of less than $100,000. Given the numbers above, it would seem that the public would clamor for better roads or at least buckle their own seatbelts more often than about

25% of the time. On the other hand, public airline safety may cost more than one million dollars per expected life saved, yet public pressure still exists for safer airline operations. It appears then, that the public rather readily accepts individuals killing themselves in their own automobiles, but views public airline safety in a very different way. Economists tend to make no distinction, but it may well be that a significant ethical difference exists between public and private safety, i.e., knowingly imposing a risk on oneself is "right," while imposing a risk on someone else is "wrong."

## Ethical Systems

Ethical systems attempt to provide a mechanism for answering the question: "Is a contemplated action right or wrong?" An ethical system can take the form of a list of rules. Examples of this class of ethical systems include such specific lists as the Ten Commandments and Kant's Categorical Imperative (1785), which states: "Act only on the maxim whereby thou canst at the same time will that it should become a universal law." Note that the Ten Commandments provide a list of specific behavioral rules while Kant provides a mechanism for generating such a list. The difficulties with lists, however, are first that some of the rules may well come into conflict (be inconsistent) under some circumstances, which as a result requires a hierarchical ordering of rules to resolve conflicts. Second, such lists, if explicit, may fail to cover certain eventualities.

An alternative specification of an ethical system takes the form of a criterion for evaluation. Thus, for example, "do unto others as you would have them do unto you," can be applied to nearly all ethical decisions. Similarly, the statements, "turn the other cheek" and "individuals should have freedom of choice where no one else is bothered" imply that ethical behavior involves not harming others under any circumstances, and yield a general criterion or decision rule.

The latter approach, ethical systems based on ethical criteria, can generally be incorporated into economic analysis by reweighting benefits and costs according to the particular criterion. The former (i.e., lists) is potentially much more difficult to treat, in that a list of rules becomes a set of mathematically specified *constraints* to a decision process such as benefit-cost analysis. Thus, in this initial exploration of ethics, economics, and risk, we focus on ethical systems which take the form of general criteria.

A second difficulty in merging ethics and economics is

the possibility that an ethical criterion and a basic assumption of economic analysis are incompatible. An example is the democratic ethic – what is "right" is what the majority approves. Arrow (1963) has shown in his impossibility theorem that majority voting may imply intransitive social preferences. Transitivity is a fundamental assumption of economic theory necessary even for the basic concept of economic efficiency. Economic analysis thus requires that "if situation A is socially preferred to situation B and B to C, then A is preferred to C." However, even if individuals are transitive in their preferences, Arrow has shown that majority votes can result in social preferences of the "situation A is preferred to B, B is preferred to C, but C is preferred to A" (intransitive) type. Thus, we also require that the ethical criteria employed be transitive.

This requirement, that an ethical system can provide a transitive criterion for social choice leaves at least four ethical systems (and probably more) for analysis. These four are described in a little more detail below.

Utilitarian (Benthamite). A Utilitarian Ethical system requires "the greatest good for the greatest number" as expressed by Jeremy Bentham (1789), John Mill (1863), and others. The social objective is to maximize the sum of the measurable utilities of all individuals in a society. Thus, the Utilitarian Ethic has a pragmatic consequentialist character which in a matter of fact way is quite appealing: if the utility gain of an action exceeds the utility loss across society, the action is "right." If the utility gain is less than the utility loss across society, the action is "wrong."

In addition to the obvious difficulty in making the requisite calculations necessary for moral choices, a fundamental problem afflicts Utilitarians – measuring utility. The problem of distributing income will serve to demonstrate the problem of measurable or cardinal utility. First, we will make the assumption, consistent, for example, with the view of Pigou (1920) that all individuals have the same utility function. Thus, turning to Figure 1, Mr. A and Mr. B have the same relationship between utility ($U_A$ and $U_B$, respectively) and income ($Y_A$ and $Y_B$, respectively). Assume the initial position of society is such that Mr. B is wealthier than Mr. A, that is, $Y_B^o > Y_A^o$; and that the traditional Utilitarian assumption of dimishing marginal utility – that the utility curves in Figure 1 "flatten" out – holds. It is easy to show that we can improve society's total utility by giving A and B the same income, $\bar{Y}$. Note that $Y_B^o - \bar{Y} = \bar{Y} - Y_A^o$, so we take the money away from B to give to A and get a gain in total utility, $U_A + U_B$, since $|\Delta U_A| > |\Delta U_B|$ or A's gain exceeds B's loss.

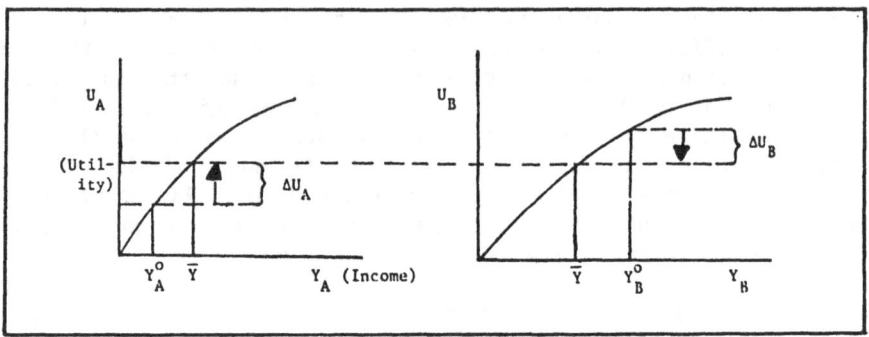

Figure 1.   Marginal utility and income

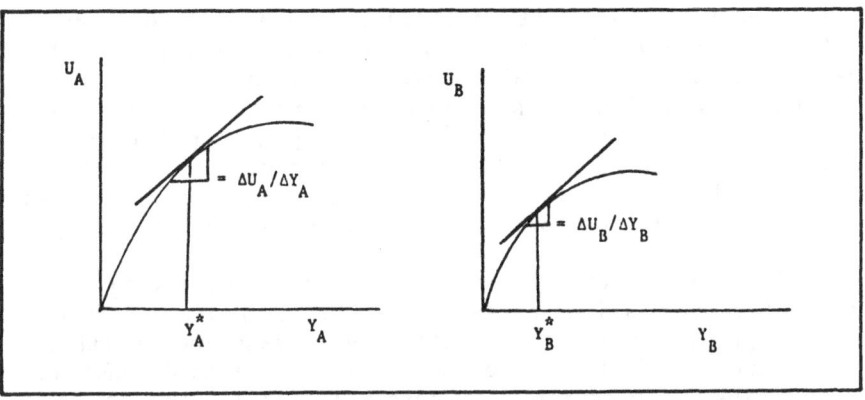

Figure 2.   Marginal utility and income

The same solution can be obtained by solving the following problem:

$$\text{maximize } U_A(Y_A) + U_B(Y_B) \tag{1}$$

$$\text{subject to } Y_A + Y_B = Y_A^o + Y_B^o \tag{2}$$

which implies at the optimum that $\Delta U_A/\Delta Y_A = \Delta U_A/\Delta Y_B$ or that the rate of increase of utility with income (marginal utility) must be equal for the two individuals. Since the two individuals in the example have the same utility function, marginal utilities are equated where incomes are the same, $Y_A = Y_B = \bar{Y}$.

If, on the other hand, we assume different individuals have different utility functions, e.g., Edgeworth (1967) argues that the rich have more sensitivity and can better enjoy money income than the poor, we end up with a situation like that shown in Figure 2. $Y_A^\star$ and $Y_A^\star$ are optimal incomes for A and B because for these incomes the marginal utilities of income are equated. Mr. A gets more income than Mr. B because he obtains more utility from income than B does. In Edgeworth's view, Mr. A, by his sensitivity, should have more money to be used in appreciated fine wine than B, who is satisfied with common ale.

Obviously, then, depending on beliefs about measurable utility functions, any distribution of income can be justified, ranging from a relatively egalitarian viewpoint (Pigou) to a relatively elitist viewpoint (Edgeworth).

_Totally Egalitarian (Rawlsian-Dantian)_. Rawls (1971) proposes that well being of a society can be measured by the well being of the worst off person in that society. This simple notion would lead, if adopted, to a totally egalitarian distribution of income. (See Arrow, 1973, for a further discussion of the Rawlsian concept.)

The Rawlsian criterion can be expressed mathematically as follows: for two individuals A and B, where utility is denoted by U, if $U_A < U_B$ we maximize $U_A$ subject to $U_A \leq U_B$; if $U_B < U_A$ then we maximize $U_B$ subject to $U_B \leq U_A$. If we can reach a state where $U_A = U_B$, then we can maximize $U_A$ subject to $U_A = U_B$. The implication of this for redistribution of income is that we begin by adding income to the worst off individual (taking income away from wealthier individuals) until he catches up with the next worst off individual. We then add income to both individuals until their utility

levels (well being) have caught up to the third worst off,
etc. Eventually, this process must lead to a state where
$U_A = U_B = U_C = U_D \ldots$ for all individuals in a society,
where all utilities are identical. This criterion can be
written more compactly for a two person society as max min
$[U_A, U_B]$, so we are always trying to maximize the utility of
the individual with the minimum utility. Implicit also in
Rawl's arguments (e.g., the veil of ignorance) is the assumption that individual's utility functions with respect to
income are about the same. Thus, a Rawlsian ethic would work
towards a relatively equal distribution of income based on
need. Rawls claims that he is a Kantian and that his criterion is consistent with Kant's Categorical Imperative as
well. Thus, we will assume that as a weighting scheme for
benefit-cost analysis, the totally Egalitarian view embodies
Kant as well.

Totally Elitist (Neitzschean). A Neitzschean criterion
can be derived as the precise opposite of the Rawlsian criterion discussed above. The well being of society is measured
by the well being of the best off individual. Every act is
"right" if it improves the welfare of the best off and
"wrong" if it decreases the welfare of the best off.

Lest the reader dismiss the Nietzschean criterion as
irrelevant for a Western democratic society, a number of
elitist arguments should be mentioned. The gasoline shortage
of the summer of 1979 moved Senator Hiyakawa of California to
comment, "The important thing is that a lot of the poor don't
need gas because they're not working." Economic productivity
can, in this sense, rationalize a defined "elite." Thus,
concepts of merit can be elitist in nature, e.g., those who
produce the most "should" have the largest merit increases
in salary (even though they may already have the highest
salaries).

Income distributional questions are a bit more complex
in that the solution is not simply to give all of society's
wealth to the best off. Obviously, it will usually be
better to keep B alive to serve A, i.e., to contribute to his
well being, than to give B nothing if A is to be best off.
Thus, subsistence is typically required for B. Similarly, if
we have two succeeding generations, it may well be "best" for
the first generation to save as much as possible to make the
next generation better off. Thus, an elitist viewpoint may
support altruistic behavior.

Libertarian (Paretian-Christian). The last of our
ethical systems is an amalgam of a number of ethical prin-
cipals embodied both in the Libertarian view (see Nozick,
1974) that any individual action is moral if no one else

is harmed, and in a Christian ethic, "turn the other cheek." Thus, we are not concerned with changing the initial position of individuals in society to some ideal state, but rather in benefiting all or at least preventing harm to others, even if they are better off. This ethic has been embodied often by economists in the form of requiring "Pareto Superiority," that all persons be made better off or at least as well off as before. Any act is then immoral or wrong if anyone else is harmed. Any act which improves an individual's or several individuals' well being and harms no one is moral or "right." The acceptance of the initial social position, even if elitist or highly unequal in income distribution as part of a Libertarian Ethic does not, however, imply consistency with an elitist ethic. Nietzsche, for example, rejects this view as a "slave mentality" in attacking Christianity.

A Libertarian Ethic does not define a best distribution of income. Rather, the criterion requires that any change from the existing social order harm no one. If, for example, Mr. A and Mr. B initially have incomes $Y_A^o$ and $Y_B^o$, we then require for any new distribution of wealth $(Y_A, Y_B)$ — for example, more wealth becomes available — that

$$U_A(Y_A) \geq U(Y_A^o) \tag{3}$$

and

$$U_B(Y_B) \geq U(Y_B^o) \, , \tag{4}$$

or each individual must be at least as well off as he was initially. Any redistribution, e.g., from wealthy to poor or vice versa, is specifically proscribed by this criterion. Thus, this criterion while seemingly weak, i.e., it does not call for redistribution, can block many possible actions if they do as a side effect redistribute income to make *anyone* worse off, however slight the effect may be. Often then, to satisfy a Libertarian criterion requires that gainers from a particular social decision must actually compensate losers (for a discussion of compensation, see Mishan, 1971).

The four ethical systems presented above are, as noted, by no means exhaustive. While some, such as a democratic ethic, have been excluded on technical grounds, others such as a Darwinian ethic — survival of the fittest — must await future treatment in our analysis. In any case, the four ethics chosen here do have the advantage of simplicity, but

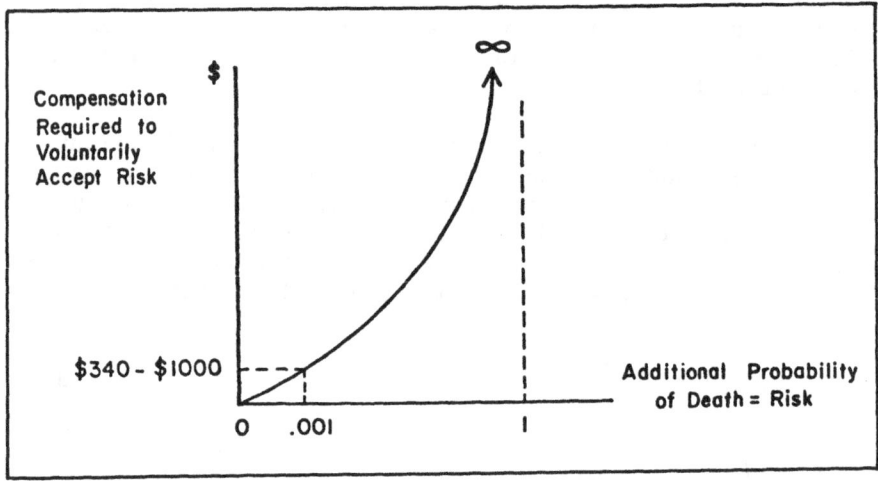

Figure 3.  Compensation versus risk

may in turn represent, at least in their mathematically specified forms, considerable oversimplifications. All ethical systems as logical constructs may, however, suffer from this charge.

## Economics, Ethics and Safety

The economics of safety has developed rapidly over the last several years. Unfortunately, earlier misguided attempts at measuring the value of safety programs have given economists a "black eye" for supposedly advocating that individual human lives could be valued as the lost economic productivity associated with a shortened life span. This view, pursued in great detail by Dorothy Rice (1966) and used by Lave and Seskin (1970) and others, implied that part of the value of the life of, for example, a 50-year-old carpenter would be the remaining earnings to retirement age. The value of the life of a retired female (somebody's grandmother) could by the same argument be taken at zero. Similarly, small children, since many years would pass before they could begin to earn productive income, were valued at next to zero, given the notion of discounting future earnings at a market rate of interest. Elaborate calculations were made for different individuals on the basis of age, occupation, sex, etc., to determine the value of remaining earnings as a measure of the "value of life." On economic theoretical grounds all of these calculations have been shown to be faulty. However, permanent harm remains in that many decisionmakers now shy away from any attempt to value the benefits of safety programs in dollar terms.

The economists' notion that individuals voluntarily trade off safety for monetary compensation in no way attempts to value life (Mishan, 1971). Rather, the question is asked, how much do individuals require as a *priori* compensation to voluntarily accept a small additional risk of death? Let us follow through on the notion of a trade-off between safety and monetary compensation.

Imagine a game of Russian Roulette in which an individual is offered sums of money to participate voluntarily. If, for example, the risk of the gun firing when the trigger was pulled were only one in ten thousand, and the compensation for accepting the risk was $1,000, current economic studies would suggest that most people would accept the risk. (This is a better proposition in terms of risk versus compensation than driving to work for a typical day's pay!) However, economic theory suggests that as the probability of death increases, monetary compensation would have to increase dramatically. Figure 3 shows that expected kind of relationship between compensation and risk. Clearly as the probability of

death approaches unity, compensation approaches infinity —
odds are that the participant won't survive the game to enjoy
the proceeds, so no amount of money is sufficient. Note,
however, that for small increases in annual risk of death
such as those associated with risky jobs (typically less than
0.001 per year) annual job compensation must be increased by
$340-$1,000, as shown in Figure 3. Thus, economists focus on
the far left hand side of Figure 3 and utilize a rather
special situation to derive estimates of the value of safety.

This method of valuing risk seems at least in part out
of accord with observed human behavior. Just as the old
value of life measure used by Rice (1966) and Lave and Seskin
(1970) leads to counter-intuitive results, the new measure
of the value of safety seems to ignore the special importance
many individuals place on involuntary or uncompensated risks.
The risks associated with nuclear reactor accidents or
nuclear waste storage, risks associated with public transportation including airlines, risks of flood, fire, earthquakes,
or other disasters, all seem to be treated differently both
in a social and individual perspective than do voluntary-
compensated risks (for a discussion on this point, see Starr,
1968 and Rowe, 1977). Economic theory, and consequently,
empirical estimates of the value of safety have notably
failed to account for these differences. Rather, economists
have argued that placing a different value on safety in different situations is economically inefficient.

The logic behind this argument is as follows: given a
fixed safety budget, if we have a program that can save one
life for $50,000 and another program which can save ten lives
for $50,000, we should pick the second program. The obvious
counter to this argument is that individuals may well value
safety differently in differing settings. Are uncompensated
risks less ethically acceptable than compensated risks? We
can use the four ethical systems presented above to analyze
uncompensated risk as follows: assume we have two identical
individuals, A and B with the same utility functions. If A
imposes a small risk on B and receives a benefit equal to
B's decremental value of safety, we have a situation which
satisfies traditional benefit-cost analysis, i.e., benefits
to A are equal to costs on B in dollar terms, so the situation is accepted. However, from an ethical perspective, A
is imposing an uncompensated risk on B.

Technically, we define A's expected utility as:

$$E_A = (1 - \Pi_A^0)U_A(Y_A^0 + G\Delta\Pi_B) \tag{5}$$

where $\Pi_A^o$ is A's risk of death, $U_A$ is A's utility which is a function of his initial income, $Y_A^o$ plus the monetary gain $G$, for imposing risk on B, times the increase in risk imposed on B, $\Delta\Pi_B$. An example of this situation would be Mr. A building a dam upstream of Mr. B for his own gain. Mr. A receives a net benefit of G for each unit of risk (of failure of the dam which could drown Mr. B) which he imposes on Mr. B. This net gain would result from the value of irrigation water net of the cost of constructing the dam. In this context, benefit-cost analysis as traditionally practiced would argue that marginal net benefits to A must exceed or equal marginal costs (of risk) to B, as we have defined the problem, so the dam is acceptable.

Mr. B's expected utility where he is not compensated for risk imposed by A, is then defined as:

$$E_B = (1 - \Pi_B^o - \Delta\Pi_B)U_B(Y_B^o) \tag{6}$$

where $\Pi_B^o$ is Mr. B's original risk of death, $\Delta\Pi_B$ is the additional risk imposed by A, and $U_B$ is Mr. B's utility, a function of his income, $Y_B^o$.

If we were to compensate Mr. B for voluntarily accepting risk from Mr. A at a rate of C dollars per unit risk, Mr. B would maximize his compensated expected utility,

$$(1 - \Pi_B^o - \Delta\Pi_B)U_B (Y_B^o + C\Delta\Pi_B), \tag{7}$$

with respect to $\Delta\Pi_B$, which implies

$$C = \left. \frac{U_B}{U_B^{'} (1 - \Pi_B^o)} \right|_{\Delta\Pi_B = 0} \tag{8}$$

or that C equals B's marginal value of safety, the definition of the right hand side of the expression above. Thus, traditional benefit-cost analysis requires that G, Mr. A's marginal gain, exceed or equal C, Mr. B's marginal loss, both valued in dollar terms. However, Mr. A does not have to actually compensate Mr. B at a rate equal to or exceeding C, as defined above.

How, alternatively would the four ethical systems described above view the situation where B's risk is uncompensated?  Where social welfare, W, for the first three criteria
is defined follows:

Utilitarian                   $W = E_A + E_B$                  (9)

Totally Egalitarian           $W = \max \min [E_A, E_B]$        (10)

Totally Elitist               $W = \max \max [E_A, E_B]$        (11)

the condition for acceptability is that $[dW/d\Pi_B]\Delta\Pi_B = 0 \geqq 0$.
If $[dW/d\Pi_B]\Delta\Pi_B = 0 < 0$, then the risk, $\Delta\Pi_B$ is rejected.  For
the Libertarian Ethic, we require:

Libertarian        $E_A \geq E_A^o \equiv (1 - \Pi_A^o)\, U_A\, (Y_A^o)$    (12)

                   $E_B \geq E_B^o \equiv (1 - \Pi_B^o)\, U_B\, (Y_B^o)$    (13)

The Libertarian Ethic, with its close relationship to
the Christian Ethic is of special importance for Western
Democracies.  This ethical system although seemingly weak in
not requiring redistribution of income, rejects all uncompensated risks, implying lexicographic preferences as described above.

It is perhaps this last point when applied in a broad
context which goes furthest in explaining the opposition that
benefit-cost analysis has received in analyzing certain
issues.  For example, in many cases, lawyers and environmentalists have argued that polluting the environment is "wrong"
and that economic policies such as selling permits for the
right to pollute or taxing pollution are unethical.  Similarly, advocates of public safety argue that no amount of
effort on the part of airlines, operators of nuclear reactors
or large hydroelectric dams is sufficient when uncompensated
risks are involved for the general public.  These attitudes,
which are reflected in enormously higher expenditures per
life saved in some safety programs as opposed to others, seem
consistent both with a Libertarian Ethic and with lexicographic preferences.

## Valuing Energy Impacts

### The Use of Survey Methods

Many environmental policy issues involve changes in
environmental attributes resulting from population growth
and energy development.  For example, coal-fired electric

power plants may significantly reduce visibility and disturb landscapes.  Strip mining coal may have substantial detrimental effects on wildlife populations both through direct impact and through the expanded demand on wildlife arising from a larger worker population.  The construction of geothermal plants adjacent to existing forest recreation areas may, through siting and noise, disturb an otherwise pristine, quiet recreation area.  If benefit-cost analysis is to be employed for decision making, techniques need to be devised to impute economic values for these and other environmental changes.

During the past few years, economists have attempted to apply a variety of techniques to reveal preferences of individuals on non-market environmental commodities (Bradford, 1970; Bohm, 1972; Randall et al., 1974; Brookshire, Ives, and Schulze, 1976).  These techniques, in general following the methodology of Davis (1963), have obtained bids from individuals which represent their maximum willingness to pay for a non-market commodity.  Almost simultaneously, other economists made substantial contributions to assessing the demand for non-market commodities and public goods (Rosen, 1974; Muellbauer, 1974; Hori, 1975).  This section presents a summary and analysis of six recent experiments which have attempted to determine the feasibility of deriving implicit prices and/or valuations for the types of environmental changes mentioned above.[1]

The techniques to be examined range from direct evaluations asking for dollar bids to hypothetical questions concerning changes in behavior.  In each case, the household was confronted with a possible change in an environmental attribute and asked for a valuation.  Since the valuation was contingent on the specific hypothetical change identified (through photographs, brochures or other means), we propose that such approaches be called contingent valuations.[2]  Individuals are queried regarding such variables as willingness to pay, minimum acceptable compensation, past and current experiences, site substitutions, potential expenditure or behavioral adjustments, etc., in order to estimate demand curves for environmental attributes.

Obtaining accurate information for individual valuation of non-market environmental commodities can be costly.  In many cases to actually derive true values, a "market" must be set in a place and operated to record prices and demands where the environmental attribute is actually purchased or sold.  However, to construct and operate such a market may not be feasible.  A more realistic approach is to use a contingent valuation study where prices can be imputed without the actual operation of an organized market. However, because of its hypothetical nature, several potential biases may occur. Clearly, asking someone what they will pay a *priori* is not the same as confronting them with a recognized and well understood market and observing what they actually pay.

## Contingent Valuation and Bias

Economists have argued that valuing public goods using a contingent market process may yield biased results. The major types of biases are: (1) strategic bias whereby the individual attempts to influence the outcome or result by not responding truthfully; (2) information bias, which is induced by lack, or type, of information given to the consumer in the contingent market; (3) instrument bias, which is bias introduced by the procedures employed to discover preferences; (4) hypothetical bias, which is the error induced by failure to confront the individual with an actual situation, i.e., an organized market with well defined prices; and (5) sampling, interviewer or non-respondent bias.[3] This section reviews our current understanding of such biases.

Strategic bias. Beginning with Samuelson's seminal work on public goods, it has been supposed that accurate estimates of consumer preferences for public goods — including environmental quality — would be impossible (Samuelson, 1954). In particular, individuals have incentives to misstate their own preferences in an attempt to impose their true preferences on others. For example, if nearby residents were asked how much they were willing to pay to clean up the air near a power plant and if they suspected that control costs would be borne by consumers and owners elsewhere, local residents would have an incentive to overstate their willingness to pay. On the other hand, if residents suspected that they would be individually taxed an amount equal to their own willingness to pay, then a clear incentive would exist to understate their own true value, hoping that others would bid more.

Empirical evidence thus far does not support the existence of strategic bias among consumers. Bohm (1972) in an experimental approach utilizing actual payments for public television failed to find strategic bias significantly affecting the outcome. Scherr and Babb (1975) utilized three different mechanisms for valuing public commodities and found little evidence supporting the existence of strategic bias. Smith (1977) in laboratory experiments also failed to find strategic bias as a significant problem. The case studies to be reported in the next section also do not find strategic bias, where tested for, to be a problem.

Information bias.  Since contingent behavior or valuation is hypothetical, it is clear that answers obtained
through surveys are not based on information similar to that
which would apply if consumers based answers on real experiences.  One is an *ex ante* response, while the other is an
*ex post* statement.[4]  Typically, consumers do re-evaluate
decisions on the basis of experience and gained knowledge.
Thus, an individual or household might respond to a hypothetical decrease in environmental quality at one location with
a low bid, thinking that other nearby sites would make good
substitutes.  However, additional information presented to
the respondent in a survey situation relating to substitution possibilities and alternative costs may well change the
stated willingness to pay.  The respondent must be made aware
of proposed alternatives in terms of quality or quantity.
Other variants of information bias might include giving the
respondent information as to how other respondents behaved
and whether in the aggregate their bid was sufficient to
achieve (or not achieve) the stated goal (i.e., possible
prevention of visibility deterioration).

Instrument bias.  Related to information bias is instrument bias whereby characteristics of the mechanism used to
obtain willingness to pay data possibly influence the outcome.  Two characteristics of the survey bidding approach
are vehicles for payment and a starting point for initiation
of the bidding process.  Studies have recognized that the
mechanism used to collect the bid or pay compensation may
influence its magnitude (Randall, et al., 1974).  That is,
a recreator's bid for an environmental attribute may depend
on whether he is asked to pay a higher park entrance fee or
some other type of tax.  Ideally, the payment mechanism
should be related to adjustments in disposable income (a wage
tax for instance), since this gives the individual the greatest latitude for potential substitution.  Practically, however, this is not always possible.  For example, surveys are
often taken at recreation sites away from the individual's
locale or state.  In this case, the recreator may not view a
wage tax as realistically payable.  Thus, in the contingent
valuation approach, there is always a tradeoff between accuracy associated with a less than ideal method of payment and
the believability of the vehicle for payment or compensation.

A second type of instrument bias is starting point bias.
The contingent valuation approach commences with questions
on payment (and/or compensation) for hypothetical changes in
environmental attributes.  Often a starting bid or minimal
level of compensation is suggested.  This procedure can give
rise to a potential bias from at least two sources.  First,
the starting bid itself may suggest to the individual a range
of "appropriate bids."  Thus the response of the individual

may depend significantly on the magnitude of the starting bid.   Second, if the individual values time highly, he may become "bored" or irritated with going through a lengthy bidding process.   Consequently, if the suggested starting bid is substantially different from his actual willingness to pay, the bidding process may terminate early, yielding inaccurate results.   The effect of these two types of starting point biases may substantially influence the accuracy of contingent valuation and therefore the usefulness of this approach for assessment of environmental preferences.

Hypothetical bias.   The discussion on information bias suggested that the contingent valuation approach produces answers which depend upon the "state of the world" as described.   Because this approach is so hypothetical in nature, it requires postulating changes in environmental attributes in such a way that they are both accurately described and believable to the individual.   The individual must understand the ramifications of a potential change and believe that his contingent valuation or behavioral changes will affect both the possibility and magnitude of the change.[5]   Otherwise, what individuals say they are willing to pay for given environmental attributes may bear little resemblance to what they would actually be willing to pay.

Other bias.   Any survey approach, including the contingent valuation approach, is subject to sampling bias, nonrespondent bias, and interviewer bias.   Any of these certainly can subject the results of an experiment to question even if all previously mentioned biases are nonexistent. Given the acknowledgement of these biases and their wide recogniton in the survey literature, we will not discuss them in detail here.   However, in discussing the case studies in the next subsection, the possible existence of these biases will be discussed in each study, where the information is available.

## Valuing Environmental Quality

### Recent Case Studies

There have been numerous efforts to value nonmarket goods: public television (Bohm, 1972); landform alterations due to strip mining (Randall et al., 1978); air pollution-induced health effects (Loehman et al., 1979); wildlife (Hammock and Brown, 1974; Bishop and Heberlein, 1979); water pollution (Gramlich, 1977); preservation of river headwaters (O'Hanlon and Sinden, 1978; Sinden and Wyckoff, 1976); urban infrastructure allocations for expenditures and taxes (Strauss and Hughes, 1976; Cummings, Schulze, and Mehr, 1978); airplane safety (Jones-Lee, 1976); and recreation (Davis, 1963).

This section will summarize in chronological order six studies which have in common the use of a survey technique, the contingent bidding survey approach, first applied by Randall et al. (1974) and Randall, Ives, and Eastman (1974). Tracing the methodology development which has occurred through these six studies aids in understanding issues relating to bias problems, replication issues and methodological cross checks.

The Four Corners Experiment. The Four Corners Experiment (Randall et al., 1974 and Randall, Ives, and Eastman, 1974) represented the first empirical application of the survey approach.[6] The roots of the effort can be traced to Davis (1963) and Bohm (1971, 1972). The focus of the study was to investigate the impacts of Navajo coal strip mines and the Four Corners electric generating plants in the Southwest region. Specifically, aesthetic benefits of abatement of environmental damage resulting from air pollution (visibility), power lines, and land disturbance from mining activities were estimated.

The Lake Powell Experiment.[7] Lake Powell, with an annual visitation now approaching two million visitor-days, is an excellent example of the trade-off between preservation and development. The lake was formed by the filling of Glen Canyon but retains the steep cliffs, rugged terrain features, and scenic vistas one associates with the Grand Canyon, and is now accessible to pleasure boaters and other recreators. Construction of the Navajo coal-fired generating station located at the southern end of Lake Powell was completed in 1976. Another larger power plant, the Kaiparowitz Project, was also proposed for construction near Lake Powell and became an issue of substantial public concern.

As part of the Lake Powell experiment, in the summer of 1974, recreators at Lake Powell were interviewed in an attempt to determine their aggregate willingness to pay to prevent construction of the proposed Kaiparowitz plant (see Brookshire, Ives, and Schulze, 1976 and Blank et al., 1977). Photographs of the existing Navajo power plant which all of the recreators had seen — stacks remain visible more than 20 miles up the lake — were shown to recreators both with visible pollution emanating from the stacks and with the stacks alone. Recreators were then asked what entrance fee they would be willing to pay to prevent construction of another similar plant, first, where only pollution would be visible from the lake itself, and second, where both stacks and pollution would be visible.

The average bid per family or recreator group was $2.77 in additional entrance fees in 1974 dollars, and the total annual bid — which can be interpreted as an aggregate marginal willingness to pay to prevent one additional power plant near Lake Powell — was over $700. An important point is that the results show impressive consistencies both with the one previous study (Randall et al., 1974) in the region as well as with the succeeding Farmington experiment discussed below. (See Table 1 for a summary of the results.)

Analysis of the data focused on strategic bias. If the recreators believed that a uniform entrance fee might actually be set on the basis of the average bid of the sample to prevent construction or believed that construction plans might be affected by the research results, then "environmentalists" might well bid very high, and "developers" might well bid zero dollars in an attempt to bias the results.[8] A theoretical model of strategic bias was constructed to explain the distribution of observed bids which would likely be bimodal rather than normally distributed if strategic bias was present. The fact that the actual distribution of bids was normally distributed was taken as evidence that strategic bias was not present. Hypothetical information and instrument biases were not addressed in this experiment.

The Farmington Experiment.[9]    This study, reported in Blank et al. (1977) and Rowe, d'Arge, and Brookshire (1980), attempted to establish the economic value of visibility over long distances. Clearly, the ability to observe long distances is almost a pure public good. In addition, efforts were made to examine the extent of certain biases which the Brookshire, Ives, and Schulze (1976) study identified. These were information, strategic, starting point, and instrument biases on compensating and equivalent surplus measures of consumer surplus.

Recreators and residents in the Four Corners Region of New Mexico and Arizona were interviewed. The interviewee was shown a set of pictures depicting visible ranges. Picture set C had a visible range of 25 miles and picture sets B and A were 50 and 75 miles, respectively. The pictures represented views in different directions from the same location — the San Juan Mountains and Shiprock. (See Table 1 for a summary of results.)

As part of the contingent bidding approach, direct tests were made for strategic bias, information bias, and instrument bias. First, to test for strategic bias, the individual was told that he would have to pay the "average" bid, not his own.[10] The presumption was that if he desired to increase the magnitude of the final aggregate bids, he would bid higher in order to shift the final bid upward. Alternatively, if his goal was to reduce the final mean bid, he would revise his bid downward.  Only in the unlikely case when the individual's minimum bid is identical to the mean bid would there be no incentive for the individual to change.  In only one case was an individual observed acting strategically and he turned out to be an economics professor from the local Junior College.  This additional information, along with the results of Brookshire, Ives, and Schulze (1976), suggests that individuals generally do not act strategically, at least not in such a way as to bias the outcome of the results.

Analysis was made of various forms of information and instrument bias.  It was observed that the higher the starting bid suggested by the interviewer, the higher the maximum willingness to pay (equivalent surplus) estimated derived from the study.  Also, the method of payment influenced the magnitude of the bid significantly.  Individuals were willing to bid higher when confronted with a "payroll tax" than with an increase in entrance fees.  Finally, it was observed that prior information given to individuals concerning average bids had a substantial impact on the maximum bid.  These results indicate that for the contingent valuation approach to be accurate, one must be very careful with the instrument used for payment and the amount and quality of information given to the interviewee upon initiation of the interview.

The Geothermal Experiment.[11]  The Jemez Mountains of New Mexico are both scenic — characterized by colored rock outcroppings and forest areas — and a major recreation resource with fishing, campgrounds, hiking trails, and hot springs all located on U.S. Forest Service lands.  However, the Jemez Mountains also contain one of the major geothermal resources in the Southwest.  Geothermal leases have been let by the U.S. Forest Service on land which is now used solely by recreators.

Both a contingent bidding and a contingent site substitution approach were used to estimate environmental damages to recreators from possible geothermal development (Thayer, forthcoming).  Recreators were shown both photographs of geothermal development in similar mountainous terrain and a map of the location of possible development relative to recreation areas.  Noise levels and emission characteristics were described in detail.  A bidding game was then conducted using a uniform entrance fee as the vehicle to prevent development.  Additionally, respondents were asked to indicate what their contingent recreation plan would be (what sites would they visit including new substitute sites and how often) if development were to occur.  The subsample which responded to the site substitution question was then also asked what they would bid in the form of a uniform entrance

Table 1. Overview of non-market valuation experiments

| Non-market valuation studies | Environmental attribute being valued | Location | Methodological cross check | Strategic bias[a] | Instrument biases | | |
|---|---|---|---|---|---|---|---|
| | | | | | Vehicle | Starting point | Information bias |
| Four Corners (Randall et al., 1974, and Randall, Ives, and Eastman, 1974) | Visibility, spoil banks, transmission lines | Four Corners area, southwest | No | N/A[b] | N/A | N/A | N/A |
| Lake Powell (Brookshire, Ives, and Schulze, 1976) | Visibility | Four Corners area, southwest | No | N/A | N/A | N/A | N/A |
| Farmington Blank et al., 1977 and Rowe, d'Arge, and Brookshire, 1980) | Visibility | Four Corners area, southwest | Yes | No | Yes[c] | Yes[c] | Yes[c] |
| Geothermal (Thayer, In press) | Noise, land disturbance | Jemez Mountains | Yes | No | N/A | No[d] | No[e] |
| Rocky Mountain Wildlife (Brookshire et al., 1977 and Brookshire, Randall, and Stoll, 1980) | Encounters with wildlife | Wyoming | Yes | No | Yes[f] | No[f] | N/A |
| South Coast Air Basin (Brookshire, d'Arge, Schulze, and Thayer, In press) | Visibility, health effects | Los Angeles Region, California | Yes | No | No[g] | No[g] | No[h] |

Table 1.  (continued)

[a]Strategic bias tests were defined in Brookshire, Ives, and Schulze (1976).

[b]N/A = not available — the experiment did not consider either structurally or analytically this form of bias.

[c]Utilizing estimated bid curves the t ratios for these variables were respectively (3.05), (7.98), and (-4.54) where the vehicle variable was 0 = utility bill, 1 = payroll deduction; starting bid variable was either $1, $5, or $10 and information variable was 0 = no prior information, 1 = prior information.  See Rowe, d'Arge, and Brookshire (1980).

[d]Utilizing an estimated bid curve the t ratio was 0.689 on the starting point variable indicating no significant influence.

[e]Information bias in this study pertained to whether the suggestion of alternative recreation cities would influence the bid.  A standard P-test was utilized with no statistical influence being observed.

[f]A T-test was conducted where the hypothesis that the final value data was influenced by the bidding vehicle (starting bids) was rejected.

[g]A T-test was conducted whereby the acceptance of the hypothesis that the mean bids for all paired areas combined for different bidding vehicles (starting points) are equal implies $1 - \alpha = 0.90$ and higher.

[h]Information bias in this study related to alternative sequencing of health and aesthetic information.  The test was as in footnote e.

fee to prevent development. Finally, starting point for the bidding game was varied from $1.00 to $10.00 in various sub-samples. Thus, the study was structured to test: (1) if contingent bidding and site substitution results were consistent; (2) if information on alternative new substitute sites would affect bidding results; and (3) for starting point bias.

A set of theoretical models were constructed to estimate a consistent measure of willingness to pay to prevent development from two measures: (1) the contingent valuation bidding, and (2) additional travel costs associated with alternative recreation plans. This was an attempt at a methodological cross check.

The results of the experiment were as follows: 32% of the respondents indicated they would no longer visit the Jemez area if development occurred. This resulted in about a 40% contingent decrease in visitation. About 65% of the respondents indicated they would visit alternative sites more frequently, usually the Pecos Forest area. Bids averaged $2.54 per visitor-party-day while the site substitution measure yielded a range of $1.85-2.59 depending on the assumed driving cost per mile. The results appear to be consistent for the two approaches and imply an annualized aggregate bid to prevent construction of about $300,000 for a 50 MW plant.

The Wildlife Experiment.[12] Through contingent bidding and site substitution approaches, this study attempted to develop a methodology for valuing wildlife experiences. The valuations were developed to enable policymakers to judge which sites should be reserved from energy developments so that energy development would not seriously impinge on wildlife. Hunters and wildlife observers were queried as to their willingness to pay for "encounters" with various types of wildlife. Encounters was chosen as the variable of perturbation. The hypothesis was that the more animals sighted the greater the satisfaction from the hunting experience.[13] The species examined were elk, cottontail, coyote, grizzly bear, bighorn sheep, trout, dipper, and brown creeper. The assumed utility function had as arguments the number of encounters and the length of activity.

A type of instrument bias was observed in that bids were recorded through license fees, access fees, and utility bill adjustments, but difficulties were encountered in convincing some respondents that competition between energy development and wildlife herds would be sufficient reason for utility bill adjustments. Starting point bias was tested for, but was not found to substantially affect the bids on species commonly hunted. Thus, this experiment appears to substantiate the comparison between the Geothermal and Farmington Experiments which led us to propose that the more clearly identified the change in environmental attribute is, the lower the probability of starting point bias.

Results indicate that, for elk, the average willingness to pay equivalent surplus measure is $54.00 per year to increase expected encounters (i.e., sightings) from 1 to 5 per day for elk hunting in Wyoming. The average willingness to accept compensating surplus measure for a reduction of 5 to 1 encounters per day of elk was $142.00. Some private clubs which specialize in elk hunting in Wyoming charge entrance fees ranging from $85.00 to $150.00 per year, roughly in the range of the compensating surplus measure for elk encounters obtained through the contingent valuation approach.

The South Coast Air Basin Experiment. (Brookshire, d'Arge, Schulze and Thayer, in press). The previous case studies reported here, while internally consistent, failed to provide a methodological cross check to actual market data. In the South Coast Air Basin Experiment, both a traditional property value study and a contingent valuation were conducted in an attempt to determine if people will *actually* pay (as exhibited by property values) what they *say* they are willing to pay.

In the south coast air basin of the Los Angeles area, deterioration in air quality in some neighborhoods has been slight, while in others, it has been relatively severe. Six pairs of neighborhoods in this basin were selected so that each pair differed in air quality, but were similar on the basis of housing characteristics, socioeconomic factors, distance to beach and services, average temperature, and subjective indicators of the "quality" of housing. The bidding game was conducted by randomly choosing homes within the paired areas. The contingent bidding and substitution approaches employed in this experiment attempted to value the components of health effects and aesthetic effects separately. Aesthetic considerations were represented by alternative levels of visibility, acute health effects by eye irritation, and chronic health effects by reduction in life span.

The property value analysis encompassed three separate, increasingly complex, approaches. First, a comparison of average housing values in sample paired communities, standardizing only for living space, was conducted. Second, a linear relationship between a home's sale price and its supply of housing and community attributes was estimated. The

value of an improvement in air quality was then deduced from
the resulting hedonic housing value equation.  Third, following Harrison and Rubinfeld (1978), a hedonic housing equation
allowing for nonlinearities in income and other household
variables, was used to estimate willingness to pay.  This
last procedure partly overcomes some of the difficulties of
more simplistic approaches such as identical preferences of
all individuals.

Accounting for factors such as distance to beach and
differences in preferences, the property value study gave an
estimated average bid of $40.00 per month per household for
a 30% improvement in air quality.  The bidding results gave
an average bid of slightly less than $30.00 per month.  Thus,
reasonable comparability was obtained between the survey and
property value estimates.  Both the bidding game and property
value studies yielded estimates ranging from $20.00 to
$150.00 per month per household for a 30% reduction in air
pollution.  These results indicate that air quality deterioration in the South Coast Air Basin has had substantial
effects on housing prices and that these negative price
effects on housing are comparable in magnitude to what people
say they are willing to pay for improved air quality.

## Conclusion

The six case studies summarized above have shown some
consistency in results and hopefully further the evaluation
of problems in structuring contingent market experiments.

Table I presents a brief summary of the characteristics
of each experiment.  The range of environmental attributes
valued is quite large — including visibility, wildlife,
health, and noise.  Four out of six attempted some internal
methodological cross check; however, only the South Coast Air
Basin Experiment utilized an observed set of market prices
for the comparison.  Biases do not appear to be an overriding
problem.  Stratetic bias was not observed in any experiment.
Vehicle and starting point bias were highly significant in
the Farmington Experiment.  Starting point bias was not found
in any other study.  Vehicle bias was significant in the
Wildlife Experiment.  A probable explanation for these
results, which offers advice for future experiments, is that
the linkage within the contingent market between the environmental attribute, institutional setting and the bidding
instrument must be realistic and be accepted by the respondent, or biased results will be obtained.  The studies further
indicate the need to establish a precise contingent market —
the "good" must be well defined.

Possibly the most important result of the studies summarized here is the replication of results utilizing a tra-

ditional property value study and a contingent bidding approach. At least for this first test case, individuals do appear to provide contingent valuations comparable to what actual market behavior implies they are willing to pay for an environmental attribute.

## Benefit-Cost Analysis for Local Impacts of Energy Development

This section discusses problems associated with valuing environmental effects of toxic trace elements in economic terms. No damage calculations are presented. Rather, this chapter focuses on two aspects of the economic quantification of toxic effects of trace elements emissions: we first treat morbidity (illness) damages, discussing both economic and ethical aspects of valuing human health risks in dollar terms; we then discuss "ecosystem effects," which imply potential economic losses to recreation (e.g., prohibition of fishing in contaminated lakes and streams), and give rise to larger questions of environmental preservation and option values as well.

### Valuing Morbidity

The valuation of morbidity is conceptually even more difficult than that of mortality. Whereas, for mortality one can focus on a simplifying construct — thè a *priori* compensation required to induce individuals to accept risk of death — morbidity has a number of diverse and difficult to quantify aspects. The easiest consequences of morbidity to quantify are lost economic productivity and increased medical care costs. Rice (1966) and others have focused on these aspects in examining the "costs of illness." Based on this approach, it is conceptually possible to associate an increase in morbidity with lost hours worked and with increased medical care costs. However, this approach will likely yield an inaccurate estimate of damages for a number of reasons. A more complete listing of the consequences of illness would include:

(1) earnings lost from time off work;
(2) increased medical care costs;
(3) pain and suffering;
(4) lost work experience;
(5) lost work productivity from physical or mental impairment; and
(6) increased leisure time.

The first two effects are included by Rice in estimates of the cost of illness while the remaining effects are excluded. Information on values for pain and suffering, (3) above,

are difficult to obtain.  Whereas some consistent estimates
of (1) and (2) have been used in, for example, court cases,
settlements for pain and suffering vary enormously from case
to case.  Ideally, one would wish to obtain the willingness
of individuals to pay to avoid pain and suffering.

Crocker et al. (1978) have found the effect of chronic
illness in *depressing* wage rates to be statistically large.
This depression in wage rates likely results from effects
(4) and (5) listed above, i.e., from losses in work experience and seniority and from debilitating effects of illness
on worker productivity.  For example, to use an extreme case,
an individual poisoned by mercury may become acutely ill and
be unable to work for a period of time.  These initial losses
would be captured by (1) and (2) above.  However, time lost
from work will likely slow occupation advancement and the
individual may suffer long term chronic mental and physical
effects from mercury poisoning which would alter the type
and intensity of future employment and consequently, wage
level.  These latter effects are captured in (4) and (5)
above, and as Crocker et al. (1978) have demonstrated with
data from the Michigan Household Survey, are quantifiable
and possibly large.

## The Ethics of Valuing Health Effects

As we pointed out earlier in discussing the valuation
of risk to life, economists value health in what may be
interpreted as a rather special set of circumstances.
Ideally, we could view a perfect world in which a *priori*
compensation takes place for all health risks.  Health risks
would be commodities traded in perfect markets.  Thus, a new
power plant locating in a previously pristine area would
purchase the "right" to emit toxic trace elements from all
individuals potentially exposed.  Such a market for risk
would, of course, require perfect information on the part of
all parties and some mechanism for overcoming common property
problems of allocating airsheds and watersheds — all of which
explains why we do not often observe such markets in the real
world.  In any case, if such a market were in place, we could
readily value health risks.  Further, since all market trans-
actions would be voluntary — the power plant would have to
pay enough to all affected parties to get them to voluntarily
accept any associated health risks — no real ethical issues
would be raised.  This conclusion holds because, in the
extreme, an individual could demand infinite payment to
accept the power plant, hence preventing its construction or
location near that individual.  Note then, that this particular arrangement protects each individual's rights — no one
is forced to accept risk involuntarily — analogous to the
perfectly competitive private market case wherein, for

example, a worker may voluntarily accept a higher wage to work at a riskier job, but is free not to accept the offered compensation and risk. (The assumption of competitive markets, of course, implies full employment with consequent free choice of occupation, i.e., no one is forced to take a risky job *or* starve. Our society, with actual unemployment, effectively prevents forced employment with welfare programs.) In the private risk case, however, if one individual in the wage market is very risk averse and does not wish to accept a risky job, then another less risk-averse individual will likely take the position. Thus, tenth story windows are washed without raising ethical questions or creating a societal crisis over *private* risk. Alternatively, our power plant example points out an unfortunate problem with public as opposed to private risks. Construction of our example power plant might be blocked by *one* very risk-averse individual objecting to the imposition of a *public* risk; that is, if the market we proposed for public health risk were in existence. The distinction between public (joint) risk and private (separable) risk is then an important one, because, if a private market existed for public risk, one risk-averse individual could then block joint action (Rowe, 1977).

Another example may be useful. Imagine that the passengers on an airliner are informed that by flying "low and fast" they will arrive at their next stop on time, making up for previous delays.[14] Clearly, a joint decision by the passengers is necessary. Those less risk averse will likely approve the divergence from standard procedures. Those fearful of flying would likely resist. Airline risk is thus a public as opposed to private risk, since risks are joint — indivisible — as opposed to separable.

Different ethical systems will view such a situation in very different ways. Democratic, Utilitarian (see Mill, 1863, and Bentham, 1789) or "Darwinian" (see Rand, 1964) ethics would all approve of "flying low and fast" if: (1) the majority voted for this alternative (Democratic), (2) the summed utility gain to those less risk-averse exceeded the utility loss to those more risk-averse (Utilitarian), or (3) the willingness to pay of those passengers wanting to fly low and fast exceeded the willingness to pay of those opting for "standard procedures" (Darwinian). The last of these criteria is identical with benefit-cost analysis in that a very risk-averse individual would be outvoted, out-"utilitied," or outpayed by other individuals. Thus these criteria in themselves — including benefit-cost analysis — do not protect individual rights against some concept of majority rule.

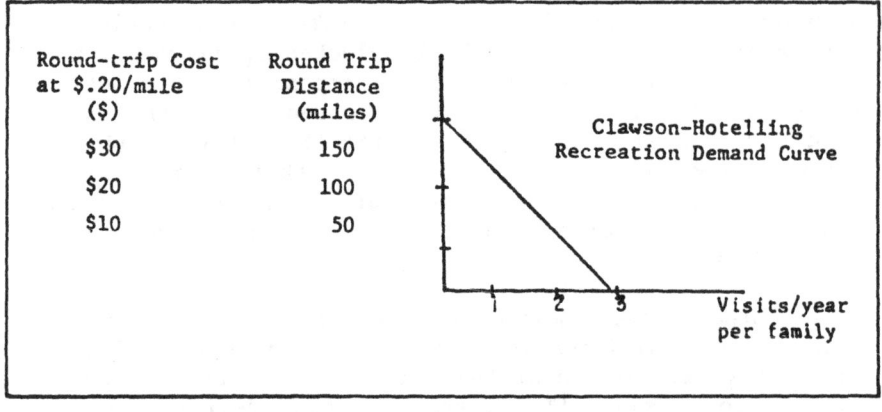

| Round-trip Cost at $.20/mile ($) | Round Trip Distance (miles) |
|---|---|
| $30 | 150 |
| $20 | 100 |
| $10 | 50 |

Clawson-Hotelling Recreation Demand Curve

Visits/year per family

**Figure 4.  Recreational demand and distance**

A number of ethical systems alternatively focus on individual rights. These include Egalitarian and Libertarian as discussed earlier. These ethical systems would reject the imposition of uncompensated risk by the majority onto an objective minority or individual. Each of these ethical systems might then reject benefit-cost analysis as it is traditionally performed. Application of these ideas would give decision makers a number of alternative outcomes in evaluating control of emissions of trace elements depending on the ethical system embodied in the analysis. Clearly, outcomes may be vastly different under ethical systems which look to the "good of the whole," as opposed to those which focus on protecting "individual rights."

## Valuing Ecosystem Effects

Recreation Damages. Although health damages can be quantified, as indicated above, use of these measures alone may, in fact, be inappropriate. For example, if a flash flood were to wash ash pond deposits into a water-course, or if a lake were polluted by stack emissions so that mercury levels in fish rose to the point where human health effects were possible from consuming the fish, fishing would likely be prohibited. Thus, possibly, no health effects would occur. Economic damage from such events would then be the lost recreation value associated with a prohibition on fishing, which would, hopefully, be less than any damages caused by health effects which would occur without the prohibition. Of course, prevention of health damages would require appropriate monitoring, the cost of which should be included in any health risk damage assessment.

The measurement of recreation damages depends on knowledge of the regional demand relationship for recreation. Two methodologies are available for determining recreation demand curves: (1) the Clawson-Hotelling travel cost approach, and (2) the survey questionnaire approach.

The Clawson-Hotelling methodology as described by Clawson and Knetsch (1966), Boyet and Tolley (1966), and Johnston and Pankey (1968), depends on knowledge of the relationship between rates of visitation to a particular site as a function of driving distance to the site. Presumably, individuals closest to a site, on average, will visit the site most frequently; the logic being that the effective price of visitation is the travel cost both in time and transportation of getting there. Thus, individuals or families closest to a site have the lowest price in travel costs, and will visit most frequently. As shown in the example demand curve in Figure 4, visits per year by family to a particular site typically decline with distance from "home" to the site.

If one assumes a fixed cost per mile for transportation, one then has the demand curve by simply translating round trip distance into cost per trip on vertical axis. This last assumption will likely lead to biased estimates of the true demand curve for a site for two reasons. First, demand will be overestimated if people enjoy the trip itself. For example, if a good lake for fishing is located in a scenic mountain area, the drive to the lake may include scenic vistas of value to fishermen. Thus, part of the travel costs are offset by the "benefits" of scenic vistas. As a result, the travel-cost based demand curve will overestimate the value of fishing alone. Second, other expenditures besides transportation costs such as food, lodging, and recreation equipment (boats, fishing poles, bait, etc.) are also associated with the recreation experience, and demand for these items would need to be included as well in approximating an overall willingness to pay measure for the benefits of fishing a particular lake or stream.

An alternative to the travel-cost approach is use of survey questionnaires. For examples, Brown, Singh, and Castle (1964) estimated the value of the Oregon salmon and steelhead fishery by postulating a hypothetical increase in costs/day for fishermen. In calculating net benefits, adjusted for inflation, their results indicate a current value of $10-$20 per fisherman-day.

Broader Ecosystem Effects. Valuing an uncontaminated or pristine environment clearly must go beyond valuing consumptive recreation alone (fishing, hunting, etc.). The recreation experience may be dramatically affected by the abundance of wildlife. Sighting of a porcupine, pronghorn antelope, marmot, elk, or other animal by a recreator on a hike or merely by travelers on a highway has some value or benefit. Perhaps even more significant is the possibility of option demand – demand by non-users for a pristine environment. Convincing evidence of option demand comes from the concern of, for example, New Yorkers over preservation of the Grand Canyon. Similarly, news articles concerning far away environmental catastrophes causes concern among environmentalists nationwide. One explanation for option demand is that even though an individual may not use a particular pristine area today, that individual may want to retain the *option* of using that area in the future and so be willing to pay for preservation.

Both types of effects noted above, subtle values associated with wildlife populations, and option value, are likely to be difficult or impossible to capture using a Clawson-Hotelling methodology. However, recent research has suggested that valid values might be obtained through survey

questionnaires wherein individuals are directly queried as
to the value of environmental attributes. This approach was
pioneered by Randall et al. (1974), and has more recently
been applied by Brookshire, Ives, and Schulze (1976). However, two new studies bear direct relevance to the problem
of valuing ecosystem effects. First, Brookshire, Randall,
and Stoll (1980) have applied survey techniques specifically
to valuing wildlife sightings and option value of wildlife
preservation. Typical values from this research are as
follows: for an encounter (sighting) with elk, hunters were
willing to pay about $44 (consumptive use); to prevent a 50%
reduction in duck and geese populations, non-hunters who used
possible affected recreation areas were willing to each pay
on the average $175 per year (non-consumptive use); as a
measure of option value, hunters, for example, were willing
to pay $21 annually today to improve, by 25%, odds of getting
a license to hunt grizzly bear in Wyoming five years hence
(no licenses are currently granted because the grizzly is
endangered). Note that the last measure, a quantification
of option value, while useful for experimental purposes, in
no way captures the broad ecosystem values which have been
postulated. In any case, the study does suggest that preservation of wildlife populations has considerable value. Thus,
toxic effects on wildlife populations could conceptually be
valued through survey research.

### Benefit-Cost Analysis for Global Energy Impacts

In recent years, benefit-cost analysis has been applied
to such long-term environmental problems as chlorofluoro-
methanes and ozone, climatic change induced by SST emissions,
and to carbon dioxide ($CO_2$)-induced climate changes (d'Arge
et al., 1975; d'Arge et al., 1976; Laurman, 1979; Bailey,
1980; Freeman, 1979). All of these studies have worked with
very uncertain estimates of both costs and benefits. However, each has had a similar set of underlying problems in
assessing results. First, in each case the process of economic discounting of the future led to small present values
for even almost catastrophic future economic losses. For
example, a complete loss of the world's GNP in 100 years,
growing at 3%, would be worth about one million dollars today
if discounted at recent prime rates (19% as of 3/21/80). If
world GNP in 100 years were the same as today's GNP, discounting would reduce the value to only approximately $70,000
at present. Thus, catastrophic losses in the distant future
are almost valueless to the present generation *if* benefit-
cost analysis, as it is generally applied, is used in valuing
the future. Second, given changing life-styles, substantial
future shifts in technologies, and probabilities of drastic
world political-social events, any quantitative measures of
benefits/costs in 100 years are not subject to better than

2-4 orders of magnitude accuracy, and may even switch sign, compared with the current economic order. For example, current estimates of the net costs of a gradual warming in the United States depend crucially on whether future increased air conditioning costs will be greater than benefits from reduced heating costs which are both sensitive to assumptions on future energy prices and location of populations in the continental U.S. (d'Arge, 1979). Given these uncertainties, perhaps the best current measure of benefits/costs to future generations is reflected by how much current generations would pay to prevent future risks. There is substantial indirect evidence that individuals are willing to pay some proportion of their current income to endow future generations with certain types of assets, e.g., National Parks, historical monuments, lack of nuclear waste materials, species preservation (see Krutilla, 1967). That is, current decisions on regulation affecting future generations should be predicted on the preferences and values of those now populating the earth's surface. Third, the ethical basis of benefit-cost analysis has not been explored to see what forms of bias are introduced when current values are imposed on future generations. It is argued in this section that the appropriate social rate of discount varies substantially depending on the underlying ethical beliefs of society. Some ethical beliefs lead to discounting future effects to zero (an implied rate of discount of infinity), while others would require valuing future effects at more than present costs or benefits.

It is the purpose of this section to explore in detail the above three problems of applying traditional benefit-cost analysis to long-term environmental choices such as the $CO_2$ problem and recommend ways that benefit-cost analysis can be altered to accommodate them. The next subsection explores the $CO_2$-economic effects problem using a qualitative approach, since actual estimates of benefits for $CO_2$ control are at this time highly uncertain. The third subsection discusses how future economic effects may be valued differently depending on underlying ethical beliefs. The final section contains a listing of research recommendations on how the $CO_2$ problem can be studied from an economic perspective, given the findings of previous sections.

## Carbon Dioxide Effects:  A Qualitative
## Economic Assessment

The $CO_2$ problem from the standpoint of an economic perspective has its most interesting elements in terms of intergenerational choice. The reason for this is the anticipated positive economic benefits accruing for several generations and the potential disasterous economic costs that may accrue to generations after that.  In the National Academy of Science (NAS) Geophysics Study Committees report, *Energy and Climate*, several potential physical and environmental effects of increasing $CO_2$ are rather dramatically proposed over a period of 170 years (NAS, 1977; Woodwell et al., 1979).  They include the "melting of glaciers" causing rises in the sea level of 3-5 m, a potential shift in agricultural zones upward in latitude in the northern hemisphere with an expansion of frost-free days, rates of photosynthesis, and production of biomass in most regions of the world along with expansion of arid and semi-arid regions.  Thus, from a qualitative perspective there may well be substantial benefits to agriculture, forestry, and other natural resources that are highly temperature dependent in terms of productivity.

In Figure 5 is a world map adapted from Kellogg (1979) indicating potential temperature changes by latitudinal zone given a doubling of atmospheric $CO_2$.  A rather arbitrary line divides the world into drier and wetter zones based on the altithermal period occurring 4-8 thousand years ago.  If this line between drier and wetter is accurate, it presents a whole series of economic difficulties in assessing benefits and costs.  For example, there is a lot of uncertainty as to where the line should pass through the continental United States and if, for example, the Northern Great Plains and Midwest were significantly drier and warmer, this would suggest a wholly different set of adaptive policies and thereby benefits or costs as contrasted to a warmer/wetter area.  The same difficulty arises for the Soviet Union in terms of wheat yields.  The line bisects the Soviet Union where only slight error in drawing it would make the winter wheat crop more or less vulnerable.  If there was more variation in the hydrologic cycle in the wetter zones identified in Figure 5, this could induce greater variations in crop yields and thereby cause substantial impacts to agrarian communities on the food threshold.  This is particularly true for the Asian cultures dependent on the monsoon season.  It would also be dependent on the possibilities of new varieties of crops which are either more drought resistant or water tolerant in their root zones (Wittwer, 1979).

A drier climate in the Northern Great Plains of the United States would cause an increase in the probability of crop failure in any one year.  This would also be true for the Midwest in terms of dry land farming.  Over a very long time, the Midwest, through development of substantial irrigation systems, could possibly even increase yields above those existing currently but at a substantial capital cost (i.e., $30-50 per acre).  In addition to the direct agricultural effects and impact on growing seasons, a substantially warmer

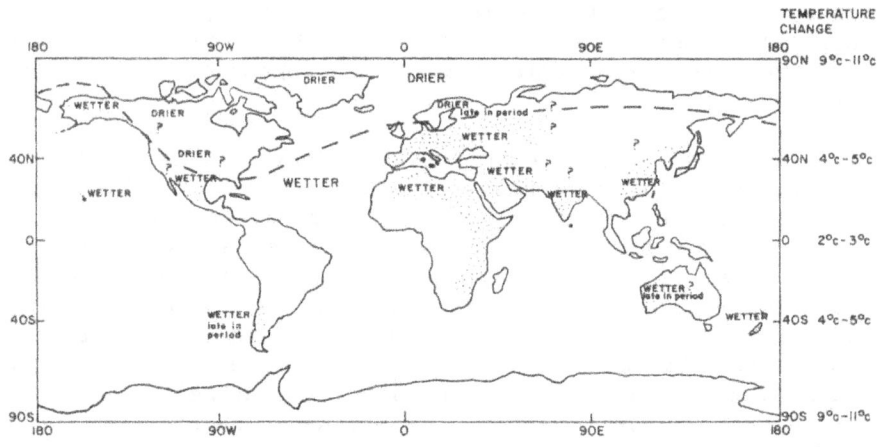

Figure 5.  Potential climatic change and the altithermal
period (4000-8000 years ago).  Temperature changes were
formulated in discussions at the Aspen Institute Workshop
on "The Consequences of a Hypothetical World Climate
Change Produced by Atmospheric Carbon Dioxide," Wye
Plantation, Maryland, February 25-29, 1980.
Source:  Kellogg, 1979.

climate would undoubtedly mean a reduction in heating costs
(Heah, 1979); a potential increase in air conditioning costs
(Heah, 1979); a movement towards or away from an optimal
urban environment depending on the initial location (Bailey,
1980; d'Arge, 1975); a potential increase in diseases (particularly in the tropical zones) such as elephantiasis and
dingue fever; and greater capital requirements for reducing
the growth of molds in relatively high humidity locations.
In addition to changes in location of agriculture, there
would be an implied movement of population and location of
urban areas. Whether such a movement would be rapid and substantial enough to induce large adjustment costs is not now
known. Neidercorn (1976) examined the capital costs involved
in a shift in the U.S. cornbelt "potentially" induced by
stratospheric effects of SST's. The cost of adjustment would
depend substantially on the depreciation rate for existing
capital assets and if the adjustment time is slow enough,
such costs might be minimal. Laurman (1979) suggests the
lead time necessary to convert to nonfossil fuels may be the
important considerations for $CO_2$-induced climate change.

A significant issue in terms of qualitative economic
assessment is that almost all of the studies completed to
date on quantitative economic impacts have examined only the
equilibrium costs of a very small long-term temperature
change in the range of less than one degree centigrade glob-
ally and there is a great deal of uncertainty as to how
measurements for such small changes can be extrapolated to
changes ranging from 4-5° centigrade in the temperate zones.

The existing set of cost and benefit estimates for a
positive temperature change of the magnitude suggested by
$CO_2$ modeling efforts has as yet to be adequately assessed.
However, in qualitative terms without substantial changes in
precipitation patterns, a warming should: (1) increase crop
yields; (2) extend growing seasons; (3) allow a greater
variety of crops over larger regions; (4) reduce heating
costs; (5) provide a more desirable urban climate in the
colder temperature zones; (6) (may) induce higher tropical
disease rates; (7) increase air conditioning costs and change
styles of living in the tropical zones; (8) require the
development of capital intensive irrigation systems or crop
adaptation in some areas; (9) reduce urban costs of snow
removal and thus, in general, transportations costs;
(10) require substantial capital investments to accommodate
a rising level of ocean; (11) reduce costs (or increase benefits) of producing fossil fuel energy. Whether all of these
taken together add up to a net positive cost to society is
unclear at this time. It appears reasonable to presume,
however, that given the existing quantitative evidence for
these sectors, that very small positive changes in global

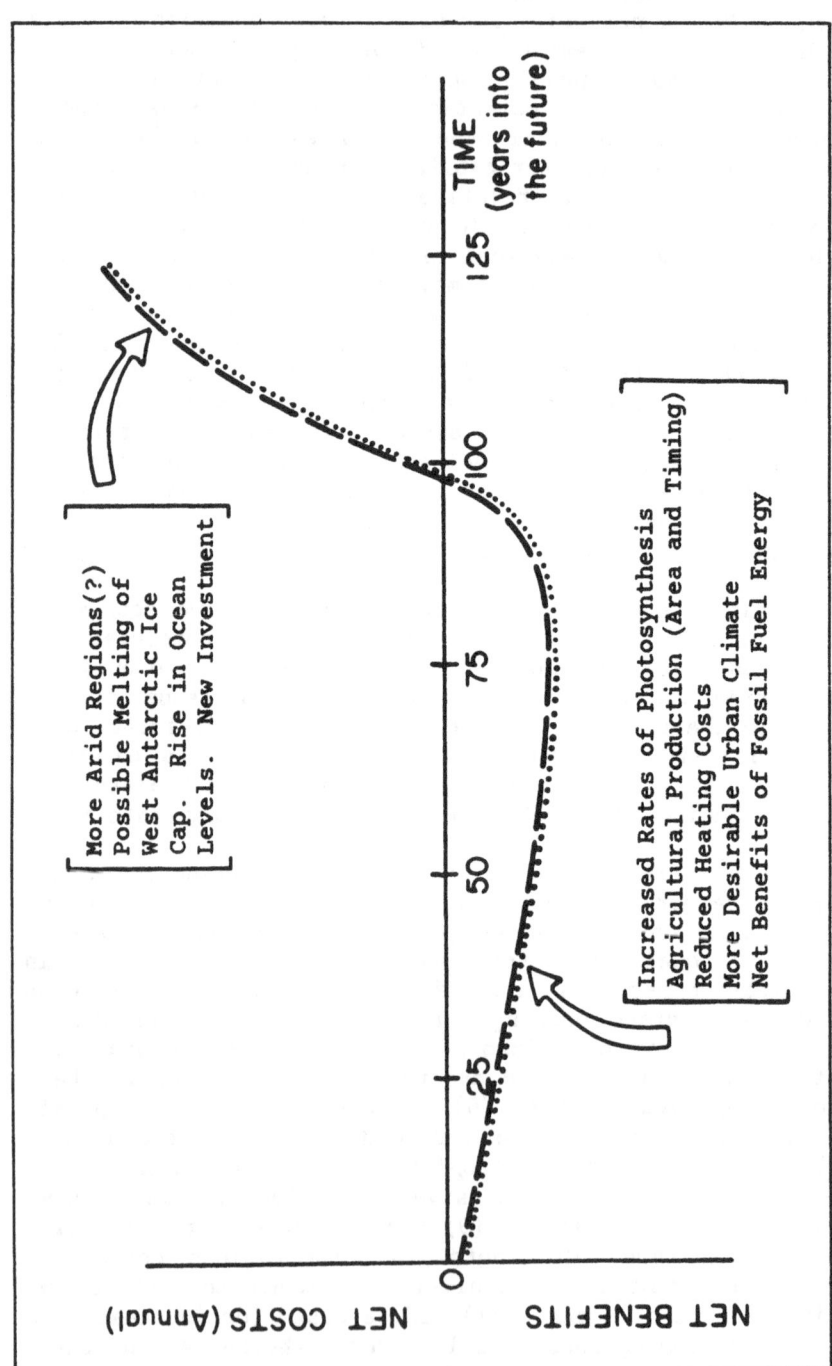

Figure 6. Long-term net costs of climatic change: a qualitative picture

temperature in the range of 0-2° centigrade, would be beneficial to at least the next several generations. Given the
highly incomplete and tentative findings on equilibrium costs
and benefits, the $CO_2$ problem might be visualized as is
depicted in Figure 6. That is, for a period of perhaps up
to 100 years, there is likely to be a net annual benefit from
increasing levels of $CO_2$ in the atmosphere. Beyond that
time, however, as the climate becomes distinctly warmer with
greater variability in precipitation patterns and a finite
probability of melting the antarctic ice caps, the potential
for very large future economic costs increases. Thus, we
visualize the $CO_2$ problem, in simple terms, as a problem of
tradeoffs between succeeding human generations where the
first few benefit substantially by imposing perhaps very
large costs on future generations. This is suggestive that
the $CO_2$ problem is really one of intergenerational choice.
That is, comparing a distinct positive benefit stream to one
set of generations with the highly uncertain but very large
potential economic cost to generations that follow. If this
paradigm is accepted, then the question arises as to whether
benefit-cost analysis, in its traditional form based on discounting of the future and not requiring compensation of
losers by the gainers, is an appropriate tool for evaluation.
This question has been raised by several authors including
Mishan and Page (1979). We believe in its present form it
is not acceptable, since even with extremely large future
costs, small current benefits will dominate the decision on
control. Thus, traditional benefit-cost analysis must be
disregarded as a valuable tool for policy making, and making
current decisions on the $CO_2$ problem. In what follows we
attempt to devise a new methodology whereby the future can be
accurately and efficiently protected given current choices.

## Ethics and Climate Change

As expressed in the introduction, one way of formulating the $CO_2$ climate problem is as an ethical question. This
section attempts to explore how alternative ethical systems
might be integrated with benefit-cost analysis. We find that
the critical parameter is the choice of discount rate.

Economists justify use of a discount rate on future
benefits and costs — weighing future economic values less
than current economic values — as follows: imagine that one
individual 100 years from now is forced to evacuate a coastal
area as a result of $CO_2$ emissions from burning coal today.
Further, let us assume that the future individual would
accept a payment of $100,000 as "fair" compensation for prop-
erty losses and any risks imposed. If we, the current generation wish to compensate that future individual, do we need
to set aside $100,000? Is the damage now the same as the

damage 100 years hence?  The usual economic answer is "no."
If we were to invest $4,979 today in a bank account paying a
3% real rate of return (over inflation) we would have
$100,000 of real value in accumulated interest and principal
100 years hence to compensate the displaced future individual.  Thus, the argument goes, a 3% discount rate would be
appropriate on damage done to future generations in making
decisions today.  For example, if scrubbing $CO_2$ from stack
emissions or finding a non-$CO_2$ emitting energy substitute
for coal — solar or nuclear for example — were to have an
excess cost of more than $4,979 today, benefit-cost analysis
would suggest not to bother, even though we will do $100,000
worth of harm 100 years hence.  Many would, of course, view
such a decision as unethical.  Page (1977), for example,
argues that compensation is likely to be only hypothetical
and not real, making the whole discounting procedure meaningless on ethical grounds since actual compensation is not
likely to be paid.

    The ethical-economic issue outlined above — that of dis-
counting — critically affects an analysis of the $CO_2$-climate
problem.  For example, Laurman (1979) concludes, based on a
benefit-cost study done for EPRI, that "since no agreement
on the correct treatment of social discounting exists, we
are unable to present conclusive estimates of present day
discounted costs for the $CO_2$-climate change problem."  Thus,
we utilize the ethical systems discussed earlier and focus on
distribution since the discount rate is the critical parameter in questions of intergenerational distribution.  We find
that differing ethical systems imply differing discount rates
(for a complete discussion, see Schulze and Brookshire,
1979).

    We explore the issue of discounting using a two period
model of climate change resulting from combustion of fossil
fuels.  The strategy is to compare the welfare or utility of
the present generation, $U_1$, with the expected utility of
future generations, $E(U_2)$.  In the Utilitarian Ethic, if
present investment to compensate future generations is possible, then the appropriate discount rate is the market rate
of return.  This occurs, because investment allows a net gain
in total utility thereby satisfying the Utilitarian criterion
of maximizing total utility.  If, however, investment as compensation is not possible, the optimal discount rate depends
on the relative marginal utilities between generations,
giving a range of discount rates from -1 to + ∞.

    In the Totally Egalitarian case, the discount rate
depends on whether or not an egalitarian solution where $U_1 =
E(U_2)$ is achievable.  There are three possible cases.  In
case (a), $U_1$ cannot be brought "up" to $E(U_2)$ so the discount

rate should be infinite, and fossil fuels should be used to the maximum desirable level in the present. In case (b), where an egalitarian solution is achieved, the discount rate exceeds or equals the market rate of return if compensation (investment) is possible but can take on any value, including negative values, if compensation is not possible. In case (c), the first generation is initially better off than the future. If investment in the future is possible, then $U_1$ can be brought *down* and $E(U_2)$ brought *up* through investment until equality is achieved so the appropriate discount rate is the market rate of return. However, if compensation is not possible and $E(U_2)$ remains below $U_1$ then no additional present use of fossil fuel should occur.

The Total Elitist criterion depends on whether the present or future can be best off. In case (a) the present can be best off. Thus, an infinite discount rate is placed on the future in all cases. "Greatness" is achieved in the present and the future is "written off." In case (b), the future is best off. If investment by the present generation is possible, then the market rate of return is the appropriate discount rate. However, if compensation is not possible, the present is written off and no additional fossil fuel use in the present should occur.

Finally, in the Libertarian Ethic, if investment is possible, then it can be used to keep the future as well off as in their initial state, i.e., as well off as before any decision to invest or deplete fossil fuels. This implies the market rate of return is an appropriate discount rate. However, if investment cannot be used to compensate the future for depletion and climate effects, then these actions are not consistent with the Paretian Ethic and our present use of fossil fuel is "unethical."

Perhaps the most important result of our analysis is that the choice of an ethical system can have a large impact on economic analysis. The traditional economic criterion of discounting future benefits and costs at the market rate of return only holds in special cases and where *actual* compensation or investment in the future is possible. Of course, by "possible" we really mean politically feasible. Economists often use the notion of "hypothetical" compensation to justify discounting. In an ethical context such arguments play no role whatsoever.

Thus, ethical weighting schemes can "resolve" the question of appropriate discount rate. However, any benefit-cost analysis then becomes conditional on the ethical system chosen. Obviously, different ethical systems will give dif-

ferent policy answers to the $CO_2$-climate problem.  An alternative interpretation of our results helps explain the diver-
sity of observed opinions on issues similar to the $CO_2$-
climate problem.  Individuals with egalitarian, elitist or
libertarian viewpoints all accepting the unlikely nature of
real compensation to future generations may in their own
"ethical" benefit-cost analysis come to differing conclusions.  This suggests that individuals in the present generation may well be able to partially internalize the intergenerational externality of climate change through their own
ethical beliefs and consequent actions.  An alternative
approach to imposing a particular ethic on a benefit-cost
analysis is then to attempt to discover directly the willingness to pay of the present generation to prevent particular
future climate change assuming that the intergenerational
externality is already internalized through individual ethical beliefs (Ben-David, Kneese, and Schulze, 1979).

To conclude, we have attempted to illustrate that the
$CO_2$ problem is one of intergenerational choice where traditional benefit-cost analysis is inappropriate.  It was suggested that depending on ethical beliefs, the structure of
benefit-cost analysis, particularly with regard to the selection of a discount rate, is altered substantially.  The
inadequacy of current estimates of economic costs or benefits resulting from 4-6° increases in global temperature and
changes in precipitation suggest that the $CO_2$ problem needs
to be analyzed in the context of uncertainty as to impacts
on future generations.  In a recent issue of *Science*, the
actual temperature changes from a $CO_2$ buildup have been estimated to be only 1/10 of previous estimates (Idso, 1980).
One method of valuing future effects is to estimate willingness to pay by present individuals to avoid environmental
risks to future generations.  Estimates of willingness to
pay embody the present generation's ethical beliefs and thus
avoid (or postpone) a decision on establishing an "optimal"
environmental ethic for future generations.

## Conclusions

In this chapter, we have attempted to demonstrate where
economic analysis can be made useful for energy policy impact
evaluation.  In so doing, a number of problems have been
demonstrated in trying to apply economic analysis to energy
impacts.  One central problem is that of selecting an appropriate ethical criterion upon which to base benefit-cost
analysis.  Secondly, a problem arises in adequately evaluating non-compensated and involuntary risks which characterize
part of many energy impacts.  Finally, there are substantial
difficulties in measuring many of the economic values associated with side effects of energy development since they are

not normally purchased or sold in organized markets (e.g., visibility). Because of these and other problems, economic evalution of energy impacts is likely to contain substantial errors, possibly of an "order of magnitude" size. However, when applied with care, economic analysis can play a useful role as one tool for valuing the positive and negative effects of energy development.

## Notes

[1]Maler (1974) has classified the possibilities for measurement of environmental goods or services into four broad categories: (1) asking individuals what they are willing to pay; (2) voting on the supply; (3) indirect methods based on observations of the relationship between private goods purchased and environmental goods; and (4) estimation of physical damage and evaluation on the basis of observed market prices. In this paper, we analyze methods only within Maler's categories (1) and (3).

[2]In the recent literature, one approach within this set has been called "bidding games," (Randall et al., 1974; Brookshire, Ives, and Schulze, 1976). However, because some types of responses are not bids but changes in behavior, e.g., site substitutions or minimum compensation, we prefer the more general "contingent valuations" to identify the set of approaches that directly query the individual for information in a series of hypothetical situations on markets.

[3]An alternative listing of explanations for bias and other problems is given in Grether and Plott (1979).

[4]See Brookshire and Crocker (forthcoming) for a discussion of the role of information in contingent markets and validity of the consumer's response.

[5]One survey of air pollution in the late 1960's for Los Angeles which we prefer not to cite asked the question "How much are you willing to pay for less air pollution?" Clearly, this question is too vague and subject to multiple interpretations as to the change in environmental attribute. Alternatively, a question "How much are you willing to pay for an annual average reduction in oxidant concentrations of 0.10 parts per million in the seven block radius around Hollywood Boulevard and Vine Street?" may be too specific and not readily understandable by the interviewee.

[6]We present this extremely brief summary of Randalls' work noting that it was the first effort, and to set the stage and focus the discussion for the remaining case studies. See Randall et al. (1974) and Randall, Ives, and Eastman (1974) for a complete discussion of the results.

[7]This research was funded by the NSF-RANN Lake Powell Research Project.

[8]The average bid concept was introduced in the survey instrument in the following manner: "Let's also assume that all visitors to the area will pay the same daily fee as you . . ." The use of the terms "environmental" and "developer" is to distinguish two groups who might have widely divergent preferences with respect to environmental commodities.

[9]This study was supported by the Electric Power Research Institute (EPRI), Palo Alto, California to the University of Wyoming. EPRI does not assume any liability for the completeness of the research, or usefulness of the results.

[10]For individuals to bid strategically to achieve a specific outcome when the respondent knows everyone must pay the final bid is extremely difficult. For instance, all previous bids by others must be known, the sample size and, if the individual is not the "last" bidder, then future bids, must be known. For more discussion see Brookshire and Eubanks (in press).

[11]The research reported here was supported by a NSF grant entitled, "An Economic and Environmental Analysis of Solar and Geothermal Energy Sources."

[12]Portions of this study were funded by the U.S. Fish and Wildlife Service contract numbers 14-61-0009-77-022 and 14-16-0009-77-003 with the University of Wyoming, and parts were subcontracted to the University of Kentucky.

[13]For a complete discussion of the study see Brookshire et al. (1977) and Brookshire, Randall, and Stoll (1980).

[14]This situation actually occurred some years ago in Texas. Passengers voted for low and fast.

## References

Arrow, K. J. 1973. Rawl's principle of just saving. *Swedish J. Econ.* 75.

Arrow, K. J. 1963. *Social Choice and Individual Values.* John Wiley and Sons, New York, N.Y.

Bailey, M. 1980. *Uncertainties and Benefit-Cost Analysis of CFC Control.* University of Maryland. Report to U.S. Environmental Protection Agency, Washington, D.C.

Ben-David, S., A. Kneese and W. Schulze. 1979. *A Study of Ethical Issues in Benefit-Cost Analysis*, study funded by the Ethics and Values in Science and Technology Program of the National Science Foundation.

Bentham, J.  1789.  *An Introduction to the Principles of Morals and Legislation.*

Bishop, R. C. and T. A. Heberlein.  1979.  Measuring values of extra-market goods:  are indirect measures biased? *Amer. J. Agr. Econ.* 61(5).

Blank. F. et al.  1977.  *Valuation of Aesthetic Preferences: A Case Study of the Economic Value of Visibility.* Research report to the Electric Power Research Institute, Resource and Environmental Economics Laboratory, University of Wyoming.

Bohm, P.  1971.  An approach to the problem of estimating demand for public goods. *Swed. J. Econ.* 73 (March).

Bohm, P.  1972.  Estimating demand for public goods:  an experiment. *Europ. Econ. Rev.* 3(2).

Boyet, W. E. and G. S. Tolley.  1966.  Recreation projection based on demand analysis. *J. Farm Econ.* 48(4).

Bradford, D.  1970.  Benefit-cost analysis and demand curves for public goods. *Kyklos* 23(4).

Brookshire, D. S. and T. Crocker.  The advantages of contingent valuation methods for benefit-cost analysis. *Public Choice* (In press).

Brookshire, D. S., R. d'Arge, W. Schulze and M. Thayer. Experiments in valuing public goods. *Advances in Applied Microeconomics* (V. Kerry Smith, ed.). JAI Press, Inc. (In press).
Brookshire, D. S. and L. Eubanks.  Contingent valuation and revealing the actual demand for public environmental commodities. *Public Choice* (In press).

Brookshire, D. S., B. Ives and W. Schulze.  1976.  The valuation of aesthetic preferences. *J. Environ. Econ. and Manage.* 3(4).

Brookshire, D. S., A. Randall et al.  1977.  *Methodological Experiments in Valuing Wildlife Resources:  Phase I.* Internal Report to the U.S. Fish and Wildlife Service.

Brookshire, D. S., A. Randall and J. Stoll.  1980.  Valuing increments and decrements in natural resource service flows. *Amer. J. Agr. Econ.* 62(3).

Brown, G., A. Singh, and E. Castle.  1974.  *Economic Evaluation of the Oregon Salmon and Steelhead Sport Fishery.* Technical Bulletin No. 78.  Agricultural Experiment Station, Oregon State University.

Cessario, F. J. and J. L. Knetsch.  1970.  Time bias in recreation benefit estimates. *Water Resources Res.* 6(4).

Clawson, M.  1959.  *Methods of Measuring the Demand for the Value of Outdoor Recreation.*  Reprint 10. Resources for the Future, Inc., Washington, D.C.

Clawson, M. and J. L. Knetsch.  1966.  *Economics of Outdoor Recreation.*  The Johns Hopkins Press, Baltimore, Maryland.

Crocker, T., W. Schulze et al.  1978.  *Experiments in the Economics of Air Pollution Epidemiology.*  EPA/600/ 5-79/001 A. U.S. Environmental Protection Agency, Washington, D.C.

Cummings, R. G., W. Schulze and A. F. Mehr.  1978.  Optimal municipal investment in boomtowns:  an empirical analysis.  *J. Environ. Econ. and Manage.* 5(3).

d'Arge, R. et al.  1975.  *Economic and Social Measures of Biologic and Transportation Changes.*  U. S. Department of Transportation, Washington, D.C.

d'Arge, R., L. Eubanks, and J. Barrington.  1976.  *Benefit-Cost Analysis for Regulating Emissions of Fluorocarbons 11 and 12.*  Final report to U. S. Environmental Protection Agency on contract 68-01-1918, University of Wyoming.

d'Arge, R.  1979.  Climate and economic activity.  Presented at *World Climate Conference*, February, 1979, Geneva, Switzerland.

Davis, R.  1963.  Recreation planning as an economic problem.  *Natur. Res. J.* 3 (May).

Eckstein, O.  1958.  *Water Resources Development:  The Economics of Project Evaluation.*  Harvard University Press, Cambridge, Mass.

Edgeworth, F.  1967.  *Mathematical Psychics:  An Essay on the Application of Mathematics to the Moral Sciences.*  A. M. Kelley, New York.

Freeman, A. M., III.  1979.  *The Benefits of Environmental Improvement:  Theory and Practice.*  The Johns Hopkins Press, Baltimore, Maryland.

Gordon, I. M. and J. L. Knetsch.  1979.  Consumer's surplus measures and the evaluation of resources.  *Land Econ.* 55(1).

Gramlich, F. M.  1977.  The demand for clear water:  the case of the Charles River.  *Nation. Tax J.* 30(2).

Grether, D. M. and C. R. Plott.  1979.  Economic theory of choice and the preference reversal phenomenon.  *Amer. Econ. Rev.* 69(4) (September).

Grubb, H. W. and J. R. Goodwin. 1968. *Economic Evaluation of Water Oriented Recreation in Preliminary Texas Water Plan*. Report 84, Texas Water Development Board (September).

Hammack, J. and G. Brown. 1974. *Waterfowl and Wetlands: Towards Bioeconomic Analysis*. The Johns Hopkins Press, Baltimore, Maryland.

Harrison, F., Jr., and D. L. Rubinfeld. 1978. Hedonic housing prices and the demand for clean air. *J. Environ. Econ. and Manage.* 5(1).

Heah, I. 1979. Climate, energy use and wages. In *Economic Aspects of Effects upon Health and Climate from the Management and Control of Ozone Depletion*. U.S. Environmental Protection Agency, Washington, D.C.

Hori, H. 1975. Revealed preferences for public goods. *Amer. Econ. Rev.* 65(5).

Idso, S. B. 1980. The climatological significance of a doubling of earth's atmospheric carbon dioxide concentration. *Science* 207 (March 28).

Inhaber, H. 1978. *Risk of Energy Production*. AECB-1119. Atomic Energy Control Board, Ottawa (May).

Johnston, W. and V. Pankey. 1968. Some considerations affecting empirical studies of recreational use. *Amer. J. Agr. Econ.* 50(5).

Jones-Lee, M. W. 1976. *The Value of Life*. The University of Chicago Press, Chicago.

Kant, I. 1785. *Fundamental Principles of the Metaphysics of Morals*.

Kellogg, W. W. 1979. Influences of mankind on climate. *Ann. Rev. Earth Planet. Sci.*

Knetsch, J. L. 1965. Economics of including recreation as a purpose of eastern water projects. *J. Farm Econ.* 46(5).

Knetsch, J. L. 1963. Outdoor recreation demand and benefits. *Land Econ.* 39(4).

Krutilla, J. V. 1964. Welfare aspects of benefit-cost analysis. In *Economics and Public Policy in Water Resource Development*. S. C. Smith and E. N. Castle (eds.). Ames, Iowa.

Krutilla, J. V. 1967. Conservation reconsidered. *Amer. Econ. Rev.* 57(4).

Lancaster, K. 1966. A new approach to consumer theory. *J. Political Econ.* 74(2).

Laurman, J.  1979.  *Economic Impact of $CO_2$–Induced Climatic Change*.  Division of Applied Mechanics, Stanford University.

Lave, L. and E. P. Seskin.  1970.  Air pollution and human health.  *Science* 109 (August).

Loehman, E. et al.  1979.  Distributional analysis of regional benefits and costs of air quality control.  *J. Environ. Econ. and Manage.* 6(3).

Maler, K. G.  1974.  *Environmental Economics: A Theoretical Inquiry*.  The Johns Hopkins Press, Baltimore, Maryland.

Mill, J.  1863.  *Utilitarianism*.

Mishan, E. J.  1971.  *Cost-Benefit Analysis: An Introduction*.  Preager Publications, New York, N.Y.

Mishan, E. J. and T. Page.  1979.  The methodology of cost-benefit analysis — with particular reference to the ozone problem.  Presented at the *Conference on Ozone Management*, U. S. Environmental Protection Agency, University of Maryland, Port Depuit, Maryland.

Muellbauer, J.  1974.  Household production theory, quality, and the "Hedonic Technique."  *Amer. Econ. Rev.* 64(6).

National Academy of Sciences (NAS).  1977.  *Energy and Climate*.  Report of the Panel on Energy and Climate, Washington, D.C.

Neidercorn, J.  1976.  The capital costs of climatically induced shifts:  the example of the American corn belt.  In *The Value Costs of Climate Modification*.  T. Ferrar (ed.).  John Wiley, New York, N.Y.

Nietzsche, F.  1886.  *Beyond Good and Evil*.

Nozick, R.  1974.  *Anarchy, State and Evil*.  Basic Books, New York, N.Y.

O'Hanlon, P. W. and J. A. Sinden.  1978.  Scope for valuation of environmental goods:  comment.  *Land Econ.* 54(3).

Page, T.  1977.  *Conservation and Economic Efficiency*.  The Johns Hopkins Press, Baltimore, Maryland.

Pigou, A.  1920.  *The Economics of Welfare*.  MacMillan, London.

Rand, A.  1964.  *The Virtue of Selfishness*.  American Library, New York, N.Y.

Randall, A.; et al.  1974.  Bidding games for valuation of aesthetic environmental improvements.  *J. Environ. Econ. and Manage.* 1(2).

Randall, A., B. Ives, and C. Eastman. 1974. *Benefits of Abating Aesthetic Environmental Damage from the Four Corners Power Plant, Fruitland, New Mexico*. New Mexico State University Agricultural Experiment Station Bulletin 618.

Randall, A. and J. Stoll. 1980. Consumer's surplus in commodity space. *Amer. Econ. Rev.* 70 (June).

Randall, A., O. Grunewald et al. 1978. Reclaiming coal surface mines in central Appalachia: a case study of the benefits and costs. *Land Econ.* 54(4).

Rawls, J. 1971. *A Theory of Justice*. Harvard University Press, Cambridge.

Rice, D. 1966. *Estimating the Cost of Illness*. U.S. Department of Health, Education and Welfare, Public Health Service, Home Economics Series No. 6 (May).

Rosen, S. 1974. Hedonic prices and implicit markets: product differentiation in pure competition. *J. Political Econ.* 82(1).

Rowe, R., R. d'Arge, and D. Brookshire. 1980. An experiment on the economic value of visibility. *J. Environ. Econ. and Manage.* 7(1).

Rowe, W. D. 1977. *An Anatomy of Risk*. John Wiley and Sons, New York, N.Y.

Samuelson, P. A. 1954. The pure theory of public expenditures. *Rev. Econ. and Statis.* 36(4).

Scherr, B. A. and E. M. Babb. 1975. Pricing public goods: an experiment with two proposed pricing systems. *Public Choice* 23 (Fall).

Schulze, W. and D. S. Brookshire. 1979. *Economics and Intergenerational Ethics: An Example Application to the $CO_2$-climate Change Problem*. Working paper. University of Wyoming (September).

Sinden, J. A. and J. B. Wyckoff. 1976. Indifference mapping: an empirical methodology for economic evaluation of the environment. *Reg. Sci. and Urban Econ.* 6(1).

Smith, R. S. 1974. The feasibility of an "Inquiry Tax" approach to occupational safety. *Law and Contemporary Problems* (Summer-Autumn).

Smith, V. K. 1977. The principle of unanimity and voluntary consent in social choice. *J. Political Econ.* 85(6).

Starr, D. 1969. Social benefit vs. technological risk. *Science* 165.

Strauss, R. P. and G. D. Hughes. 1976. A new approach to the demand for public goods. *J. Public Econ.* 6(3).

Thaler, R. and S. Rosen. 1976. The value of saving a life: evidence from the labor market. *Household Production and Consumption* (N. E. Terleckyj, ed.). Columbia University Press, New York, N.Y.

Thayer, M. Contingent valuation techniques for assessing environmental impact: further evidence. *J. Environ. Econ. and Manage.* (In press).

Willig, R. D. 1976. Consumer's surplus without apology. *Amer. Econ. Rev.* 66(4).

Wittwer, S. 1979. *Remarks to the National Academy of Sciences Workshop on Critical Future Environmental Issues.* Washington, D.C.

Woodwell, G. et al. 1979. *The Carbon Dioxide Problem: Implications for Policy in the Management of Energy and Other Resources.* Report to the Council on Environmental Quality. Washington, D.C.